Health Status and Well-being of the Elderly

Health Status and Well-being of the Elderly

National Health and Nutrition Examination
Survey-I Epidemiologic Follow-up Study

Edited by
JOAN C. CORNONI-HUNTLEY, Ph.D., M.P.H.
ROBERT R. HUNTLEY, M.D.
JACOB J. FELDMAN, Ph.D.

Foreword by
MANNING FEINLEIB, M.D., Dr.P.H.

New York   Oxford
OXFORD UNIVERSITY PRESS   1990

Oxford University Press

Oxford New York Toronto
Delhi Bombay Calcutta Madras Karachi
Petaling Jaya Singapore Hong Kong Tokyo
Nairobi Dar es Salaam Cape Town
Melbourne Auckland

and associated companies in
Berlin Ibadan

Copyright © 1990 by Oxford University Press, Inc.

Published by Oxford University Press, Inc.,
200 Madison Avenue, New York, New York 10016

Oxford is a registered trademark of Oxford University Press

Library of Congress Cataloging-in-Publication Data
Health status and well-being of the elderly: National Health and
Nutrition Examination Survey-I Epidemiologic Follow-up Study/ edited by
Joan C. Cornoni-Huntley, Robert R. Huntley, Jacob J. Feldman;
foreword by Manning Feinleib.
p. cm.
ISBN 0-19-504962-4
1. Aged—Health and hygiene—United States—Statistics.
I. Cornoni-Huntley, Joan. II. Huntley, Robert R. III. Feldman, Jacob J.
[DNLM: 1. National Health and Nutrition Examination Survey (U.S.)
Epidemiologic Follow-up Study. 2. Aged. 3. Follow-up Studies.
4. Health Surveys—United States. 5. Nutrition Surveys—United States. WT 30 H4353]
RA564.8.H455 1990 614.4′273′0846—dc20 DNLM/DLC
for Library of Congress 89-9212 CIP

Printing 9 8 7 6 5 4 3 2 1

Printed in the United States of America
on acid-free paper

Foreword

The National Health and Nutrition Examination Survey-I Epidemiologic Follow-up Study (NHEFS) is a landmark accomplishment in the venerable history of the national health statistics system of the United States. Never before has any nation established a nationally representative cohort of examined individuals and successfully followed them for more than a decade to elucidate in astonishing detail the predictors of good health as well as the risk factors for illness, disability, and institutionalization.

This volume presents the association of a variety of physiologic measures, personal behaviors, and nutritional factors with the occurrence of acute and chronic illnesses over a period of 10 years. It also describes changes within individuals in dietary patterns, physical functioning, and personality characteristics during this period. Many of the results confirm, on a national level, findings obtained in more circumscribed samples. But some of the findings are at variance with those obtained previously and reinforce the dictum that localized findings cannot always be extrapolated to an entire country as heterogeneous as the United States.

Longitudinal studies are essential for understanding the process of change in individuals, including the relation between physiologic and behavioral characteristics and the subsequent development of illness and disability, or their complements, fitness, and longevity. Although much is known about the health of the aged from many diverse cross-sectional studies, only longitudinal studies can relate outcomes in later years to precursors at earlier ages.

The First National Health and Nutrition Examination Survey (NHANES I) provides a wealth of baseline data to relate to subsequent health outcomes. Because the cross-sectional NHANES I was designed to assess the health status of the American population in a way that would be comparable to previous National Health Examination Surveys and was also to serve as a reference standard, a great deal of attention was devoted to standardizing the measurements to provide the most accurate data that the state of the art would permit.

The NHANES I sample was chosen in a complex but statistically valid manner to be representative of the entire United States population. Those over the age of 25, who formed the base sample for the NHANES I Epidemiologic Follow-up Study (NHEFS), constitute the first nationally representative cohort to be followed for the elucidation of general risk factors related to longevity and a wide variety of health and functional outcomes.

In addition to the substantive results reported in this volume, and to be reported elsewhere, the NHEFS is also of great methodological import. It demonstrated that it is feasible to follow up a large national sample economically despite the mobility of the U.S. population and to obtain reliable, complete information on a variety of health issues through continuing mail and telephone contact. By linking the NHANES I files to other national data bases such as the National Death Index and Medicare beneficiary files, it is possible to obtain continuing information on essential health outcomes in an unobtrusive and "passive" manner. However, NHEFS has also demonstrated the importance of face-to-face contact and the value of obtaining direct measurements over time. It has given much impetus to developing examination methods that are portable and relatively easy to use.

It is apparent from the wide variety of health issues covered in this volume that a large cadre of experts contributed to the design, maintenance, and analysis of the NHEFS. Although the survey is fairly expensive to conduct, by combining a wide array of research issues into a common protocol there was an appreciable economy over what even a few separate limited studies would have cost. These broad-based objectives provided for efficient use of available resources while greatly enhancing the value of the data base for exploring the associations among a wide collection of factors.

National policies will no doubt be guided by the results obtained from the NHEFS. Educating the public regarding risk factors for cardiovascular diseases, cancer, and arthritis will be strengthened by knowledge of how these factors operate in a nationally representative sample. The common patterns, as well as the diversity, of changes in functional ability, personality factors, and individual behaviors will help us understand the aging process and the normal needs of the aging. New areas of research will be addressed and new insights as to how individual changes affect subsequent health will enable us to prevent and delay some of the costly effects of imprudent behaviors. The initial successes of the NHEFS have encouraged the National Center for Health Statistics to make a commitment to the continued follow-up of this cohort and to design subsequent NHANES to allow for establishment of new longitudinal cohort studies.

The data tapes from the NHEFS are publicly available for all researchers to use. Although many have contributed to the continuing success of this survey, no one has proprietary rights to it and all persons interested in the health of this country are encouraged to use the data.

I am pleased to acknowledge the fine work of the editors and authors of this book in making so much of the data available in a single volume. But I would also like to give special credit to Joan Cornoni-Huntley, who pioneered the NHEFS and whose unfailing dedication brought together the array of resources that made the study feasible. And finally, I would like to express appreciation to the late Dr. Robert S. Gordon, who chaired the Publications Committee for the NHEFS and enabled so large and diverse a group of experts to work together harmoniously.

Manning Feinleib

Acknowledgments

For support during the formative phase of the NHANES I Epidemiologic Follow-up Study, the editors wish to acknowledge the contribution of Dorothy P. Rice, former Director of the National Center for Health Statistics, Robert N. Butler, former Director of the National Institute on Aging, and Jacob A. Brody, former Associate Director for Epidemiology, Demography and Biometry, National Institute on Aging.

For their intellectual leadership, understanding, and encouragement during the implementation phase, we also wish to acknowledge Manning Feinleib, Director of the National Center for Health Statistics, T. Franklin Williams, Director of the National Institute on Aging, Robert S. Gordon, Special Assistant to the Director of the National Institutes of Health, and the Directors of the Institutes and Agencies that provided financial support.

The original NHANES I, conducted between 1971 and 1975, provides the infrastructure upon which the present Epidemiologic Follow-up is based. The Division of Health Examination Statistics of the National Center for Health Statistics, under the direction of Arthur J. McDowell, was responsible for the design, execution, and analysis of NHANES I. While we recognize our debt to the many individuals from the Division of Health Examination Statistics and from various other components of the National Center for Health Statistics for their prodigious accomplishments in maintaining high scientific standards in the face of a survey of the size and complexity of NHANES I, we wish to accord special recognition to Robert S. Murphy, the current Director of the Division of Health Examinations Statistics, and Dale C. Hitchcock, Dorothy C. Blodgett, and Mary A. Dudley of that division who not only participated in the original survey team but made major contributions to the Epidemiologic Follow-up.

The contribution of Westat, the contractor for the data collection phase of the survey, is also gratefully acknowledged. Directed by Thomas McKenna and Diane Cadell, Westat's dedicated survey research staff carried out their assignments with expertise and creativity.

The Office of Analysis and Epidemiology of the National Center for Health

Statistics was responsible for the design of the survey and exercised oversight responsibility for the field operations, editing, coding, and data tape preparation. Helen Barbano, Bruce Cohen, Christine Cox, Fanchon F. Finucane, Joel C. Kleinman, and Jennifer H. Madans played major roles in these stages of the survey.

Finally, the editors wish to express particular gratitude to Josephine Cruz, Betty Knapp, Sally Ham, and Mary Adams for their dedication and superior work in the preparation of the manuscript.

Contents

Contributors

Helen E. Barbano, M.S.P.H.   Special Assistant for Follow-up Studies, Division of Analysis, Office of Analysis and Epidemiology, National Center for Health Statistics, Centers for Disease Control

Lawrence G. Branch, Ph.D.   Professor of Public Health, Boston University School of Public Health

Louise A. Brinton, Ph.D.   Chief, Environmental Studies Section, Environmental Epidemiology Branch, Epidemiology and Biostatistics Program, Division of Cancer Etiology, National Cancer Institute, National Institutes of Health

Dwight B. Brock, Ph.D.   Chief, Biometry Office, Epidemiology, Demography, and Biometry Program, National Institute on Aging, National Institutes of Health

Christine L. Carter, Ph.D., M.P.H.   Staff Fellow, Cancer Prevention Studies Branch, National Cancer Institute, National Institutes of Health

Bruce B. Cohen, Ph.D.   Statistician, Division of Epidemiology and Health Promotion, Office of Analysis and Epidemiology, National Center for Health Statistics, Centers for Disease Control

James Colliver, Ph.D.   Senior Analyst, Alcohol Epidemiology Data System, CSR Incorporated

Joan C. Cornoni-Huntley, Ph.D., M.P.H.   Special Assistant to the Director, Office of the Director, National Institute on Aging, National Institutes of Health

Paul T. Costa, Jr., Ph.D.   Chief, Laboratory of Personality and Cognition, Gerontology Research Center, National Institute on Aging, National Institutes of Health

Christine S. Cox, M.A.   Statistician, Division of Analysis, Office of Analysis and Epidemiology, National Center for Health Statistics, Centers for Disease Control

Connie M. Dresser, R.D.P.H., L.N.   Public Health Nutrition Analyst, Division of Cancer Prevention and Control, National Cancer Institute, National Institutes of Health

Mary C. Dufour, M.D., M.P.H.   Chief, Epidemiology Branch, Division of Biometry and Epidemiology, National Institute of Alcohol Abuse and Alcoholism, National Institutes of Health

Donald F. Everett, M.A. Statistician, Epidemiology, Demography and Biometry Program, National Institute on Aging, National Institutes of Health

Jacob J. Feldman, Ph.D. Associate Director for Analysis and Epidemiology, National Center for Health Statistics, Centers for Disease Control

Manning Feinleib, M.D., Dr. P.H. Director, National Center for Health Statistics, Centers for Disease Control

Fanchon F. Finucane, M.H.S. Statistician, Division of Analysis, Office of Analysis and Epidemiology, National Center for Health Statistics, Centers for Disease Control

Daniel J. Foley, M.S. Statistician, Epidemiology, Demography, and Biometry Program, National Institute on Aging, National Institutes of Health

M. Beth Grigson, M.A. Research Analyst, Alcohol Epidemiology Data System, CSR Incorporated

Jack M. Guralnik, M.D., Ph.D. Senior Staff Fellow, Epidemiology, Demography and Biometry Program, National Institute on Aging, National Institutes of Health

Tamara B. Harris, M.D., M.S. Medical Officer, Office of Analysis and Epidemiology, National Center for Health Statistics, Centers for Disease Control

Richard J. Havlik, M.D., M.P.H. Special Assistant for Biomedical Applications, Office of Planning and Extramural Programs, National Center for Health Statistics, Centers for Disease Control

Marc C. Hochberg, M.D., M.P.H. Associate Professor of Medicine, Professor of Rheumatology, Division of Molecular and Clinical Rheumatology, Division of Molecular and Clinical Rheumatology, Johns Hopkins School of Medicine

Robert N. Hoover, M.D., Sc.D. Chief, Environmental Epidemiology Branch, Epidemiology and Biostatistics Program, Division of Cancer Etiology, National Cancer Institute, National Institutes of Health

Robert R. Huntley, M.D. Professor and Chairman Emeritus, Department of Community and Family Medicine, School of Medicine, Georgetown University

Lillian M. Ingster-Moore, M.H.S. Statistician, Epidemiology and Biometry Program, Division of Epidemiology and Clinical Applications, National Heart, Lung, and Blood Institute, National Institutes of Health

D. Yvonne Jones, Ph.D. Staff Fellow, Cancer Prevention Studies Branch, National Cancer Institute, National Institutes of Health

Joel C. Kleinman, Ph.D. Director, Division of Analysis, Office of Analysis and Epidemiology, National Center for Health Statistics, Centers for Disease Control

Andrea Z. LaCroix, Ph.D., M.P.H. Epidemiologist, Epidemiology, Demography, and Biometry Program, National Institute on Aging, National Institutes of Health

Reva C. Lawrence, M.P.H. Epidemiology and Data Systems Program Officer, National Institute of Arthritis and Musculoskeletal and Skin Disease, National Institutes of Health

Paul E. Leaverton, Ph.D. Professor and Chairman, Department of Epidemiology and Biostatistics, College of Public Health, University of South Florida

Steven Lipson, M.D., M.P.H. Medical Director, Hebrew Home of Greater Washington, Associate Professor of Community and Family Medicine, Georgetown University School of Medicine

Ben Z. Locke, M.S.P.H.   Chief, Epidemiology and Psychopathology Research Branch, National Institute of Mental Health, National Institutes of Health

Katalin G. Losonczy, M.A.   Statistician, Epidemiology, Demography and Epidemiology Program, National Institute on Aging, National Institutes of Health

Jennifer H. Madans, Ph.D.   Deputy Director, Division of Analysis, Office of Analysis and Epidemiology, National Center for Health Statistics, Centers for Disease Control

Diane Makuc, Dr. P.H.   Branch Chief, Analytical Coordination Branch, Division of Analysis, Office of Analysis and Epidemiology, National Center for Health Statistics, Centers for Disease Control

Robert R. McCrae, Ph.D.   Research Psychologist, Laboratory of Personality and Cognition, Gerontology Research Center, National Institute on Aging, National Institutes of Health

Suzanne P. Murphy, Ph.D., R.D.   Assistant Research Nutritionist and Lecturer, Department of Nutritional Sciences, University of California at Berkeley

Mitchell B. Pierre, Jr., B.S.   Statistician, Division of Analysis, Office of Analysis and Epidemiology, National Center for Health Statistics, Centers for Disease Control

Arthur Schatzkin, M.D., Dr. P.H.   Staff Fellow, Cancer Prevention Research Program, Cancer Prevention Studies Branch, National Cancer Institute, National Institutes of Health

Frederick Stinson, Ph.D.   Senior Analyst, Alcohol Epidemiology Data System, CSR Incorporated

Philip R. Taylor, M.D., Dr. Sc.D.   Chief of Cancer Prevention Studies Branch, National Cancer Institute, National Institutes of Health

Lon R. White, M.D., M.P.H.   Chief, Epidemiology Office, Epidemiology, Demography, and Biometry Program, National Institute on Aging, National Institutes of Health

T. Franklin Williams, M.D.   Director, National Institute on Aging, National Institutes of Health

Philip A. Wolf, M.D.   Professor of Neurology, Research Professor of Medicine (Preventive Medicine, and Epidemiology), Department of Neurology, Boston University School of Medicine

Regina G. Ziegler, Ph.D., M.P.H.   Nutritional Epidemiologist, Environmental Epidemiology Branch, Epidemiology and Biostatistics Program, Division of Cancer Etiology, National Cancer Institute, National Institutes of Health

Introduction

The purpose of this volume is to provide practitioners, planners, and researchers concerned with the health of older people detailed information on the first large prospective study ever conducted on a probability sample of the aging population of the United States. It is possible, because of the nature of this sample, to generalize from findings of this study to the general population of the United States.

From 1971–1975 the National Center for Health Statistics (NCHS) carried out a national survey, which included a health questionnaire and physical measurements, on a sample of the population of the United States. This survey is known as the National Health and Nutrition Survey-I (NHANES I).

In 1980 scientists at the NCHS and at the National Institute on Aging (NIA) recognized the possibility of doing a follow-up on the cohort examined in NHANES I to determine both the incidence of new diseases and the morbidity, disability, death, and institutionalization resulting from the diseases discovered in the NHANES I survey. To investigate the feasibility of finding those individuals from whom cross-sectional data had been gathered in NHANES I, a pilot project was carried out in the Baltimore area. It confirmed that the great majority of the NHANES I cohort probably could be found. Therefore, investigators designed a survey that included many of the questions asked during NHANES I, with additional questions relating especially to mental status, physical disability, nutrition, and life-style. This survey sample included all individuals who were 25 years old or older when they participated in NHANES I. The follow-up study is known as the NHANES I Epidemiologic Follow-up Study (NHEFS). This volume reports findings from NHEFS for participants who were 55–74 years old when NHANES I was conducted, approximately 10 years earlier, and relates these findings to observations at NHANES I.

In addition to involvement and support from NCHS and NIA, scientists at the National Cancer Institute; the National Heart, Lung, and Blood Institute; the National Institute of Arthritis, Diabetes, Digestive, and Kidney Diseases; the National Institute of Allergy and Infectious Diseases; the National Institute for Neurological and Communicative Diseases and Stroke; the National Institute of Alcohol Abuse and Alcoholism; and the National Institute of Mental Health participated in the NHEFS, and these agencies provided additional funding.

The detailed NHEFS data are now available for the first time, and they provide information on both prevalence and incidence of disease and the ability to link outcomes to risk factors. They thus provide a valuable resource to health care providers in the community as well as to health planners who are designing systems to meet the health needs of the rapidly aging population of the United States. The usefulness of this research is enhanced by continued surveillance of the NHEFS population; periodic telephone contact and the National Death Index are used for detection of new incidents (morbidity, mortality, and institutionalization). These additional data will strengthen the power of future analyses.

As already noted, this volume reports findings on NHEFS participants who were 55 through 74 years old approximately 10 years earlier, when they participated in NHANES I. The authors provide information on the design of the research and information on the content of the data set, which is in the public domain. They also perform a limited number of analyses in each area. This work, therefore, serves both to characterize the cohort and to demonstrate the potential for further research provided by the data set resulting from this epidemiologic follow-up.

Previously available data on prospective community studies of aging populations have been limited to relatively small geographic areas (e.g., the Framingham Heart Study) or have been limited in scope (e.g., the Surveillance, Epidemiology, and End Results Project [SEER] of the National Cancer Institute). However, most data sets on older populations have, in fact, come from cross-sectional studies. Even more limiting, most data sets combine people 65 years of age and older into a single category, which makes the data useless for analysis of the effects of aging beyond 65. Morbidity and disability are most highly correlated with age among those older than 65 years; therefore, classification of the over-65 NHEFS population by 5-year age groups (i.e., 65–69, 70–74, etc.) permits examinations of the health effects of aging in the elderly that were not possible previously.

Even the present study, with a total of over 14,000 subjects at baseline aged 25 and older and almost 5700 subjects aged 55 and older, has numbers too small for analysis in some of the areas of interest. However, the study is already yielding many health-related incidents (1700 deaths and 10,000 episodes of institutionalization, mostly in acute care hospitals) that make it possible to do hitherto impossible analyses. Furthermore, with continuing telephone follow-up and with continuing surveillance through the National Death Index, the number of incidents will continue to grow, thereby permitting more accurate and refined analyses in the future.

Another limitation, which this study shares with all cohort studies, is that the information obtained at baseline is limited to those items considered important, and measurable, at the time the study was conceived, during the late 1960s. For example, in retrospect, it would have been very useful to have obtained more detailed information on cognitive functioning. This would have permitted detailed analyses relating the level of cognitive function at baseline to subsequent outcomes in an aging population. Such analyses would clearly have been useful to those responsible for planning services for the very old, the most rapidly growing segment of the U.S. population.

The three sections of this book are devoted to research design, to specific common disease conditions, and to life-style, personality, and disability.

Section I gives details of study design and data collection. In testing the representativeness of the study cohort, it was found that the probability of survival of the cohort was quite similar to that of the general population of the United States during that period. The distribution of causes of death recorded for the study cohort was also quite similar to that found in the vital statistics of the United States for the same period. Thus, although follow-up is not complete, tracing rates are very high and there do not seem to be any strong biases in the mortality data (see Chapter 2).

Section II deals with diseases common in the elderly: infection, coronary heart disease and hypertension, cancer, stroke, and arthritis. Baseline health status and risk factors are examined in relation to the incidence of new disease.

In Chapter 3 the authors examine hospital admissions and deaths associated with selected infectious diseases. They also compare rates of selected infections according to gender and age and examine the concordance between the reporting of infections on hospital discharge records and on death certificates. They found that the incidence of both hospitalization and death were higher in men and that both increased with age in both sexes. Rates of hospitalization for pneumonia were much higher for both men and women than the rates for any other infection.

The diagnosis of pneumonia was used to test the degree of concordance in recording infections on hospital discharge records and death certificates in those cases with a fatal outcome. In a little less than half the cases a diagnosis was found on both documents. In one third of the cases the diagnosis appeared only on the hospital discharge record; in 18% it appeared only on the death certificate. This suggests that there may be substantial underreporting of pneumonia, and possibly other infections, as causes of death in the elderly.

For coronary heart disease (CHD) the risk factors identified in the Framingham Heart Study and other local studies are confirmed in this population, although cholesterol is less strongly associated with risk.

As additional incidents are accumulated with continuing follow-up, it may become possible to examine reliably such issues as ethnic differences in hospitalizations and sudden deaths. Table 4-2 suggests some intriguing possibilities: black men are shown to sustain only 83% as many coronary events as white men but 93% as many deaths, with only 72% as many hospitalizations. Does this mean that coronary events are less likely in black males but more lethal, or is this a reflection of poorer access to medical care, or simply poorer ascertainment of incidents? Perhaps further follow-up will shed additional light on such questions.

In Chapter 5 the authors analyze the NHEFS data set to test hypotheses relating to alcohol consumption and breast cancer, dietary fat consumption and breast cancer, and serum cholesterol and cancer at all sites and at certain specific sites. They confirmed a positive association between risk of breast cancer and alcohol intake, with a modest dose–response relationship. They were not able to confirm a positive association between dietary fat and breast cancer. They did observe an inverse relationship between serum cholesterol level and cancer, especially smoking-related cancers. With further follow-up and an increase in the number of incidents, additional studies relating cancer to other biochemical parameters and to specific intakes of various dietary components should become increasingly fruitful.

In Chapter 6 White et al. point out that, although cerebrovascular disease is a less common cause of death now than in years past, it is still a very significant cause of both death and long-term disability among the elderly. In this cohort, of those who were 65–74 years of age at baseline, 21% had a cerebrovascular accident during the subsequent 10 years. For those with thromboembolic stroke or ill-defined cerebral vascular disease, the short-term (0–6 months) death rate was approximately 40%; however, of those who survived with various levels of disability, approximately half were still alive 7 years later.

In Chapter 7 Lawrence et al. examine the power of symptoms of knee pain and roentgenographic evidence of osteoarthritis of the knee to predict subsequent disability and mortality. Symptoms of osteoarthritis of the knee at baseline were shown to be highly predictive of subsequent disability in this cohort. In the group aged 55 through 59 years at baseline, x-ray changes of osteoarthritis in the knee did appear to predict an increase in mortality in subsequent years. This issue remains unresolved, but further follow-up may yield a definitive resolution.

A variety of health practices and health states can be considered both causes and consequences of disease and death. A few of these complex interactions are examined in Section III.

In Chapter 8 the authors examine differences in mortality by educational attainment, marital status, and place of residence (geographic regions and rural–urban). They demonstrate an inverse relationship between mortality and educational attainment among white men and women aged 65–74 and for white men aged 55–64. Additional years of mortality follow-up should provide incidents enough to permit analysis for other age, race, and gender groups.

The authors confirm previous observations that the unmarried state is a risk factor for subsequent mortality, especially in men. They also confirm previously observed geographic differentials in mortality.

The health effects of smoking and drinking are examined in Chapter 9. An important observation is that 61% of all male respondents were abstainers at the time of NHANES I, and only 7.7% were heavy drinkers (defined as those having two or more drinks a day). These percentages were remarkably stable at NHEFS. The proportion of subjects who were smokers was substantially higher, although among participants aged 70–74 years at NHANES I only 30% had ever smoked and only 3% were still smokers at NHEFS.

Data from the two surveys show a pattern of decreasing consumption of alcohol over time in this aging population, and smoking and drinking practices appear to be related. Persons who abstain from one tend to abstain from the other. Furthermore, those who had been smokers at baseline and had become nonsmokers by NHEFS also tended to change their drinking profile to one resembling that of nonsmokers. Although rates of drinking and smoking were not high, heavy consumption of alcohol and any past cigarette use were both shown to have increased the risk of mortality from several diseases (e.g., lung cancer, cirrhosis) known to be related to these risk factors.

In Chapter 10 Murphy et al. identify several changes in dietary intake between NHANES I and NHEFS. Individuals who had been diagnosed as diabetic or as having diverticulitis were shown to have modified their diet in a manner to be expected for patients with these problems, and obese patients were found actually to record fewer food servings and to choose less calorically dense foods than their nonobese counterparts. It was also found that there had been a general increase in daily servings of fruits, vegetables, cereals, and legumes/nuts as well as an increased number of servings of fish by this cohort during the decade. There also had been an increase in servings of dairy products and a decreased number of servings of sweets. The authors speculate that these changes may be related to dietary guidance offered by national health organizations. However, fat and sodium intakes had not been reduced at NHEFS.

In Chapter 11 Costa et al. examine personality characteristics and look for changes over time. Twenty-seven percent of those who reported depression at NHANES I also reported depression at NHEFS. Of the 875 persons not depressed at baseline, 6.7% reported depression at follow-up. Depression at NHANES I was not found to be a predictor of death in the subsequent follow-up. Basic personality characteristics of openness, neuroticism, and extraversion were found to be quite stable with aging, a finding that contradicts the common assertion that the elderly become more introspective and withdrawn with advancing age.

Chapter 12 examines some of the determinants of physical disability. The differences in the level of physical functioning between men and women constituted a salient finding. Not only did men show less difficulty in activities of daily living than women at every age, but the disability of women increased exponentially with age, whereas that of men was more gradual. A strong relationship between perceived state of health and disability was observed in both men and women at every age.

The findings highlighted here exemplify some of the analyses that can be done with data from a cohort study to elucidate the magnitude of associations between common health problems in an aging population and a variety of risk factors. The chapters contain descriptions of detailed analyses that have already been performed, suggest further lines of research with this data set, and indicate that continuing follow-up of this aging cohort by repeated telephone interviews and through the Death Index will make possible even more detailed analyses.

I

STUDY DESIGN AND IMPLEMENTATION

1

Objective, Design, and Implementation

HELEN E. BARBANO, BRUCE B. COHEN,
JOEL C. KLEINMAN, JENNIFER H. MADANS,
JACOB J. FELDMAN, AND JOAN C. CORNONI-HUNTLEY

The first National Health and Nutrition Examination Survey (NHANES I) collected data on a national probability sample of the noninstitutionalized civilian population between the ages of 1 and 74 years. NHANES I included a standardized medical examination and questionnaires covering various health and demographic topics. The survey took place between 1971 and 1974 and was augmented by an additional national sample (1974–1975) that increased the size of certain subpopulations receiving a detailed physical examination. The total NHANES I sample included 23,808 persons 1–74 years of age (National Center for Health Statistics 1973; 1977a; 1978).

Although NHANES I provided a wealth of information on prevalence of conditions and risk factors, the cross-sectional nature of the survey limits its usefulness for the study of the health effects of clinical, environmental, and behavioral factors and of the natural history of disease. Therefore, a follow-up study was designed to investigate the relationship between factors measured at baseline and the development of specific health conditions. The NHANES I Epidemiologic Follow-up study (NHEFS) was jointly initiated by the National Center for Health Statistics and the National Institute on Aging, in collaboration with other agencies of the National Institutes of Health and Public Health Service. The goal of NHEFS is to examine the relationship of baseline clinical, nutritional, and behavioral factors assessed in NHANES I to subsequent morbidity, disability, and mortality. The size and scope of the population in NHEFS provide a unique opportunity not only to replicate more limited studies but also to examine etiologic relationships in a large, heterogeneous, nationally representative population.

The NHEFS population comprises all 14,407 participants who were 25–74 years of age when they were first examined in NHANES I (1971–1975). The follow-up includes personal interviews with those traced (or with a proxy for those who were incapacitated or deceased); measurements of pulse rate, weight, and blood pressure for surviving participants; collection of diagnostic information from

3

hospital and nursing home records; and collection of death certificates for decedents.

By convention, in this chapter the term *subject* refers to the individual examined as a participant in NHANES I, and the *respondent* is the person who provides the information at follow-up (i.e., the subject or a proxy).

To comprehend NHEFS fully, the reader needs to understand the design, content, and procedures of NHANES I. This chapter gives a basic overview of the salient aspects of both NHANES I and NHEFS.

NHANES I

Design of the NHANES I Sample

The NHANES I is based on a multistage, stratified, probability sample of clusters of households. The successive sampling elements were the following: a primary sampling unit, an enumeration district, a segment (a cluster of households), a household, and finally a sample person. A randomly selected subset of the sample persons received a more detailed examination and additional questionnaire items. The design was further complicated by the oversampling of certain population subgroups: low-income persons, women of childbearing age (25–44 years old), and the elderly (65 years old and over).

The first-stage sample consisted of primary sampling units (or "stands") selected from approximately 1900 such units into which the co-terminous United States had been divided. Each primary sampling unit represented a county or small group of contiguous counties. The 65 selected units consisted of 15 self-representing large metropolitan areas with populations of more than 2 million, plus 2 units from each of 25 other strata that were based on geographic region and population density.

Between July 1974 and September 1975 the original 65 primary sampling units were supplemented with an additional sample consisting of 35 units (stands 66–100, known as the Augmentation Survey), which would also constitute a national probability sample. The Augmentation Survey did not involve oversampling of any population subgroups.

Specially equipped mobile examination centers were set up in a central location of each primary sampling unit. Subjects were brought from their homes to the mobile centers for examinations. In each unit the examinations were conducted over a period of approximately 6 weeks. Then the mobile centers moved on to another stand. In northern primary sampling units examinations were scheduled in the summer, whereas in southern units they were done during the winter. Thus, most examinations were conducted during moderate weather.

Content of NHANES I Questionnaire and Examination (1971–1974)

NHANES I included an interview, a medical examination, and laboratory tests. A summary of the content for adults 25–74 years of age appears in Table 1–1.

Table 1-1 Components of NHANES I, as Administered to Subjects 25 to 74 Years of Age (1971–1975)

Recipients	Questionnaires
All households in the sample	Household Questionnaire
All households containing one or more sample persons	Food Programs Questionnaire*
All sample persons	General Medical History*
	Dietary Intake, 24-Hour Recall*
	Dietary Intake, Food Frequency*
Additional for all sample persons in the detailed component	General Medical History Supplement
	Supplement A, Arthritis; Supplement B, Respiratory; Supplement C,
	Cardiovascular. (Supplements A, B, and C depend on certain positive responses in other history questionnaires.)
	Health Care Needs Questionnaire
	General Well-being Questionnaire
	Depression Scale†
	Water Usage Supplement†
	1975 NHIS Questionnaire items on hearing, visual acuity, reading, and hypertension†
	Examination procedures and measurements
All sample persons	General medical examination
	Dental examination*
	Dermatological examination*
	Ophthalmic examination
	Anthropometric measurements
	Laboratory determinations:

Hemoglobin	Serum iron
Hematocrit	Iron binding capacity
Red cell count	Serum folates
White cell count	Cholesterol
Sedimentation rate	Glucose qualitative
MCV	(urine)
MCH	Albumin qualitative
MCHC	(urine)
Vitamin A	Occult blood qualitative (urine)
Vitamin C	tive (urine)
Magnesium	Creatinine (urine)
Total protein	Thiamine (urine)
Albumin	Riboflavin (urine)
	Iodine (urine)

Recipients	Questionnaires
Additional for all sample persons in the detailed component	Extended medical examination
	X-rays of chest and major joints (hand–wrist, knee, hip)
	Audiometry (air and bone)
	Electrocardiography
	Goniometry
	Spirometry

(*continued*)

Table 1–1 (Continued)

Recipients	Questionnaires
Additional for all sample persons in the detailed component (continued)	Pulmonary diffusion Tuberculin test‡ Speech test† Vision test† Laboratory determinations:

	Bilirubin	Phosphorus
	SGOT	W.B.C. differential
	Alkaline phosphatase	count
	Uric acid	Serological tests for
	Calcium	amebiasis, mea-
	Thyroid (T-3, T-4)	sles, tetanus, diph-
	Serology for syph-	theria, rubella,
	ilis†	polio
		Blood urea nitrogen†

*Locations 1–65 only. †Locations 66–100 only.
‡Locations 1–35 only.

The examination began with a general physical examination that emphasized nutritional status. After measurement of blood pressure and pulse, the physician examined the head and neck, looking particularly for lesions associated with nutritional deficiencies, especially the lack of vitamins A, B complex, and C and of minerals. The chest, abdomen, and neurological and musculoskeletal systems were then evaluated in such a way that other vitamin and mineral deficiencies would be detected. Venipuncture was performed on all subjects. Those in the subsample selected for detailed examination received a comprehensive cardiovascular and musculoskeletal examination, and the appropriate supplemental Medical History Questionnaire. Then, for persons in stands 1–35, a thorough ophthalmologic examination was given. Next, the dermatologic and dental examinations were performed in stands 1–65.

Laboratory and health technicians were responsible for the rest of the examination. Tests included hematology and urine analyses, and measurements of height, weight, anthropometric, and skinfold. All persons 1–17 years of age were given x-rays of the hand and wrist. Examinees given detailed examinations had an audiometric test, electrocardiogram, spirometric and single-breath diffusions capacity tests, goniometry, and x-rays of the chest, hand, wrist, hips, and knees.

Information on nutritional status was collected in several ways. The first was an assessment of food intake through a 24-hour Dietary Recall Questionnaire and a Food Frequency Questionnaire. Second, nutritional deficiency or malnutrition was appraised clinically by a trained physician. Third, the nutritional biochemistry section of the examination consisted of determinations of serum levels of vitamins A and C, magnesium, iron, folate, total protein, albumin, and cholesterol. Iron-binding capacity of serum was also measured. Fourth, information about family participation in food stamp and commodity programs was obtained through a Food

Programs Questionnaire. A fifth set of data addressed the relationship of body build and composition to nutritional status. Measurements in this area included height, weight, triceps, and subscapular skinfolds (measures of obesity); elbow and bitrochanteric breadth (bone structure); and sitting height (measure of trunk length). The final component of NHANES I related to nutrition was the dental examination. Gums were examined for manifestations of malnutrition and related diseases. The relationship between dietary intake and dental conditions was determined by responses to questions about the chewing of foods.

The NHANES I Augmentation Survey (1974–1975)

The augmentation survey was similar to the first part of NHANES I except for some changes in the content and sample design of the detailed examination. The dietary questionnaires as well as the dental, dermatologic, and opthalmologic examinations were eliminated. Three new procedures were added: a hearing test to understand conversational speech, a vision test, and a household water sample study (conducted in collaboration with the National Institutes of Health and the Environmental Protection Agency). In addition, several new sets of questions were asked. The relationship between response to the survey and clinical findings was evaluated by use of questions on vision and hearing from the 1975 National Health Interview Survey (NHIS) (National Center for Health Statistics 1985). Questions from the 1975 NHIS dealing with hypertension were added for comparison of the participants' responses with their blood pressure measurements. A 20-question depression scale developed at the National Institute of Mental Health (the CES-D) was also administered to participants (Radloff 1977). Because of interest in monitoring the prevalence of venereal disease, serologic tests for syphilis were added to the survey.

As a result of these design features, not all NHEFS participants received the same questionnaires or examination components at baseline. Only 6913 of the total of 14,407 examinees who were 25–74 years of age at the time of NHANES I received the detailed medical examination. Those respondents receiving the detailed examination may have also received one of the supplementary questionnaires on arthritis, cardiovascular, or respiratory problems: administration of these questionnaires was based on the responses to screening questions. Only 11,348 persons in the NHEFS cohort received the nutritional questionnaires described previously.

NHANES I EPIDEMIOLOGIC FOLLOW-UP STUDY

Objectives of NHEFS

The NHEFS had four major objectives. The first and major goal was to detect and measure the association, if any, between suspected risk factors and subsequent morbidity, disability, and mortality.

At baseline information was gathered on risk factors such as blood pressure, smoking, cholesterol levels, alcohol consumption, nutritional deficiencies, estrogen use, impaired pulmonary function, weight, and psychological characteristics. Morbidity, disability, and mortality data at NHEFS were obtained from responses of subjects and proxies to the interview, from hospital and from nursing home records and, for those who died between NHANES I and NHEFS, from death certificates.

The second objective of NHEFS was longitudinal surveillance of mortality for the purpose of correlating suspected risk factors with patterns of mortality. The data obtained on risk factors at both baseline and follow-up will be related to mortality and cause of death for subjects who die after their follow-up interview. These deaths will be ascertained through the National Death Index (United States Department of Health and Human Services 1981) and by continued tracing and follow-up.

Measurement of changes in participants' characteristics between NHANES I and NHEFS was a third important objective of NHEFS. The follow-up questionnaire was designed to permit ascertainment and study of changes in risk factors between baseline and follow-up.

Examination of the natural history of chronic disease and functional impairments was another goal of NHEFS. Since a substantial number of respondents reported having a chronic disabling condition and/or loss of visual acuity or hearing in the NHANES I interview, the degree of progression or remission of these conditions over time can be studied by comparison of responses at follow-up to the same questions as were used in NHANES I. For example, it is important to attempt to understand why certain individuals with radiologic evidence of osteoarthritis (as determined in the baseline NHANES I examination) develop functional impairment whereas others with the same severity of disease do not. Extensive data on arthritis were collected in both NHANES I and NHEFS. Furthermore, a scale of performance of activities of daily living was specifically developed for NHEFS to measure functional status.

Design of NHEFS

The design of NHEFS specified five steps for obtaining information on the NHANES I cohort: ((1) tracing the subjects or their proxies to a current address; (2) performing in-depth, in-person interviews with the subject (or with a proxy if the subject is incapacitated or deceased); (3) taking pulse, blood pressure, and weight measurements; (4) obtaining hospital records and nursing home information to specify diagnoses and gather pathology reports and electrocardiograms; and (5) acquiring death certificates to establish dates and causes of death. Although each component represents a separate survey activity with its own set of procedures for data collection, processing, and reporting, the information gathered in any one part of the survey was used in fielding other components. In addition, the intent is for data from the different components to be used together when appropriate.

Tracing Procedures

The first phase of the project involved the tracing and locating of the NHANES I subjects. A variety of sources was used in tracing and locating the subjects and proxies: telephone contact, direct mail, post office change of address service, State

Department of Motor Vehicle files of licensed drivers, State Vital Statistics files, field visits to neighbors at subjects' last known address, and other low-yield procedures. Attempts were made to trace all subjects in the cohort and to determine their vital status (i.e., whether dead or alive). Date of death and the state in which the death occurred were obtained for subjects who had died. This information was used to obtain a copy of the death certificate from the appropriate state vital statistics office. The tracing process was also used to obtain the current address of living subjects as well as to identify a knowledgeable proxy respondent for deceased subjects. Respondents identified and located through the tracing procedure were then contacted and asked to participate in a personal interview. In a few ($n = 65$) cases, respondents who had been traced successfully could not be relocated for the interview. Only vital status as of the tracing date is available for those subjects.

For tracing to be considered confirmed, certain information had to be verified with the subject him- or herself, or in the case of a deceased subject, with someone who knew him well. The name was verified and two of the following three criteria had to be satisfied to consider that the NHANES I subject had been located. (1) The date of birth was considered verified if the year of birth obtained in the NHEFS tracing was the same as that reported during NHANES I, or if the month and day were the same, then birth year could fluctuate ($\pm$ 2 years). (2) The subject's address at date of NHANES I examination was considered verified if at the date of the initial examination the street name, city, and state matched. The street number did not need to match. (3) Household composition at the time of NHANES I examination was considered verified if the subject or proxy recalled the name and relationship of at least one household member correctly. The household composition was asked only if date of birth or address was not verified.

Interview Procedures

About 2 weeks before interviewing was to start in an area, all subjects in the NHANES I were sent a letter describing the study. Interviewers then called the subject to set up an appointment for the interview. If the subject was not accessible by telephone, the interviewer made an in-person visit to obtain the interview or to set up an appointment for interview.

Most in-person interviews were conducted at the subject's residence. However, some interviews were conducted in nursing homes, prisons, mental health facilities, or occasionally at some other convenient location such as a parent's home. Proxies for the deceased were usually interviewed by telephone. The interview lasted an average of 2 hours. Blood pressure and pulse and weight measurements were included. At the close of the interview the subject was asked to sign a form authorizing the National Center for Health Statistics to obtain information from medical records. Upon completion of the physical measurements, the individuals examined were given reports of the measurements. Subjects were paid $10 for participating.

Thorough quality control procedures were instituted. Field edits were conducted by the interviewer and the field office. Respondents were contacted again if there were discrepancies or missing sections in key items. Fifteen percent of the questionnaires were randomly selected for validation, which was usually done by telephone and, if necessary, by mail. Additional questionnaires were selected to be validated when there was reason to believe that the data might be false. Ten percent of the telephone interviews were also validated.

In planning for the follow-up study, the 100 primary sampling units comprising the NHANES I national sample were grouped into four approximately equal workload regions representing the Northeast, South, Midwest, and West. Each region had a central field supervisor and three field offices staffed by a supervisor and an assistant; these supervisory personnel maintained close contact with interviewers in each region.

Interviewing carried out in the North region, a pilot phase, began in May 1982 and was followed by the main data collection, which began about 3 months after completion of the pilot study interviews.

The success of an interview study such as NHEFS depends in great part on the skill of the interviewers in obtaining the needed information from respondents in a consistent manner. Therefore, in each of the four regions, 50 to 60 local interviewers were trained to meet the precise standards of the study. Interviewer candidates had to complete successfully the 3-day physical measurements training session before they were accepted for the intensive 8-day interview training session. Interviewers were trained and certified to take blood pressure measurements in accordance with the guidelines of the American Heart Association (Kirkendall et al. 1967) and the National Heart, Lung and Blood Institute (Hypertension Detection and Follow-up Program Cooperative Group 1978).

The field supervisors in each region maintained close contact with the interviewers by telephone, and they made observational visits to monitor each interviewer in the field. The physical measurements technique of each interviewer was retested early in the interviewing phase.

Tracing was carried out centrally throughout the survey period; the field work was conducted regionally. Thus, some subjects who were located after field work was completed in a particular region were interviewed by a small cadre of traveling interviewers. However, it was not possible to conduct in-person interviews with all surviving members of the cohort who were traced, particularly those in remote areas who were located at the end of the field period. So that as much information as possible would be obtained without extreme cost, these subjects were interviewed by telephone; they did not receive those portions of the questionnaire that required in-person interview. Also, certain sections were omitted to shorten the length of the telephone interview. Telephone interviews were completed for 131 subjects. (Telephone interviews were also conducted with 1206 proxy respondents.)

When a subject could not be contacted by telephone, a survey form was sent by mail. This form was designed to obtain the information necessary for verification of the subject's identity and for future tracing, as well as to obtain the names of hospitals to which the subject had been admitted and the dates of each stay. Mail forms were also used for proxy respondents for deceased subjects in cases where the proxy could not be reached by telephone and the expense associated with the in-person interview exceeded the funds budgeted. Although the receipt and return of a mail form does not constitute an interview, the information was important for other survey components such as verifying vital status and collecting hospital records and death certificates.

The personal interview was designed to gather information on selected aspects of the subject's health history since the NHANES I baseline examination. The data sought included a history of the occurrence or recurrence of selected medical conditions; an assessment of behavioral, social, nutritional, and medical risk factors believed to be associated with these conditions; and an assessment of various aspects of functional status. A basic aim in the design of the questionnaire was retention of item comparability between baseline and follow-up so that change over time could be measured. Whenever possible, the questions used at baseline were repeated in the follow-up questionnaire. However, questionnaire items were modified, added, or deleted when necessary to take advantage of advances in biomedical knowledge and improvements in questionnaire methodology. The questionnaire also included a complete history of hospital and nursing home utilization during the interval between the NHANES I examination and the NHEFS interview.

An attempt was made to interview all respondents identified during tracing. The interview consisted of two sections: a detailed questionnaire and a physical measurement section. The actual content of the interview was determined by the vital status of the subject and whether or not the respondent was the subject or a proxy. For incapacitated subjects unable to respond to the questionnaire, a proxy responded to a subset of the Subject Questionnaire. For deceased subjects a proxy responded to a separate questionnaire, that is, the proxy interview.

After the pilot phase was completed, the questionnaire and field procedures were evaluated. It was decided that, in most instances, proxy interviews for deceased subjects could most efficiently be conducted by telephone, except when the proxy had no telephone or the proxy also was a subject in the study. In the latter circumstances an in-person interview was conducted with the subject and a proxy interview was conducted for the deceased spouse.

The Questionnaires

Two versions of the interview questionnaire were developed: the Subject Questionnaire and the Proxy Questionnaire (Appendix A). The vital status of the subject determined which version of the questionnaire would be administered. The Proxy Questionnaire was used only for deceased subjects. In most cases Proxy Questionnaires were administered by telephone, whereas Subject Questionnaires were administered in person.

The Subject Questionnaire was used whenever the subject was alive at the time of interview. The questionnaires were administered by trained interviewers, with the exception of more sensitive sections of the Subject Questionnaire (female medical history and psychological questions), which were self-administered. If a subject was unable to take part in the interview, selected portions of the Subject Questionnaires were administered to a proxy respondent. This version of the Subject Questionnaire is referred to as the "boxed" questionnaire. The questions on the Subject Questionnaire that are included in the "boxed" questionnaire are identified by the shaded boxes in which the questionnaire numbers are enclosed. In general, only questions that would elicit objective responses are included in the "boxed" questionnaire. Questions relating to feelings, opinions, or perceptions are omitted. On some occasions when the subject needed help answering some questions, an assistant was used and the Subject Questionnaire was answered. It is important to keep in mind the distinction between a proxy respondent and the Proxy Questionnaire. Proxy respondents were used when the subject was deceased or was unable to participate in the interview because of disability. However, Proxy Questionnaires were administered only when the subject was deceased.

Both the Subject and the Proxy Questionnaires are divided into sections according to general topic. Certain questions on the Subject Questionnaire were omitted from the Proxy Questionnaire where appropriate. General topics as well as specific question batteries were developed collaboratively by the participating agencies.

Part A includes questions on the subject's household composition and the first part of the Mental Status Questionnaire (MSQ) to be administered only to subjects aged 60 and over (Kahn et al. 1960). The MSQ is used to identify dementia and was placed in this section to screen those subjects who could not respond to the questionnaire. If the subject received a score of less than 3, the interviewer immediately administered the second part of the battery, which is located in Part H. If the subject scored less than 8 on the total MSQ, he or she was asked the questions in Parts I, J., and P, but the interviewer was instructed to try to have a family member or close friend assist the subject with the rest of the questionnaire. However, if the interviewer felt that the subject could provide valid responses, or if a proxy respondent could not be located, the interviewer continued to ask the questions of the subject. One hundred seventy-three subjects scored less than 8 on the MSQ, and in 81 of these cases another person assisted the subject in responding to the questions.

Part B of the questionnaire contains information on the composition and vital status of the subject's family of origin and on the history of cancer in parents and siblings. Questions on parents' vital status were omitted from the subject telephone interview.

Part C contains the female medical history, which includes questions on menstrual and pregnancy history, exposure to estrogens, and status of reproductive organs. Some questions on status of reproductive organs found in Part C of the Subject Questionnaire are found in Part G of the Proxy Questionnaire.

Part D contains a self-reported history of selected medical conditions. The conditions were selected on the basis of prevalence and clinical importance. They include hypertension, angina, myocardial infarction, claudication, stroke, gall bladder disease, cancer, and respiratory problems. The questions on angina and coronary heart disease are those developed by Dr. Geoffrey Rose of the University of London (Rose 1965; Rose et al. 1982), and the respiratory scale was adapted from that recommended by the American Thoracic Society–National Heart, Lung and Blood Institute, Division of Lung Disease Joint Project (National Heart, Lung and Blood Institute 1978). A diagram was included in the Self-administration Booklet so that the subject could identify the location of anginal pain. Each set of questions on a particular condition also included a question on whether or not the subject had been hospitalized for the condition since 1970. If a hospitalization had occurred, information on the name and address of the facility, the year of the stay, and the reason for the stay was recorded. Also included in this section is a battery of questions on exposure to sunlight and the occurrence of bedsores after confinement to bed. Questions pertaining to symptoms were omitted from the "boxed" questionnaire and the Proxy Questionnaire.

Part E of the Subject Questionnaire concerns arthritis. The battery of questions is adapted from the Arthritis Supplement used in NHANES I. The questions on symptoms meet the diagnostic criteria for rheumatoid and osteoarthritis of the American Rheumatism Association (*Dictionary of Rheumatic Diseases* 1982). The battery includes a scale that is found in the Self-administration Booklet and that is designed to measure the amount of joint pain experienced by the subject. The battery of arthritic questions was not included in the Proxy Questionnaire, but a global question on arthritis was added to Part G in the questionnaire. The questions in Part E relating to the experience of pain or other symptoms were omitted from the "boxed" questionnaire.

Part F concerns functional impairment. The battery represents an adaptation of selected items from the Fries Functional Disability Scale for arthritis (Fries et al. 1980), the Rosow–Breslau Scale (Rosow ad Breslau 1966), and the Katz Activities of Daily Living Scale (Katz and Akpom 1976). The questions are designed to measure how much difficulty the subject has in performing a set of everyday activities without the help of another person and without mechanical aid. Information is also collected on whether or not help is received and how this help affects the person's ability to perform the activity. Thus, these questions can be used to measure the impact of disease on functional ability. They can also be used to determine the effect on functional level of the receipt of help or use of aids. The items can be grouped in different ways to investigate different aspects of functional status. Part F is omitted from the Proxy Questionnaire, and a shorter version was used for the Subject Telephone Questionnaire.

Part G is a checklist designed to provide information on diseases and conditions not identified in other parts of the questionnaire. Conditions identified in NHANES I as having a high probability of being reported or required for proposed analyses were included in the list. Information was collected on whether or not the subject had ever been told by a doctor that he or she had a specified condition, the year of initial diagnosis of the condition, and whether or not the subject had been hospitalized since 1970 for the condition. Information was also gathered on any hospitalization or stays in other health facilities that was not obtained previously. Questions on the subject's use of selected prescription medicines, aspirin, antacids, vitamins, minerals, and other nutritional supplements are also found in Part G. The final question in Part G obtains the subject's social security number.

Part H contains the second portion of the Mental Status Questionnaire. Its use was described in the explanation of Part A.

Part I includes the CES-D Depression scale (Radloff 1977) and selected items from the General Well-being Scale (National Center for Health Statistics 1977b), which correspond to Negative Affect, Positive Affect, and Health Concern. Both scales were designed for self-administration and therefore are included in the Self-administration Booklet. Questions on social support are also included in this section.

Part J. concerns bowel and bladder functioning. This section was included in the Self-administration Booklet because of the possible sensitivity of these questions.

Part K contains questions on changes in the subject's weight over time.

Part L. was designed to obtain a smoking history that identifies periods of commencement and cessation of smoking, the average number of cigarettes smoked, the current amount smoked, and the use of cigars, pipes, snuff, and chewing tobacco.

Part M concerns consumption of alcoholic beverages. The questions were designed to obtain the subject's lifetime pattern of usual drinking. Information on binge drinking during the past year and on the period of heaviest drinking during the subject's lifetime was also collected.

Part N contains an extensive battery of questions designed to identify aspects of the subject's usual diet. The section includes questions on how frequently specific foods are consumed. The questions cover the major food groups: meat, fish, poultry, grains, fruits, vegetables, dairy products, sweets, and snacks. The main criteria for inclusion of individual food items in this expanded listing was whether the item is frequently consumed and whether the food is high in fat, cholesterol, fiber, vitamin A, or vitamin C. The food frequency list also includes items on condiments, coffee, tea, soda, and alcohol. Questions on food preparation, use of prepared food, special diets, frequency of eating meals and snacking, use of salt, and eating problems are also included in Part N. Part N was not included in the Proxy Questionnaire or the Subject Telephone Questionnaire.

Part O gathers information on sleep problems and changes in sleep patterns. The questions used were adapted from those used in the Stanford Sleep Study (Karacan et al. 1983). These questions were not included in either the "boxed" or Proxy Questionnaires.

Part P includes two scales that measure the traits of extroversion and "openness to experience" (Costa and McCrae 1980). Measures of type A personality are also included in this section. Part P is not included in either the "boxed" or Proxy Questionnaires.

Part Q contains a limited number of questions on physical activity. This part includes physical activity items used in NHANES II plus added items on jogging. Neither the "boxed" nor the Proxy Questionnaire contains these items (National Center for Health Statistics 1981).

Part R contains questions on the extent of tooth loss, the use of dental plates, and the use of flouridated toothpaste. The items used are repeated from NHANES I. The Proxy Questionnaire does not contain this section but these questions are included in the "boxed" questionnaire.

Part S contains questions that measure the subject's ability to hear, and Part T contains questions measuring ability to see. The scales in both sections are the same as those used in NHANES I. Neither Part S nor Part T is included in the Proxy Questionnaire, and only parts of the each section are included in the "boxed" questionnaire.

Part U obtains background information on race; marital status; where the subject lived most of his or her life; usual occupation; current activity; exposure to dust, fumes, or vapors during work or hobbies; and sources of income.

Part V in the Proxy Questionnaire includes questions concerning the circumstances surrounding the subject's death. It is found only in the Proxy Questionnaire. Items seek information on whether the subject was confined to home or an institution prior to death, cause of death, who was present at the time of death, the experience of pain at death, and place of death (i.e., home or hospital).

Physical Measurement

At the end of the household interview, the interviewer measured the pulse rate, took three consecutive blood pressure readings, and weighed the subject. All measurements were obtained according to a specific protocol. Arm cuffs in child, adult, and large sizes were available so that the interviewer could select the correct size. There was an interval of at least 30 seconds between the three readings. The cuff bladder was fully deflated between readings. Procedures for blood pressure measurement were adapted from those of Kirkendall (Kirkendall et al. 1967) and the Hypertension Detection and Follow-up Program (Hypertension Detection and Follow-up Program Cooperative Group 1978).

Health Facilities and Data Collection

Parts D, E, and G of the Subject and Proxy Questionnaires contain items that ask about any overnight stays in a health care facility since 1970. If a stay was reported, information on the name and address of the facility, the date of the stay, and the reason for the stay was recorded on a special chart on the back cover of the Self-administration Booklet.

A list of all subjects who reported a stay in a particular hospital was compiled. As field interviewing in a region neared completion, all hospitals and nursing homes in the region that had stays reported by study subjects were sent a medical records survey packet. Although information on hospitalizations was elicited from subjects for the entire period from 1970 to the time of follow-up, the request to the hospital did not include the specific dates of hospitalization, but asked for all admissions from January 1 of the year of the NHANES I examination to the date of the follow-up interview.

At the conclusion of the interview, subjects were asked to sign a Medical Authorization Form that requested hospitals to release data to the study. The signed forms were retained on file, and a photocopy was made for each hospital identified by the subject during the interview.

A letter was mailed to the administrator of the hospital advising that a request for information was being sent to the hospital's medical records department. Some hospitals did not have the staff to answer the requests. In those cases, an abstractor, usually someone at the hospital, was hired by the NHEFS project to collect the data. In only two cases did the National Center for Health Statistics provide an abstractor to collect the data.

Very limited data were requested on the Hospital Abstract form (Appendix B). The dates of admission and discharge and the diagnoses were the major data requested. In addition, photocopies of the "face sheet" and "discharge summary" for each hospital episode in the specified time period were requested. For diagnoses of myocardial infarction (ICD9, 410 codes) a photocopy of the third-day ECG was requested. For any admission where a malignancy was initially diagnosed, a photocopy of the pathology report was requested. All medical records were recoded by trained medical coders using ICD9-CM.

Similarly, a request was made to each nursing home identified during the interview. Abstracts were mailed to the nursing home administrators (Appendix C), who were asked for information on the dates and reasons for admission for each nursing home stay.

Collection of Death Certificates

Deaths identified by the National Death Index (United States Department of Health and Human Services 1981) or other tracing methods were verified by obtaining the death certificate from the state where the subject had died. These death certificates were coded by using ICD9 multiple cause-of-death codes (World Health Organization 1977).

REFERENCES

Costa, P. T., Jr., and R. R. McCrae. 1980. "Still stable after all these years: Personality as a key to some issues in aging." In *Life Span Development and Behavior,* vol. 3. P. B. Baltes and O. G. Brim, eds. New York: Academic Press, pp. 68–74.

Dictionary of the Rheumatic Diseases. 1982. Prepared by the American Rheumatism Association Glossary Committee. New York: Contact Associates International, Ltd.

Fries, J. F., P. Spitz, R. G. Krains, and H. R. Holman. 1980. "Measurement of patient outcome in arthritis." *Arthritis Rheum* 23:137–145.

Hypertension Detection and Follow-up Program Cooperative Group. 1978. "Variability of blood pressure and the results of screening in the Hypertension Detection and Follow-up Program." *J Chronic Dis* 31:651–667.

Kahn, R. L., A. I. Goldfarb, M. Pollack, and A. Peck. 1960. "Brief objective measures for the determination of mental status in the aged." *Am J Psychiatry* 117:326–328.

Karacan, I., J. I. Thornby, and R. L. Williams. 1983. "Sleep disturbance: A community survey." In *Sleep/Wake Disorders: National History, Epidemiology and Long Term Evolution.* C. Guilleninault and E. Lugaresi, eds. New York: Raven Press, pp. 37–71.

Katz, S. C., and C. A. Akpom. 1976. "Index of ADL." *Med Care* 14(supp.):116–118.

Kirkendall, W. M., A. C. Burton, F. H. Epstein, and E. D. Freis. 1967. "Recommendations for human blood pressure determination by sphygmomanometer." *Circulation* 36:980–988.

National Center for Health Statistics. 1973. Plan and Operation of the Health and Nutrition Examination Survey, United States, 1971–1973. *Vital and Health Statistics.* Series 1,

No. 10a. DHEW Publication No. (PHS) 79-1310. Washington, DC: U.S. Government Printing Office.

National Center for Health Statistics. 1977a. Plan and Operation of the Health and Nutrition Examination Survey, United States, 1971–1973. *Vital and Health Statistics.* Series 1, No. 10b. DHEW Publication No. (PHS) 79-1310. Washington, DC: U.S. Government Printing Office.

National Center for Health Statistics. 1977b. A Concurrent Validational Study of the NCHS General Well-Being Schedule. *Vital and Health Statistics.* Series 2. No. 73. DHEW Publication No. (HRA) 78-1347. Washington, DC: U.S. Government Printing Office.

National Center for Health Statistics. 1978. Plan and Operation of the NHANES I Augmentation Survey of Adults 25–74 Years, United States, 1974–1975. *Vital and Health Statistics.* Series 1, No. 14. DHEW Publication No. (PHS) 78-1314. Washington, DC: U.S. Government Printing Office.

National Center for Health Statistics. 1981. Plan and Operation of the Second National Health and Nutrition Examination Survey, 1976–1980. *Vital and Health Statistics.* Series 1, No. 15. DHHS Publication No. (PHS) 81-1317. Washington, DC: U.S. Government Printing Office.

National Center for Health Statistics. 1985. M. G. Kovar and G. S. Poe, The National Health Interview Survey Design, 1973-1984, and Procedures, 1975–1983. *Vital and Health Statistics.* Series 1, No. 18. DHHS Publication No. (PHS) 85-1320. Washington, DC: U.S. Government Printing Office.

National Heart, Lung and Blood Institute. 1978. B. F. Ferris, *Epidemiology Standardization Project.* Contract No. 1-HR-5-3028 (Report No. HR-53028-F). Division of Lung Diseases, pp. 7–54.

Radloff, L. S. 1977. "The CES-D scale: A self-report depression scale for research in the general population." *Appl Psychol Measurement* 1(3):385–401.

Rose, G. A. 1965. "Chest pain questionnaire." *Milbank Mem Fund Q* 43(2):32–39.

Rose, G. A., H. Blackburn, R. F. Gillum, and R. J. Prineas. 1982. "Cardiovascular survey methods." In *Cardiovascular Survey Methods.* Geneva: World Health Organization pp. 162–165.

Rosow, I., and N. Breslau. 1966. "A Guttman health scale for the aged." *J Gerontol* 21(4):556–559.

United States Department of Health and Human Services, 1981. *User's Manual: The National Death Index.* DHHS Publication No. (PHS) 81-1148. Washington, DC: U.S. Government Printing Office.

World Health Organization. 1977. *Manual of International Statistical Classification of Diseases, Injuries, and Causes of Death.* Based on recommendations of 9th Revision Conference. Geneva: World Health Organization.

2

Effectiveness of Field Operations:
Data Collection and Tracing

JENNIFER H. MADANS, JOEL C. KLEINMAN,
CHRISTINE S. COX, AND FANCHON F. FINUCANE

The NHANES I Epidemiologic Follow-up Study (NHEFS) is composed of several separate data collection activities: tracing, interviewing, collection of death certificates, and collection of hospital records. These procedures are described in detail in Chapter 1. Analyses can be based on data from any one of these components, or data from all components can be combined. This chapter contains a summary of the results of each of these data collection activities and provides a description of the mortality experience of the cohort.

DATA COLLECTION

Collection of data for the 1982–84 follow-up (NHEFS) was officially completed in August 1984. Data were included in the follow-up files if the report of the event (e.g., tracing report, completed questionnaire, hospital record, death certificate) was received at the home office by August 31, 1984. Events such as deaths and hospitalizations that occurred after the interview date were not included in this wave of data collection but are part of the data collection for a continued follow-up of the cohort. On the basis of the data received, the "last date known alive" was determined for each subject. For deceased subjects, this is the date of death; for living subjects who were successfully interviewed it is the date of the interview; for subjects traced but not interviewed it is the date of last tracing contact; and for those lost to follow-up, it is the date of the NHANES I examination. Length of follow-up for those still alive is the period between date of initial examination and date of follow-up interview or tracing date if not interviewed. The average length of follow-up for traced surviving subjects is 10 years (range = 6–13 years). Five percent of the subjects were followed up for less than 8 years; 35%, for 8 to 9 years; 32%, for 10 years; and 27%, for 11 or 12 years.

Figure 2–1 is a flow chart of the data collection activities for NHEFS subjects

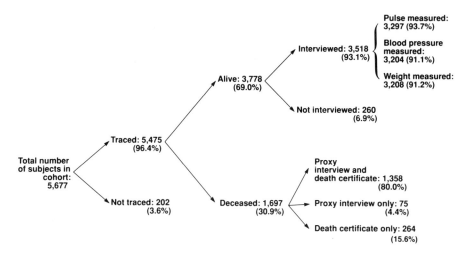

Fig. 2–1. NHEFS data collection procedures, initial follow-up (1982–1984).

aged 55 years or older at baseline. The number of respondents participating in each component of the survey is provided, as are the results of each data collection activity. The figure also illustrates the relationship between the survey's various activities. Detailed results for each data collection activity follow. All results are based on respondents 55 years of age or older at baseline.

Tracing

Until the initiation of NHEFS, NHANES I examinees had not been contacted in any way by the National Center for Health Statistics or any of the collaborators at the National Institutes of Health. Since the validity of longitudinal studies is dependent on completeness of follow-up, extensive and varied efforts were made to trace and establish the vital status of all NHEFS subjects. A person was considered successfully traced if the person or a proxy (in the case of those deceased or incapacitated) correctly responded to a set of verification questions establishing the person's identity. All persons not traced were considered lost to follow-up. In addition, the fact of death had to be corroborated by either a death certificate or a proxy interview. In some cases, information about the death of a subject was obtained from neighbors or other tracing contacts. Although this information was noted in the record, these persons were considered lost to follow-up unless the information was confirmed by a proxy interview or by a death certificate.

As of August 1984, 96% of the study population (aged 55 years or older at NHANES I examination) was successfully located. However, the success of the tracing efforts varied by age, race, and gender (third column of Table 2–1). To summarize how demographic factors were related to success of tracing, a multiple logistic model was fitted to the cross-classification of age, race, and gender, with the proportion lost to follow-up as the dependent variable. Because of the small

Table 2–1 Percentage Distribution of Status at Follow-up (NHEFS) According to Race, Gender, and Age at Baseline (NHANES I)

Race, gender, and age at baseline	Percentage with indicated status at NHEFS			Total no.
	Alive	Dead	Lost	
All races	66.5	29.9	3.6	5677
Men				
55–64 years	75.8	21.3	2.9	860
65–74 years	50.9	45.5	3.6	1836
Women				
55–64 years	86.1	10.4	3.5	964
65–74 years	67.5	28.7	3.8	2017
White	68.2	29.0	2.7	4739
Men				
55–64 years	77.3	20.1	2.6	741
65–74 years	52.6	45.0	2.4	1501
Women				
55–64 years	86.9	10.4	2.7	819
65–74 years	69.1	27.8	3.2	1678
Black	58.2	33.9	7.8	893
Men				
55–64 years	63.8	30.5	5.7	105
65–74 years	44.1	46.3	9.6	313
Women				
55–64 years	81.7	10.6	7.7	142
65–74 years	59.8	33.3	6.9	333
Other	53.3	42.2	4.4	45
Men				
55–64 years	85.7	14.3	*	14
65–74 years	27.3	68.2	4.5	22
Women				
55–64 years	66.7	*	33.3	3
65–74 years	66.7	33.3	*	6

Note: The sampling frame for NHANES I included persons aged 1–74 years at the time of the interview. Several subjects reached their 75th birthday between the interview and the examination. In addition, date of birth was incorrectly coded for several subjects. This error was corrected in the follow-up. As a result, three subjects were over 75 but were retained in the analysis.

*There were no individuals in these categories.

number of subjects of "other" races, this analysis was limited to whites and blacks. Terms were deleted from the saturated model until the simplest model that fit the data was obtained. The smallest p-value for a deleted term was 0.17. The final model includes only a main effect for race ($p < 0.001$). Loss to follow-up is higher for blacks than for whites (odds ratio for blacks relative to whites = 2.99).

The design of NHANES I included oversampling of residents of "poverty areas" (i.e., a sampling segment in which a substantial percentage of the population has income below the poverty level) (National Center for Health Statistics 1973, 1977, 1978). Residence in a poverty area did not substantially affect rates of loss to follow-up.

Another indicator of sociodemographic differentials is education. Since educational differentials in mortality are analyzed in Chapter 8, the relationship between education and loss to follow-up was investigated by fitting a multiple logistic model to the cross-classification of race, gender, and education, with the proportion lost to follow-up as the dependent variable. Since number of years of education varies significantly by age, separate models were fit for those 55–64 years old and those 65 years or older. Loss to follow-up does not vary by educational attainment among black persons or white persons aged 65 years or older. However, among whites 55–64 years old there is a significant gender–education interaction. Women with 12 or more years of education were least likely to be lost. Odds ratios relative to women with 12 or more years of education are 1.35 for males with less than 12 years, 2.15 for men with 12 or more years, and 2.78 for women with less than 12 years. The number of black persons aged 55–64 years is too small to investigate the relationship between education and tracing status.

To ascertain whether those lost to follow-up were at relatively high risk of death, a multiple logistic regression analysis was done with tracing status as the dependent variable. Six baseline health characteristics (in addition to age, race, and gender) that have been established as risk factors for mortality were tested as independent variables. These included high blood pressure (systolic blood pressure of 140 mmHg or higher), high serum cholesterol (260 mg/100 ml or more), overweight (for men, body mass index greater than or equal to 27.8 kilograms/meter and for women, body mass index greater than or equal to 27.3 kilograms/meter),* history of heart attack, history of diabetes, and smoking (smoker, nonsmoker, unknown). Table 2–2 shows the results. Three of the risk factors were inversely associated with loss to follow-up: high blood pressure, high serum cholesterol levels, and a history of heart attack. Overweight examinees and those with a history of diabetes were more likely to be untraced. None of these differences was statistically significant. Smoking was most strongly associated with loss to follow-up: smokers were more than twice as likely as nonsmokers to be untraced ($p = 0.003$). These results suggest that those lost to follow-up are somewhat more likely to have died than those successfully traced. It should be noted, however, that the proportion lost to follow-up among those aged 55 years or older is quite small relative to the proportion deceased. There should be relatively little bias in mortality findings as a result of loss to follow-up.

Interview Data

Interviews with the subject or a proxy were completed for 87% of the original cohort (4951 persons), or 90% of those successfully traced. Of the 1433 proxy interviews for decedents, 1002 were completed by telephone. In 35 cases, interviews for living subjects were conducted by telephone rather than in person. Telephone interviews

---

*These cut points were used because they represent the sex specific 85th percentile for persons 20–29 years of age in the 1976–1980 National Health and Nutrition Examination Survey. Pregnant women were not included (National Center for Health Statistics 1981).

Table 2–2 Relationship of Health Characteristics at NHANES I on Loss to Follow-up at NHEFS

Characteristic	Odds ratio*	95% Confidence interval*	p-value*
High blood pressure	0.88	0.64, 1.19	0.406
High cholesterol	0.89	0.65, 1.21	0.456
Overweight	1.12	0.82, 1.53	0.481
Heart attack	0.89	0.53, 1.51	0.674
Diabetes	1.42	0.90, 2.24	0.131
Smoker	2.20	1.40, 3.46	0.003

*Based on multiple logistic regression including age, gender, and race and all health characteristics listed.

were used if the respondent lived in a remote area or if the respondent was traced too late in the field period for an in-person interview. Nonresponse rates for the interview, by age, race, gender, and vital status are given in Table 2–3. Seven percent of the traced, living subjects were not interviewed; proxy interviews could not be obtained for 16% of the decedents. The lower rate of success for interviewing the deceased as compared with surviving subjects was apparent in all age, gender, and race groups. This is due in part to the fact that many of the decedents were located from vital statistics files and that no proxy could be identified.

The relationship between demographic factors and interview status was summarized by use of multiple logistic models that were fit to the cross-classification of age, race, and gender. The proportion of respondents not completing the interview was the dependent variable. Separate models were fitted for living and deceased persons. After deleting nonsignificant terms from the saturated model (the smallest p-value for a deleted term was 0.16), the final model for deceased persons includes a main effect for race ($p < 0.001$) and a marginally significant interaction between age and gender ($p = 0.06$). Nonresponse rates for the proxies of black decedents are substantially higher than those for whites (odds ratio = 2.43). Response rates are lowest for females 55–64 years old and highest for males 55–64 years old (odds ratios are 1.84 for men 55–64, 1.56 for women 65–74, and 1.36 for men 65–74 relative to women 55–64). The final model for surviving subjects includes an age–gender interaction ($p = 0.06$) but no race effect. All other terms deleted from the model had p values greater than 0.14. Noninterview rates were highest for men 65 years and older and lowest for men 55–64 years of age (odds ratios relative to men 55–64 are 2.29 for men 65–74, 1.90 for women 65–74, and 1.43 for women 55–64).

Physical Measurements

During the personal interview, interviewers attempted to take pulse, blood pressure, and weight measurements for each subject. Interviewers had extensive training in physical measurements and were reevaluated in the course of the field period. The physical measurements were not attempted for the 35 persons interviewed by telephone or for the 140 who were incapacitated and did not take part in the interview at all. Sixty-seven other incapacitated persons did not act as respondents to the interview but did participate in the physical measurement section. Another six re-

Table 2–3 Percentage of Traced NHEFS Cohort Without Completed Interview According to Race, Gender, Age at Baseline, and Vital Status at NHEFS

Race, gender, and age at baseline	Percentage without completed interview*	
	Alive	Deceased
All races†	6.9	15.6
Men		
55–64 years	4.3	18.6
65–74 years	8.8	14.6
Women		
55–64 years	5.8	12.0
65–74 years	7.5	16.6
White	6.7	12.9
Men		
55–64 years	3.7	15.4
65–74 years	8.5	12.7
Women		
55–64 years	6.0	7.1
65–74 years	7.5	13.5
Black	7.5	26.7
Men		
55–64 years	7.5	34.4
65–74 years	10.9	22.8
Women		
55–64 years	4.3	40.0
65–74 years	7.0	27.9

Note: The sampling frame for NHANES I included persons aged 1–74 years at the time of the interview. Several subjects reached their 75th birthday between the interview and the examination. In addition, date of birth was incorrectly coded for several subjects. This error was corrected in the follow-up. As a result, three subjects were over 75 but were retained in the analysis.

*Percentages are based on subjects who were successfully traced.

†Includes races other than white or black.

spondents terminated the interview before the physical measurement section. Thus, none of the physical measurements were attempted for 181 of the 3518 NHANES I survivors who completed an interview in NHEFS.

In addition to these 181, pulse was not measured for another 40 participants. (Note that if pulse measurement is missing for an individual, blood pressure or weight measurements also may be missing.) The pulse measurement was not attempted for 36 of the 40 because of refusal (seven cases), medical contraindications (18), or other reasons (11). No valid physical measure was obtained for the other four persons. Thus, the overall failure rate for obtaining a pulse measurement was 6.3%. A multiple logistic model was used to summarize the age-, gender-, and race-

Table 2–4 Percentage of Interviewed NHEFS Cohort Without Completed Physical Measurements According to Race, Gender, and Age at Baseline

Race, gender, and age at baseline	Percentage without successfully completed physical measurements*		
	Pulse	Blood pressure†	Weight‡
All races§	6.3	8.9	8.8
Men			
55–64 years	5.0	6.1	5.8
65–74 years	6.5	9.3	8.8
Women			
55–64 years	2.8	5.5	4.5
65–74 years	9.0	12.2	13.0
White	5.9	8.3	8.2
Men			
55–64 years	5.1	6.2	6.2
65–74 years	6.1	8.3	7.7
Women			
55–64 years	2.5	5.4	4.0
65–74 years	8.3	11.3	12.2
Black	8.9	13.1	12.9
Men			
55–64 years	4.8	6.5	3.2
65–74 years	8.9	15.4	15.4
Women			
55–64 years	4.5	6.3	7.2
65–74 years	13.0	17.8	17.8

Note: The sampling frame for NHANES I included persons aged 1–74 years at the time of the interview. Several subjects reached their 75th birthday between the interview and the examination. In addition, date of birth was incorrectly coded for several subjects. This error was corrected in the follow-up. As a result, three subjects were over 75 but were retained in the analysis.

*Percentages are based on the total number of traced, living subjects with a completed subject interview. This includes 35 cases who were interviewed by telephone and on whom no measurements were attempted.

†Completed blood pressure measurement is defined as the successful completion of either the second or the third measurement.

‡Completed weight measurement is defined as a successful measurement taken on either of two attempts.

§Includes races other than white or black.

specific failure rates shown in Table 2–4. The final model contains a significant age–gender interaction ($p = 0.002$) and a main effect for race ($p = 0.015$). Relative to women 55–64 years of age, the odds ratios for pulse measurement failure were 1.96 for men 55–64, 3.59 for women 65 and older, and 2.50 for men aged 65 and older. In addition, blacks were 54% more likely than whites to have no pulse measurement recorded.

Three blood pressure measurements were attempted. Failure to obtain a reading was considered an attempt and could not be repeated. Either the second or the third of the three blood pressure measurements had to be successful for the procedure to be considered complete. Blood pressure of 133 subjects was not measured (in addition to the 181 noted earlier). The blood pressure procedure was not attempted for 99 of the 133 persons (eight refusals, 68 medical contraindications, and 23 other reasons). The procedure was attempted but not successfully completed on another 34 subjects. (As noted previously, individuals with missing blood pressure measurements may have no pulse or weight measurement recorded.)

Therefore, 8.9% of the NHEFS subjects with a completed interview had no blood pressure measurement (Table 2–4). The final multiple logistic model contained a marginally significant age–gender interaction ($p = 0.08$) and showed an effect of race ($p = 0.001$). The odds ratios for no blood pressure measurement relative to women 55–64 years of age were 1.18 for men 55–64 years old, 2.46 for women 65 years and older, and 1.80 for men 65 years and older. Blacks were 63% more likely than whites to have no blood pressure measurement recorded.

In addition to the 181 subjects for whom no physical measurements were attempted, weight was not measured for another 129 participants. (As was the case for individuals whose blood pressure or pulse measurements are missing, those whose weight was not recorded may also be missing one of the other two measurements.) Measurement of weight was not attempted for 123 subjects (16 refusals, 95 medical contraindications, and 12 others). No valid measure was obtained for another six persons (Table 2–4). The final multiple logistic model contains a marginally significant age–race–gender interaction ($p = 0.06$). Persons under 65 years of age were more likely to have a weight measurement as were those of the white race. White women younger than 65 years were most likely to have a measurement, and black women 65 years or older were least likely. Black women over 65 years of age were five times more likely not to have a weight measurement than were white women younger than 65 years.

Death Certificates

Tracing activities identified 1697 deaths among those 55 years old or older at baseline. A subject is considered deceased only if a death certificate was received or death was verified by a proxy interview. Death certificates have been obtained for almost 96% of all decedents. Table 2–5 presents the percentage of decedents by age, race, and gender and the percentage for whom no death certificates were available. There was little difference by age or race in the percentage of decedents for whom no death certificate was obtained, but death certificates were 59% more likely to be available for women than for men.

Facility Records

One of the objectives of the NHEFS interview was to obtain a complete history of overnight stays in health care facilities such as hospitals and nursing homes. Respondents were asked to sign a form authorizing the facility to release records to the study. Any health care facility named in the interview that could be located was

Table 2–5 Number of Deaths Among NHEFS Cohort and Percentage of Decedents for Whom a Death Certificate Was Not Obtained

Race, gender, and age at baseline	No. of deaths	Decedents without death certificate (%)
*All races**	1697	4.4
Men		
55–64 years	183	2.2
65–74 years	835	3.8
Women		
55–64 years	100	6.0
65–74 years	579	5.7
White	1375	4.1
Men		
55–64 years	149	2.0
65–74 years	675	3.3
Women		
55–64 years	85	4.7
65–74 years	466	5.8
Black	303	6.3
Men		
55–64 years	32	3.1
65–74 years	145	6.9
Women		
55–64 years	15	13.3
65–74 years	111	5.4

Note: The sampling frame for NHANES I included persons aged 1–74 years at the time of the interview. Several subjects reached their 75th birthday between the interview and the examination. In addition, date of birth was incorrectly coded for several subjects. This error was corrected in the follow-up. As a result, three subjects were over 75 but were retained in the analysis.

*Includes races other than white or black.

contacted and information was requested on each stay that occurred between the date of the NHANES I examination and the date of the NHEFS interview for surviving subjects and between the NHANES I examination and the date of death for decedents. Further contacts were attempted with other hospitals mentioned on death certificates or discharge abstracts.

Hospital records (9575) and nursing home records (416) were received for 3070 participants aged 55 years and older. Table 2–6 shows the results of the collection of records from health care facilities. Both the proportion of respondents with at least one facility report and the average number of facility reports received per person increase with age. These patterns are similar to those found in national hospital discharge statistics (National Center for Health Statistics 1984a).

Although these patterns are encouraging, there are indications that the hospital file is not complete. First, 190 of the 2557 hospitals and 59 of the 409 nursing homes contacted for records refused to participate. Second, several hospitals had

Table 2–6 Receipt of Records from Hospitals and Nursing Homes for NHEFS Cohort by Race, Gender, and Age at Baseline Examination

Race, gender, and age at baseline	Subjects with at least one episode report received		No. of episode reports received		
	Total	Percent of traced	Total	Average for traced subjects	Average for subjects with at least one report
All races	3070	(56.1)	9991	1.82	3.3
Men					
55–64 years	456	(54.6)	1417	1.70	3.1
65–74 years	1059	(59.9)	3459	1.96	3.3
Women					
55–64 years	444	(47.7)	1231	1.32	2.8
65–74 years	1111	(57.2)	3884	2.00	3.5
White	2660	(57.7)	8759	1.90	3.3
Men					
55–64 years	402	(55.7)	1268	1.76	3.2
65–74 years	892	(60.9)	2971	2.03	3.3
Women					
55–64 years	393	(49.3)	1095	1.37	2.8
65–74 years	973	(59.9)	3425	2.11	3.5
Black	394	(47.9)	1204	1.46	3.1
Men					
55–64 years	48	(48.5)	138	1.39	2.9
65–74 years	158	(55.8)	472	1.67	3.0
Women					
55–64 years	51	(38.9)	136	1.04	2.7
65–74 years	137	(44.2)	458	1.48	3.3

Note: The sampling frame for NHANES I included persons aged 1–74 years at the time of the interview. Several subjects reached their 75th birthday between the interview and the examination. In addition, date of birth was incorrectly coded for several subjects. This error was corrected in the follow-up. As a result, three subjects were over 75 but were retained in the analysis.

closed and no information about the disposition of their records was obtainable; thus, these facilities were not contacted. Third, some facilities did not send records, either because the records were inaccessible or because the search for them was unsuccessful. Finally, authorization forms were not obtained for 3% of surviving subjects and 12% of decedents.

It is difficult to measure precisely the extent to which the health care facility record file is complete. To do so requires that reported stays and facility records be matched on the basis of date and reason for the stay. The accuracy of such a search is dependent on the respondent's ability to recall these events for the average follow-up period of 10 years. Since this kind of recall is prone to error, such a match was not attempted. It is possible, however, to identify one group of missing records. No hospital records were obtained for 813 persons who reported at least one hospitalization after the NHANES I examination. In 13% of these cases the respondents refused to sign the authorization, and in another 47% the hospital refused or was not contacted for other reasons. In the remaining cases, records were not found by the hospital, perhaps because of reporting errors by respondents. The name of a facility could have been misreported or the date of a hospitalization might have been reported as occurring after the examination when in fact it occurred prior to NHANES I and, therefore, the stay would be excluded from consideration by NHEFS. A more extensive analysis designed to evaluate the completeness of the record collection is currently under way.

MORTALITY EXPERIENCE OF THE COHORT

Analysis of the mortality experience of the NHEFS cohort according to baseline characteristics is one of the major objectives of NHEFS. If tracing was successful, the mortality experience of the cohort should be similar to that of the entire population of the United States. Large deviations from national data would suggest bias in the database and limit the validity of the results. This part of the chapter compares the mortality experience of the NHEFS cohort with vital statistics of the United States.

Methodology for Analysis of Mortality Data

Comparisons of the mortality experience of the NHEFS cohort with vital statistics for the entire nation need to be evaluated with use of both separate age groups and survival analysis techniques that take into account variation in length of follow-up. Controlling for length of follow-up is particularly important in this sample, because the sample design of the NHANES I changed over the course of the survey and the sampling probabilities used were based on factors, such as residing in a poverty area, that are related to survival (see Chapter 1 and referenced reports [National Center for Health Statistics 1973, 1977, 1978] for a description of the NHANES I design). For example, a much larger proportion of low-income people was examined in 1971–1972 than in 1974–1975. Those examined earlier had a greater chance of dying merely because they were under observation for a longer period of time. Thus, the relationship between income and mortality would be distorted if length of follow-up were not properly controlled for in the analysis.

Cumulative survival rates and standard errors for 12 age-, race-, and gender-specific subgroups were calculated by use of the Kaplan–Meier product limit method (SAS Institute, Inc. 1985). Both graphs of survival curves and tables of survival probabilities at 5 and 8 years are presented. Five-year survival was chosen since it is the approximate midpoint of the follow-up period. Eight-year survival is also presented because over 90% of the cohort were followed for at least 8 years. Survival rates beyond 8 years become highly unstable, especially for small subgroups. Five-year age groups were used. Race was categorized as white or black. Persons of other races were omitted from this analysis.

Persons who could not be traced (2.5% of white men, 3.0% of white women,

8.6% of black men, and 7.2% of black women) were excluded from the survival calculations. In effect, this assumes that mortality among those lost to follow-up is identical to that for persons successfully traced. Those found alive were censored at last date known alive (usually the date of the follow-up interview).

Survival among persons in each age group of the NHANES I sample was compared to survival probabilities derived from life tables for the United States using the midpoint of the age interval. For example, survival for persons aged 55–59 years at the time of NHANES I (baseline) was compared to the U.S. survival probability for persons aged 57 years. For each age, race, and gender group, the U.S. life table for 1973 provided the expected probability of surviving 1 year after the baseline examination. (The year 1973 was selected because it is the midpoint of the examination period.) Information from U.S. life tables for the years 1974–1982 was used for calculation of the probabilities of surviving 2–10 years after the baseline examination. For each age, race, and gender group, the expected proportion surviving n years is given by the following formula:

$$\prod_{i=0}^{n-1}\left(1 - {}_1q_{a+i,\ 1973+i}\right)$$

where

$_1q_{x,y}$ = probability that persons in a given race–sex group alive at age x will die within 1 year according to U.S. life table for year y.

a = midpoint of age interval at baseline (1973).

Expected survival probabilities were calculated from successive life tables rather than from just the initial (1973) life table in order to take into account the decrease in U.S. death rates that occurred over this time period. However, the U.S. life tables still only approximate the expected survival of the NHANES I sample. Differences in survival probabilities between the NHANES I sample and the U.S. population are expected because of the sample design of NHANES I. Because NHANES I was a sample of noninstitutionalized persons, higher survival probabilities would be expected than those for the entire U.S. population, which includes institutionalized persons. This effect would be greatest among elderly persons and would decrease over time as the sample approaches the institutionalization patterns of the U.S. population. On the other hand, because income is inversely related to mortality, the oversampling of persons with low income in NHANES I would lead to a counterbalancing expectation of lower survival probabilities in the NHANES I sample than in the entire U.S. population. Women of childbearing age and the elderly were also oversampled, but since results are presented by age and gender, the mortality comparisons would not be affected by this aspect of the design.

For assessment of the effect of sample design on the mortality experience of the cohort, survival probabilities were calculated separately for three subgroups. The NHANES I design oversampled residents of poverty areas (i.e., geographic units with substantial percentage of the population below the poverty level). The rate of oversampling by residence in a poverty area was greatest during 1971–1972, reduced during 1973–1974, and eliminated entirely for those selected as part of the augmentation sample (1974–1975). For white men and white women aged 65–69 and 70–74 years at baseline, cumulative survival probabilities were calculated for those examined between 1971 and 1974 residing in poverty areas, for those examined between 1971 and 1974 residing in nonpoverty areas, and for those examined as part of the augmentation sample.

To determine whether the patterns of mortality among the four race and gender groups were comparable to what would be expected on the basis of national vital statistics, proportional hazard models (SAS Institute, Inc. 1983) were estimated for two age groups (55–64 and 65 years and older). Each model included three dummy variables for comparison of the race and gender groups (relative to white women) and a continuous variable that adjusted for age.

Finally, the distributions of causes of death for decedents in NHEFS were compared to those for all U.S. deaths, as recorded in national vital statistics, by use of four race and gender groups. Because the age distribution of NHEFS sample is different from that of the entire U.S. population, the comparisons were adjusted for age by the indirect method. For each race and gender group, the expected number of deaths for each cause in the NHEFS population was calculated by applying the percentage of deaths for that cause in vital statistics to the number of NHEFS deaths in each age group:

$$e_c = \sum_{a=1}^{7} p_{ac}\, d_a$$

where e_c = expected number of deaths for cause c

p_{ac} = proportion of deaths from cause c in age group a (from U.S. vital statistics)

d_a = number of NHEFS deaths in age group a

a = age groups 30–44, 45–54, 55–64, 65–69, 70–74, 75–79, or 80–84.

Note that deaths were tabulated according to age at death rather than age at NHANES I. The survival comparisons are done according to age at NHANES I. U.S. vital statistics for 1979 (National Center for Health Statistics 1984b) were used as the basis for comparison, since this was the closest year to the midpoint of the follow-up period in which deaths were coded according to ICD9 (World Health Organization 1977). Underlying cause of death was coded from the death certificate for 1622 decedents (death certificates have not yet been located for the other 4.4% of decedents).

Causes of death were initially aggregated into the NCHS standard 34-cause list (National Center for Health Statistics 1984b). Causes with fewer than five expected deaths (for whites) were combined, so that the final list included 19 causes for men and 20 causes for women. (The additional cause for women is breast cancer.) Observed and expected deaths for each race and gender group were compared by the standard χ^2 statistic.

Because of the several differences between the NHEFS cohort and the U.S.

population (i.e., oversampling of certain population subgroups and exclusion of institutionalized persons), precise agreement between mortality experience of this NHEFS population and the U.S. population would not be expected. The comparisons presented here are designed to help determine whether the mortality experience of the NHEFS sample is reasonably close to that of the U.S. population. Although standard errors and significance tests were used for comparison of NHEFS results with expected values based on U.S. vital statistics, modest departures from the null hypotheses are to be expected. Such "significant" differences need to be interpreted carefully with respect to their magnitude and implications for deriving useful results in future epidemiologic studies. It should also be noted that standard errors and significance tests are based solely on the sample sizes in each group and do not reflect the effects of the complex survey design.

Mortality Finding for NHEFS Cohort Survival

Cumulative survival probabilities and their associated standard errors for 5 and 8 years of follow-up for each age, race, and gender group of the NHEFS cohort and for the U.S. population are presented in Tables 2–7 and 2–8. In general, the survival of each group of the NHEFS cohort corresponds quite closely to that expected on the basis of the survival probabilities given in U.S. life tables. Differences between observed and expected survival probabilities are generally greatest among blacks. However, the smaller number of blacks in the sample make these estimates less stable particularly in the younger age groups. The only group with

Table 2–7 Cumulative Survival Probabilities for Men After 5 and 8 Years of Follow-up: Comparison of U.S. Vital Statistics with NHEFS Sample

	5 years			8 years		
Race and age	U.S.	NHEFS*	Standard error (NHEFS)*	U.S.	NHEFS*	Standard error (NHEFS)*
White						
55–59 years	0.910	0.938	0.012†	0.847	0.869	0.017
60–64 years	0.867	0.873	0.019	0.778	0.782	0.023
65–69 years	0.806	0.814	0.013	0.683	0.695	0.016
70–74 years	0.724	0.766	0.017	0.569	0.584	0.020
Black						
55–59 years	0.860	0.880	0.044	0.772	0.767	0.057
60–64 years	0.828	0.837	0.056	0.722	0.744	0.067
65–69 years	0.762	0.793	0.032	0.625	0.664	0.037
70–74 years	0.682	0.698	0.042	0.536	0.521	0.046

Note: The sampling frame for NHANES I included persons aged 1–74 years at the time of the interview. Several subjects reached their 75th birthday between the interview and the examination. In addition, date of birth was incorrectly coded for several subjects. This error was corrected in the follow-up. As a result, three subjects were over 75 but were retained in the analysis.

*Estimated by Kaplan–Meier product limit method (SAS Institute, Inc. 1985).

†Difference between U.S. and NHEFS rates are significant at the 0.05 level.

Table 2–8 Cumulative Survival Probabilities for Women After 5 and 8 Years of Follow-up: Comparison of U.S. Vital Statistics with NHEFS Sample

Race and age	5 years			8 years		
	U.S.	NHEFS*	Standard error (NHEFS)*	U.S.	NHEFS*	Standard error (NHEFS)*
White						
55–59 years	0.956	0.970	0.008	0.922	0.926	0.013
60–64 years	0.936	0.954	0.011	0.889	0.912	0.014
65–69 years	0.902	0.910	0.009	0.829	0.835	0.012
70–74 years	0.843	0.859	0.013	0.734	0.756	0.016
Black						
55–59 years	0.920	0.946	0.026	0.866	0.918	0.032
60–64 years	0.899	0.947	0.030	0.832	0.895	0.040
65–69 years	0.845	0.896	0.023†	0.747	0.809	0.029†
70–74 years	0.768	0.780	0.037	0.652	0.637	0.043

Note: The sampling frame for NHANES I included persons aged 1–74 years at the time of the interview. Several subjects reached their 75th birthday between the interview and the examination. In addition, date of birth was incorrectly coded for several subjects. This error was corrected in the follow-up. As a result, three subjects were over 75 but were retained in the analysis.

*Estimated by Kaplan–Meier product limit method (SAS Institute, Inc. 1985).

†Difference between U.S. and NHEFS rates are significant at the 0.05 level.

survival significantly different from that expected at both 5 and 8 years of follow-up is that composed of black women aged 65–69 years.

Graphs of the cumulative probabilities of survival for the three subgroups related to residence in a poverty area among white men and white women 65–69 years old are presented in Figs. 2–2 and 2–3. Residence in a poverty area is clearly related to survival among white men in the 65–69-year age group. Persons examined from 1971–1974 who resided in poverty areas experienced significantly higher mortality than the population residing in nonpoverty areas. Survival for the total NHEFS cohort falls between the rates for the other two subgroups. Although white women 65–69 years old residing in nonpoverty areas also experienced lower mortality than those in poverty areas, the difference is not as large as that found for men 65–69 years old and is not statistically significant. There are no differences among the three subgroups for those 70–74 years of age.

Comparison of Race and Gender Groups

Table 2–9 presents the results of proportional hazards models designed to assess the relative risk of death for each race and gender group (white women were used as the base comparison). In each age group white women have the lowest and black men the highest death rates. There is a decline with increasing age in the relative risk for men. These patterns are remarkably similar to those seen by examination of age-specific death rates recorded in U.S. vital statistics (National Center for Health Statistics 1984b).

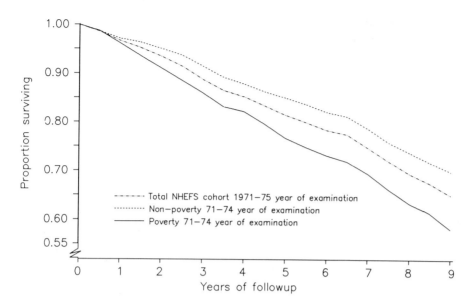

Fig. 2–2. Survival of NHEFS cohort according to place of residence (poverty or non-poverty) for white men 65–69 years of age at baseline (NHANES I).

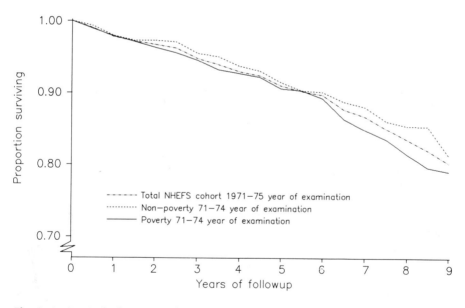

Fig. 2–3. Survival of NHEFS cohort according to place of residence (poverty or non-poverty) for white women 65–69 years of age at baseline (NHANES I).

Table 2–9 Relative Risk of Death (95% Confidence Interval) for Race–Gender Groups of NHEFS Sample by Age at Baseline

Race–gender group	55–64 years	65–74 years
White men	2.14 (1.63,2.79)	1.87 (1.66,2.10)
Black men	3.50 (2.35,5.24)	2.14 (1.77,2.57)
White women	1.00	1.00
Black women	1.13 (0.66,1.93)	1.28 (1.04,1.58)

Cause of Death

Table 2–10 compares the distribution of causes of death of male decedents in NHEFS to the numbers expected on the bases of national vital statistics for 1979. There are no significant differences between the observed and expected distributions for white ($p = 0.199$) or black ($p = 0.371$) men. In fact, there are only three causes for which the individual standardized deviates are close to 2: excess numbers of deaths from pneumonia and influenza for white men (28 deaths observed vs. 17.26 expected), from chronic obstructive pulmonary diseases for both whites (52 vs. 39.47) and blacks (8 vs. 4.25), and from motor vehicle accidents for whites (1 vs. 5.55).

There were also no significant differences between the observed and expected distributions for white ($p = 0.116$) or black ($p = 0.334$) women (Table 2–11). For white women only three causes of death had a discrepancy close to two standard deviations: infectious diseases (8 observed deaths vs. 3.37 expected), diabetes (20 vs. 13.22), and accidents other than motor vehicle (2 vs. 8.88). Cerebrovascular disease, or stroke, was the only cause of death among black women that had a standardized deviate of close to 2; black women had a higher number of deaths from cerebrovascular diseases than expected (26 vs. 15.77).

Overall, the cause-of-death distributions among NHEFS participants appear to be quite similar to what would have been expected from national vital statistics. Inspection of age-specific cause-of-death distributions generally revealed the same level of agreement.

In conclusion, the NHEFS results presented in this chapter show that rates of successful tracing of potential participants (i.e., all persons examined in NHANES I) were high, as were the rates at which interviews were obtained, physical measurements taken, and death certificates acquired.

Comparisons of the mortality experience of the NHEFS cohort with national survival data provide another perspective on the completeness of the NHEFS tracing activities. Some differences in survival probabilities between the NHANES I sample and the U.S. population were expected because of the sample design of NHANES I. However, the observed and expected survival curves were similar, and differences could be explained by variation in sampling. Furthermore, the distribution of causes of death recorded for the NHEFS cohort was quite similar to that found in U.S. vital statistics. Thus, although follow-up is not complete, tracing rates are very high and there do not seem to be any strong biases in the mortality data.

Table 2–10 Observed and Expected Numbers of Deaths in the NHEFS Cohort: Data for Men 55–84 Years of Age at Death

	White			Black		
	Observed	Expected	Standardized deviate*	Observed	Expected	Standardized deviate*
Infectious diseases	6	5.26	0.32	4	2.12	1.29
Cancer						
Digestive organs	45	51.54	−0.91	14	11.88	0.62
Respiratory organs	61	68.48	−0.90	6	12.93	−1.93
Genital organs	18	21.95	−0.84	11	8.70	0.78
Urinary organs	15	10.98	1.21	1	1.57	−0.45
Leukemia	8	7.00	0.38	2	0.96	1.06
All other	28	32.80	−0.84	3	6.30	−1.31
Diabetes	10	11.88	−0.54	1	3.23	−1.24
Cardiovascular diseases						
Ischemic heart disease	283	277.83	0.31	44	39.32	0.75
Other heart diseases	68	68.25	−0.03	19	23.06	−0.84
Cerebrovascular diseases	66	60.54	0.70	16	17.24	−0.30
Other cardiovascular diseases	22	24.78	−0.56	5	4.36	0.31
Pneumonia and influenza	28	17.26	2.59	3	3.95	−0.48
Chronic obstructive pulmonary diseases	52	39.47	1.99	8	4.25	1.82
Chronic liver disease and cirrhosis	9	9.71	−0.23	3	1.54	1.17
Nephritis, nephrotic syndrome, and nephrosis	6	6.16	−0.06	4	2.60	0.87
Symptoms, signs, and ill-defined conditions	11	7.10	1.46	5	4.04	0.48
All other diseases	45	51.24	−0.87	13	12.09	0.26
Motor vehicle accidents	1	5.55	−1.93	0	1.21	−1.10
All other accidents and adverse effects	15	18.45	−0.80	3	4.63	−0.76
		$\chi^2_{19} = 23.96$			$\chi^2_{19} = 20.17$	

*$(O − E)/\sqrt{E}$.

Table 2–11 Observed and Expected Numbers of Deaths in the NHEFS Cohort: Data for Women 55–84 Years of Age

	White			Black		
	Observed	Expected	Standardized deviate*	Observed	Expected	Standardized deviate*
Infectious diseases	8	3.37	2.52	1	1.44	-0.36
Cancer						
Digestive organs	37	38.46	-0.24	10	7.89	0.75
Respiratory organs	15	17.99	-0.70	0	2.52	-1.59
Breast	21	20.49	0.11	1	2.85	-1.10
Genital organs	11	14.40	-0.90	4	3.27	0.40
Urinary organs	8	4.40	1.72	0	0.74	-0.86
Leukemia	6	4.33	0.80	1	0.60	0.52
All other	23	23.44	-0.09	5	4.26	0.36
Diabetes	20	13.22	1.86	5	4.72	0.13
Cardiovascular diseases						
Ischemic heart disease	154	162.77	-0.69	31	28.94	0.38
Other heart diseases	51	52.77	-0.24	12	18.12	-1.44
Cerebrovascular diseases	61	57.11	0.51	26	15.77	2.58
Other cardiovascular diseases	18	14.14	1.03	1	3.45	-1.32
Pneumonia and influenza	8	10.05	-0.65	0	1.94	-1.39
Chronic obstructive pulmonary diseases	10	12.15	-0.62	1	0.90	-0.95
Chronic liver disease and cirrhosis	4	4.85	-0.39	1	0.81	0.21
Nephritis, nephrotic syndrome, and nephrosis	7	4.30	1.30	2	2.04	-0.03
Symptoms, signs, and ill-defined conditions	5	4.08	0.46	3	2.59	0.25
All other diseases	39	39.79	-0.13	7	8.83	-0.62
Motor vehicle accidents	6	3.03	1.70	0	0.36	-0.60
All other accidents and adverse effects	2	8.88	-2.31	4	1.96	1.45
		$\chi^2_{20} = 27.75$			$\chi^2_{20} = 22.12$	

*$(O - E)/\sqrt{E}.$

REFERENCES

National Center for Health Statistics. 1973. Plan and Operation of the Health and Nutrition Examination Survey. *Vital and Health Statistics.* Series 1, No. 10a. DHEW Publication No. (PHS) 79-1310. Washington, DC: U.S. Government Printing Office.

National Center for Health Statistics. 1977. Plan and Operation of the Health and Nutrition Examination Survey. *Vital and Health Statistics.* Series 1, No. 10b. DHEW Publication No. (PHS) 79-1310. Washington, DC: U.S. Government Printing Office.

National Center for Health Statistics. 1978. Plan and Operation of the NHANES I Augmentation of Adults 25–74 Years. *Vital and Health Statistics.* Series 1, No. 14. DHEW Publication No. (PHS) 78-1314. Washington, DC: U.S. Government Printing Office.

National Center for Health Statistics. 1981. Plan and Operation of the Second National Health and Nutrition Examination Survey, 1976–1980. *Vital and Health Statistics.* Series 1, No. 15. DHHS Publication No. (PHS) 81-1317. Washington, DC: U.S. Government Printing Office.

National Center for Health Statistics. 1984a. R. Pokras and L. J. Kozak, Adjustment of Hospital Rates, United States, 1965–80. *Vital and Health Statistics.* Series 13, No. 81. DHHS Publication No. (PHS) 85-1742. Washington, DC: U.S. Government Printing Office.

National Center for Health Statistics. 1984b. *Vital Statistics of the United States, 1979. Vol. II, Mortality, Part A.* DHHS Publication No. (PHS) 84-1101. Washington, DC: U.S. Government Printing Office.

SAS Institute, Inc. 1983. *SAS Supplemental Library User's Guide, 1983 Edition.* Cary, NC: SAS Institute, Inc.

SAS Institute, Inc. 1985. *SAS User's Guide: Statistics, Version 5 Edition.* Cary, NC: SAS Institute, Inc.

World Health Organization. 1977. *Manual of International Statistical Classification of Diseases, Injuries, and Causes of Death.* Based on recommendations of 9th Revision Conference. Geneva: World Health Organization.

II

THE ASSOCIATION OF RISK FACTORS WITH MORBIDITY AND MORTALITY FROM SPECIFIC DISEASES

3

Infectious Diseases

ANDREA Z. LaCROIX, STEVEN LIPSON,
AND LON R. WHITE

The changes in host defenses that accompany aging have been a topic of active research in recent years. Declines in physical defenses, such as epithelial atrophy, decreased activity of respiratory tract cilia, and lower levels of cellular and humoral immunity, have been demonstrated (Finkelstein 1984; Yoshikawa 1987). Despite the increase in host susceptibility that one might expect would accompany these changes, there is little data supporting an increased incidence of infection in the absence of chronic illness.

Even so, increased incisence rates of all infectious diseases, ranging from tuberculosis to influenza, are generally accepted as an accompaniment of aging, although we do not completely understand the mechanisms that increase risk. In addition to declines in immune function and alterations in physical defenses, the presence of disabling chronic conditions is likely to play an important role in increasing the risk of infectious diseases in older people. As a whole, the problem of infectious diseases was seen as so significant among older people that reduction of their occurrence was established as a national goal by the Surgeon General of the Public Health Service (U.S. Public Health Service 1979; National Center for Health Statistics 1986).

Nevertheless, quantitative data on rates and risk factors for infectious diseases are remarkably sparse. As noted by Schneider (Schneider 1983), previous studies have been largely restricted to retrospective and cross-sectional reports of selected populations, such as hospital or nursing home residents, or those with bacteriologic or serologic documentation of specific infections. By their design such studies are subject to selection biases related to higher prevalences among the elderly of chronic conditions that place the individual older person under medical care or in a health care institution. Definition of the population at risk is generally impossible.

For those infections that appear on hospital records or death certificates, the National Health and Nutrition Examination Survey-I Epidemiologic Follow-up Study (NHEFS) provides a unique opportunity to quantify the relationship between age and risk. Since a wide range of potential risk factors was assessed at baseline, their contribution may be estimated in a representative, noninstitutionalized population. Utilizing this unique resource, the present investigation had the following objectives: (1) to determine hospitalization and mortality rates associated with selected infectious diseases in an older cohort; (2) to compare rate of infectious diseases in men and women, and to compare rates by age within each gender group; (3) to examine the proportion of all deaths associated with selected infectious diseases by age among those who died during the follow-up period in order to determine whether the contribution of infectious diseases to death increases with age; and (4) to evaluate the strengths and limitations of hospital discharge records and death certificates as data sources for investigating infectious diseases in an epidemiologic study.

ANALYTIC METHODOLOGY

The study population for this investigation included 2605 men and 2869 women aged 55 and older who were initially examined in the First National Health and Nutrition Examination Survey (NHANES I) during 1971–1975. In this age range, 5677 subjects were eligible for repeated interview and examination in 1982–1984 as part of NHEFS. Vital status was known for 96.4% of the baseline cohort (all but 203 subjects). The only subjects excluded from the analytic sample were those lost to follow-up.

During the 7- to 12-year follow-up period, 1019 and 679 deaths occurred among men and women, respectively. Death certificates were obtained for all but 37 deaths among men and 39 deaths among women. The data file on multiple causes of death was the basis of the rates of infection associated with mortality. Cases of infectious diseases were extracted by ICD9 codes (World Health Organization 1977) from death certificates, if the infection was reported as the underlying cause of death, immediate cause of death, or as any other contributing cause of death on the death certificate. Most infections identified on the death certificate were listed as immediate or contributing, rather than underlying, causes of death. Since the total number of deaths associated with any particular infectious disease was anticipated to be small, no attempt was made to distinguish between immediate, contributing, and underlying causes of death.

Rates of hospitalization associated with selected infectious diseases were based on diagnoses recorded in hospital or nursing home discharge records. These records were obtained from hospitals and nursing homes when study subjects (or proxy informants) reported any hospitalization or nursing home admission during the follow-up period (Chapters 1 and 2). Up to six diagnoses were recorded for each hospitalization or nursing home discharge. As with death certificates, cases of infectious diseases were extracted from the list of diagnoses on the discharge records using specified ICD9 codes. Although repeated admissions for the same kind of infection were possible, rates reported in this study were based upon the first documented episode and date of that episode. In this regard, rates reported in this

Table 3–1 Infectious Disease Categories: Definitions and ICD9 Codes

Category, specific subcategory	ICD9 codes
Miscellaneous infectious diseases	001–139.8
Intestinal infections	008–009.3
Septicemia	038–038.9
Bacterial infections of unspecified site	041–041.9
Herpes zoster	053–053.9
Respiratory infections	Not grouped
Acute bronchitis	466–466.1
Pneumonia	480–486
Influenza	487–487.8
Chronic bronchitis	490–491.9
Kidney and urinary tract infections	590–590.9; 595–595.9
Kidney infections	590–590.9
Cystitis	595–595.9
Skin and wound infections	Not grouped
Cellulitis	681–682.9
Gangrene	785.4

study should be viewed as "cumulative incidence" rates rather than "attack" rates of infectious diseases. For the infections studied, 97% or more of the cases were identified on hospitalization discharge records, with the remaining cases identified on nursing home records (3% or less). Therefore, in this report rates are henceforth referred to as hospitalization rates. As described in Chapter 2, an unknown number of hospitalization events are not captured in the NHEFS data base because of refusal on the part of the participant or the hospital to provide access to records of the admission, or the inability to locate such records. For this reason, the rates of hospitalization reported in this investigation are likely to be conservative.

The choice of infections to study in this investigation was based on two sources of information about clinical infections in older populations: (1) data from the National Hospital Discharge Survey on numbers of diagnoses for inpatients aged 65 and older discharged from short-stay nonfederal hospitals in 1985, by ICD9 code (National Center for Health Statistics 1987); (2) a computerized literature search that identified published clinical and research reports from 1975 to the present on infections in older persons.

The combination of both sources of information allowed the selection of several infections that were likely to occur in adequate numbers for investigation in the present study and that would also be of greater public health and clinical importance. The infections chosen are listed in numerical order by ICD9 code in Table 3–1. Three broad categories of infectious diseases were defined: (1) respiratory infections, including acute and chronic bronchitis, pneumonia, and influenza; (2) kidney and urinary tract infections; (3) skin and wound infections, including cellulitis and gangrene. In addition, infections classified within the broad category of "Infectious and Parasitic Diseases" defined in the ICD9 (001-139.8) were examined as a group denoted in Table 3–1 by the label "miscellaneous infectious diseases." Within this grouping several specific infections were chosen by the preceding criteria for individual investigation; these included intestinal infections, bacterial infections of unspecified site, septicemia, and herpes zoster.

Several limitations are inherent in the use of death certificates and hospital discharge records as indicators of incidences of infectious diseases. Both sources are subject to vagaries of recording, including errors of omission (unreported cases) and commission (incorrectly recorded cases). With respect to errors of commission, it was not possible in the present study to determine whether diagnoses of infectious diseases had been verified by cultures of blood, sputum, or other biologic specimens or if the organisms responsible for diagnosed clinical infections had been identified. With respect to errors of omission, the use of hospitalization records as a basis for monitoring cases of infectious diseases is subject to the many selection biases that exist for hospital admission. The factors predisposing to hospital admission may not be solely related to the severity of the infectious disease episode. The decision to hospitalize may be more strongly influenced by the presence and severity of co-existing chronic conditions, the living situation and/or the age of the subject, or the availability of third-party reimbursement. Likewise, the recording of infectious disease diagnoses on the death certificate is subject to several influences that cannot be directly quantified. Neither record source is sensitive to the occurrence of infections in community-dwelling older people that do not result in hospitalization or death. Therefore, rates presented in this investigation represent only a fraction of the totality of infections occurring in this population and should be interpreted within the context of the record sources from which they originate.

Mortality and hospitalization rates associated with the selected infectious diseases were computed separately for men and women from Kaplan–Meier Product Limit curves (Kaplan and Meier 1958). For all rates computed, subjects who died during the follow-up contributed person-years from the date of their baseline examination until the time of death. All other subjects contributed person-years for the length of follow-up between the baseline examination and the follow-up interview, or the last date on which they were known to be alive. For hospitalization rates, subjects who were hospitalized with the infectious disease under consideration contributed person-years from the time of their baseline examination until the date of their first hospitalization with that infection. The rates reported are cumulative event rates at 12 years of follow-up; unequal follow-up time was taken into account for all participants. For each gender group, rates were also computed for two age groups (55–64 years and 65 years and older) on the basis of age at the baseline examination. Similarly, proportionate mortality ratios were examined by gender and age among NHEFS participants who had died during the follow-up interval. Proportionate mortality ratios were calculated as the percentage of all deaths in the gender and age category that were related to the specified infectious disease.

Consistency of reporting infectious diseases on the death certificate and hospital discharge record was evaluated among a subset of the cohort who had died in the hospital during the follow-up period and for whom hospitalization records and death certificates had been obtained. Among these decedents agreement in the recording of pneumonia on each record source was ascertained.

INFECTION, HOSPITALIZATION, AND DEATH: OBSERVED INCIDENCE AND MORTALITY RATES

Cumulative mortality rates per 1000 at 12 years of follow-up for deaths associated with infectious diseases are presented in Table 3–2. Of the infections selected for investigation, pneumonia was the one most frequently listed as a cause of death. Cumulative mortality rates among men were twice those among women (55.2 vs. 22.7 per 1000). Among men, older age was associated with a twofold higher pneumonia-related mortality rate as compared to younger age (68.7 vs. 29.4 per 1000 in older and younger men, respectively). Although rates were lower in women, the influence of age on risk was more dramatic than that for men; the mortality rate among older women was approximately fivefold that for younger women (31.2 vs. 6.2 per 1000).

Mortality rates for septicemia-related deaths were the second highest among the infections examined. For septicemia-related deaths, no marked gender differences were observed in total rates or in either age group. For both men and women, septicemia-related mortality was much higher in the older as compared to the younger age group.

Mortality rates for deaths related to herpes zoster, kidney and urinary tract infections, and gangrene were low for both men and women: below 5.0 per 1000 with fewer than ten deaths in each gender group associated with any one of these infections. Deaths related to other infections listed in Table 3–1 are not presented because they occurred too infrequently for the computation of rates. Mortality rates for the composite ICD9 category of "infectious and parasitic diseases" indicated that a contribution of one or more of these infections to death was not uncommon among older people, with rates in the older age group reaching 151.4 per 1000 for men and 89.0 per 1000 for women aged ≥65 at baseline. The patterns of mortality rates for this composite infectious disease category by gender and age were similar to those observed for pneumonia.

Since death is a prerequisite for the recording of infections on death certificates, the marked gender and age patterns noted for infection-related mortality rates in Table 3–2 are strongly influenced by the rates of total mortality in each group. As can be seen, total mortality rates were also higher among men than among women, and higher among older than younger subjects of both genders. For this reason, examination of age trends in proportionate mortality ratios is particularly enlightening, since these are not directly influenced by total mortality rates. Proportionate mortality ratios for the same infections just discussed are shown in Table 3–3 by gender and age. In contrast to the age trends noted in mortality rates, for each of the infections examined age differences in proportionate mortality ratios were absent or slight. For example, 10.3% of all deaths among men aged 65 and older were related to pneumonia, a figure quite similar to the 10.0% of all deaths noted for men aged

Table 3–2 Mortality Rates for Deaths Associated with Infectious Diseases at 12 Years of Follow-up According to Gender and Age at Baseline (NHANES I)*

Type of infection/ICD9 code	Men			Women		
		Age group			Age group	
	Total	55–64	≥ 65	Total	55–64	≥ 65
(Sample size)	(2605)	(836)	(1769)	(2869)	(927)	(1942)
Pneumonia 480–486	55.2 (101)	29.4 (18)	68.7 (83)	22.7 (35)	6.2 (4)	31.2 (31)
Septicemia 038–038.9	13.0 (23)	2.8 (2)	18.5 (21)	15.9 (25)	5.6 (5)	20.9 (20)
Herpes zoster 053–053.9	4.1 (9)	2.6 (2)	4.9 (7)	3.0 (6)	1.1 (1)	3.8 (5)
Kidney 590–590.9	3.6 (6)	0 (0)	5.5 (6)	2.7 (7)	1.2 (1)	3.5 (6)
Gangrene 785.4	3.4 (6)	1.3 (1)	4.5 (5)	3.1 (6)	3.2 (1)	3.1 (5)
Miscellaneous infectious diseases 001–139.8	120.0 (224)	57.9 (39)	151.4 (185)	71.7 (141)	35.4 (26)	89.0 (115)
Total mortality all causes†	486.1 (1019)	249.2 (184)	564.4 (835)	305.7 (679)	134.3 (100)	378.0 (579)

*Rates presented are cumulative event rates at 12 years of follow-up computed from Kaplan–Meier survival curves; number of events are in parentheses.
†Includes 37 deaths among men and 39 deaths among women, where no death certificate has been obtained.

Table 3-3 Percentage of All Deaths with Selected Infectious Diseases Recorded on the Death Certificate According to Gender and Age at Baseline (NHANES I)

	Men			Women		
		Age group			Age group	
Type of infection	Total	55–64	≥ 65	Total	55–64	≥ 65
(Number of deaths)	(982)	(180)	(802)	(640)	(94)	(546)
Pneumonia	10.3	10.0	10.3	5.5	4.3	5.7
Septicemia	2.3	1.1	2.6	3.9	5.3	3.7
Herpes zoster	0.9	1.1	0.9	0.9	1.1	0.9
Kidney and urinary tract	0.6	0	0.7	1.1	1.1	1.1
Gangrene	0.6	0.6	0.6	0.9	1.1	0.9
Miscellaneous infectious diseases	22.8	21.7	23.1	22.0	27.7	21.1

Note: Number in parentheses is number of deaths in indicated group. This number excludes deaths in the study population where no death certificate has been obtained.

47

Table 3–4 Rates of Hospitalization for Selected Infectious Diseases During 12 Years of Follow-up According to Gender and Age at Baseline (NHANES I)*

	Men			Women		
		Age group			Age group	
Type of infection	Total	55–64	≥ 65	Total	55–64	≥ 65
(Sample size)	(2605)	(836)	(1769)	(2869)	(927)	(1942)
	Rate per 1000 (number of cases)					
Intestinal infections	5.6 (12)	5.6 (4)	5.6 (8)	7.8 (19)	3.1 (2)	10.3 (17)
Septicemia	19.5 (31)	14.1 (6)	22.2 (25)	17.4 (29)	7.8 (7)	22.2 (22)
Bacterial infections un-specified site	20.3 (36)	13.1 (9)	24.2 (27)	26.4 (54)	16.5 (13)	31.1 (41)
Herpes zoster	3.4 (7)	1.3 (1)	4.6 (6)	4.6 (10)	4.6 (10)	4.5 (6)
Miscellaneous infections	75.1 (141)	58.5 (35)	83.4 (106)	70.6 (146)	44.5 (34)	83.5 (112)
Acute bronchitis	25.2 (49)	11.2 (8)	32.8 (41)	28.2 (67)	18.4 (15)	33.0 (52)
Pneumonia	109.2 (191)	68.4 (42)	130.6 (149)	78.0 (165)	51.1 (34)	91.3 (131)
Influenza	12.8 (28)	7.6 (7)	15.6 (21)	16.3 (40)	7.1 (4)	21.0 (36)
Chronic bronchitis	40.1 (77)	30.3 (19)	45.4 (58)	34.1 (80)	29.4 (22)	36.5 (58)
Kidney and urinary tract	29.5 (57)	17.4 (12)	35.9 (45)	40.7 (94)	24.1 (19)	49.0 (75)
Kidney	11.8 (23)	9.6 (7)	12.9 (16)	16.9 (38)	8.4 (7)	21.3 (31)
Cystitis	18.6 (36)	7.8 (5)	24.4 (31)	26.4 (62)	17.9 (14)	30.4 (48)
Cellulitis	23.4 (35)	43.0 (18)	13.5 (17)	22.0 (46)	9.8 (8)	27.8 (38)

*Rates presented are cumulative event rates at 12 years of follow-up computed from Kaplan–Meier curves; numbers of events are in parentheses.

55–64 years. The gender differences observed in pneumonia-related mortality rates were also reflected in proportionate mortality ratios for pneumonia, with pneumonia contributing to 5.5% of deaths among women as compared with 10.3% of deaths among men. For the other infections examined, no consistent patterns of gender differences were observed in the proportionate mortality ratios.

Cumulative event rates during the 7–12-year follow-up for hospitalizations with infectious disease diagnoses listed on the discharge summary are presented in Table 3–4. Consistent with the mortality rates, rates of pneumonia-related hospitalization were by far the highest of rates for any of the infections examined (109.2 and 78.0 per 1000 for men and women, respectively). Of the respiratory infections studied, hospitalization because of acute and chronic bronchitis also was relatively common on the discharge records. Rates of hospitalization with influenza were the lowest among the respiratory infections, with 12.8 and 16.3 cases per 1000 among men and women, respectively. Older age was associated with higher rates of hospitalization of both men and women for respiratory infections. Gender differences, with higher rates among men, were observed only for pneumonia.

Rates of hospitalization with kidney and urinary tract infections were higher among women than among men (40.7 vs. 29.5 per 1000, respectively). The cumulative rates of hospitalization with kidney and urinary tract infections were plotted by age for men and women in Fig. 3–1. In both genders, older age was associated with approximately twice the rate of hospitalization with clinically diagnosed kidney and urinary tract infections. Aside from slightly higher rates among women for hospitalization with bacterial infections of unspecified site, no consistent

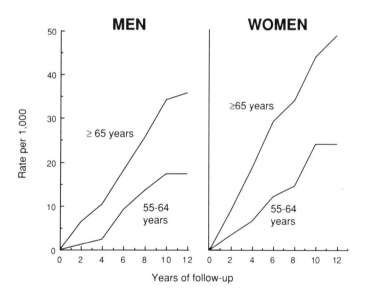

Fig. 3–1. Cumulative rates of hospitalization with kidney and urinary tract infection during the follow-up interval.

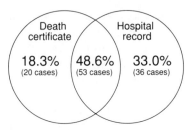

Fig. 3–2. Percentage of subjects who died in the hospital and who had pneumonia recorded on either death certificate or hospital discharge record.

gender differences in hospitalization rates for these selected infections were observed.

One issue raised by the use of death certificates and hospital discharge records as a means of classifying cases of infectious disease in an epidemiologic study is the degree of concordance between the two record sources in identifying cases. As described in the section on methodology, this issue was investigated among a subset of subjects for whom both record sources were available—those who died in a hospital during the follow-up period. Because pneumonia is a major clinical infection in older populations and a leading cause of mortality, and because pneumonia was the most frequently recorded infection on both types of records in the present study, we chose to examine the consistency in recording pneumonia on the hospital discharge records and death certificates of these decedents. Figure 3–2 summarizes the results. Among subjects who died in a hospital, a total of 109 cases of pneumonia were recorded on either hospital discharge summaries or death certificates. For 48.6% of these cases, pneumonia was recorded on both records. One third (33.0%) of the cases were recorded only on the hospital discharge summary, and 18.3% were recorded only on the death certificate. These findings suggest that case groups of subjects who developed pneumonia, as defined in hospital records, are likely to differ substantially from case groups classified by death certificates, although substantial overlap would also be anticipated.

CONCLUSIONS

In conclusion, data from this national cohort demonstrated that rates of death attributable to infectious diseases increased with age among both men and women and that rates for men were higher. In contrast, among those who died, proportionate mortality ratios showed no or only slight increases from younger to older ages. One interpretation of the lack of association of proportionate mortality ratios with age is that this finding fails to support any substantial clinical importance for declining immune function with age, as distinct from the effect of an increased burden of chronic illness preceding death. Nevertheless, persistent increases in rates of hospitalization with age were observed for many of the selected infectious dis-

Table 3–5 Examples of Potential Risk Factors for Clinical Infections: Characteristics Identified in NHANES I Available for Investigation in NHEFS

History of chronic conditions
    Chronic obstructive pulmonary disease
    Tuberculosis
    Pleurisy
    Chronic cough
    Heart attack
    High blood pressure
    Congestive heart failure
    Stroke
    Diabetes
    Cancer
    Hip fracture
Nutritional status indicators
    Hemoglobin
    Serum albumin
    Anthropometric measurements
    Dietary intake
    Serum vitamin levels
Health habits
    Alcohol consumption
    Cigarette smoking

eases examined here. Such increases may be a result of declines in immune function, or alternatively may reflect a greater likelihood of diagnosis of infectious diseases in older people who are hospitalized for one or more major chronic conditions. Therefore, the role of age-related declines in immune function in increasing the vulnerability of the elderly to a variety of clinical infections remains an open question that could be examined only indirectly in the present study.

The demonstrated differences in reporting pneumonia on death certificates and hospital discharge records illustrate a limitation of these data sources in determining the incidence of infectious disease events. Nevertheless, these findings raise interesting possibilities for further investigation within the context of NHEFS. Outstanding among these possibilities is the identification of baseline characteristics within this population that are associated with increased risk of the common infectious diseases. Table 3–5 summarizes baseline attributes that might alter susceptibility to clinical infections: the existence of prevalent chronic conditions at baseline, indicators of nutritional status, and health habits. The identification of risk factors found to be important in predicting the occurrence of future infections in this national cohort could provide a basis for hypotheses in future studies.

These results emphasize the need for future investigations in which quantified changes in cellular and humoral immunity, declines in physical defenses, and presence of disabling chronic conditions are examined prospectively to determine their relative roles in the development of clinical infections in older people.

REFERENCES

Finkelstein, M. S. 1984. "Defenses against infection in the elderly: The compromises of aging." *Triangle* 23:57–64.

Kaplan, E. L., and P. Meier. 1958. "Nonparametric estimation from incomplete observations." *J Am Stat Assoc* 53:457–481.

National Center for Health Statistics. 1986. Health, United States, 1986. DHHS Pub. No. (PHS) 87-1232. Public Health Service. Washington, DC: U.S. Government Printing Office.

National Center for Health Statistics. 1987. R. Pokras. *Detailed Diagnoses and Procedures for Patients Discharged from Short-Stay Hospitals, United States, 1985.* Vital and Health Statistics. Series 13, No. 90. DHHS Pub. No. (PHS) 87-1751. Washington, DC: U.S. Government Printing Office, April 1987.

Schneider, E. L. 1983. "Infectious diseases in the elderly." *Ann Intern Med* 98:395–400.

U.S. Public Health Service. 1979. Healthy People: The Surgeon General's Report on Health Promotion and Disease Prevention.

World Health Organization. 1977. *Manual of International Statistical Classification of Disease, Injuries, and Causes of Death.* Based on recommendations of 9th Revision Conference. Geneva: World Health Organization.

Yoshikawa, T. T. 1987. "Impact of aging on host response to infectious disease." In *Geriatric Clinical Pharmacology,* W. G. Wood and R. Strong, eds. New York: Raven Press, pp. 107–113.

4

Coronary Heart Disease
and Hypertension

PAUL E. LEAVERTON, RICHARD J. HAVLIK,
LILLIAN M. INGSTER-MOORE, ANDREA Z. LaCROIX,
AND JOAN C. CORNONI-HUNTLEY

Coronary heart disease (CHD) and stroke (Chapter 6) represent the important components of cardiovascular disease, the major cause of morbidity and mortality in older persons (National Center for Health Statistics 1987). The various risk factors for CHD have been well defined for younger populations but are less so for the older age groups (Kannel and Gordon 1978).

Hypertension has been identified as a major risk factor for CHD and stroke and is known to be related to other forms of heart disease and to renal failure. Because of the frequency and importance of hypertension, epidemiologic data on this disorder in the elderly are very relevant to any discussion of their overall health (Kannel 1985).

The NHANES I Epidemiologic Follow-up Study (NHEFS) provides an excellent opportunity to investigate both the strength of the known risk factors for CHD, including high blood pressure, in a nationally representative population and, specifically, to explore the prevalence and incidence of hypertension as well as trends in frequency of treatment. Detailed studies of these latter hypertension-related issues have been published recently (Cornoni-Huntley et al. 1989; Havlik et al. 1989). In the section of this chapter devoted to hypertension we present data on prevalence and incidence and its role as a risk factor for CHD.

CORONARY HEART DISEASE

Coronary heart disease (CHD) continues to be the leading cause of death in the United States (National Center for Health Statistics 1985). Although age-adjusted mortality has been declining consistently and dramatically at the rate of about 2% each year since the late 1960s (Feinleib et al. 1982), the absolute number of deaths due to CHD has remained high because of the aging of the U.S. population (Rosenberg and Klebba 1979). Age-specific death rates for all causes and for cardiovascular disease in particular rise exponentially with increasing age; two thirds of all deaths involve persons aged 65 years or older. National figures indicate that 50–75% of these deaths are due to cardiovascular disease, and the two major contributors are stroke and coronary heart disease (or ischemic heart disease, as it is termed in the International Classification of Diseases ICD9 [World Health Organization 1977]). Those over 65 have achieved almost the same percentage decline in CHD mortality as younger members of the population, but because of the originally very high death rate among the elderly, the absolute increase in the numbers of survivors has been even more impressive.

Interventions designed to reduce these rates further must be based on an understanding of the CHD risk factors as they affect incidence in the older population. Most of the evidence for risk factors in the elderly, as in younger groups, will come from carefully conducted epidemiologic investigations. Although several epidemiologic studies of cardiovascular disease in older persons have been conducted (Kannel and Gordon 1980; 1978; Harris et al. 1985; Kannel and Brand 1985; Rowe 1983; Barrett-Conner et al. 1984; Jajich et al. 1984), none have been on the scale of NHEFS, the follow-up of the National Health and Nutrition Examination Survey-I. With over 5600 men and women over age 55 in the original cohort, this opportunity to assess the risk factors in a probability sample of the United States population is unique.

Results from various smaller studies have suggested that blood pressure, especially systolic blood pressure, continues to be predictive of CHD mortality and morbidity at older ages. The Hypertension Detection and Follow-up Program (HDFP) (HDFP Cooperative Group 1982) has shown that antihypertensive therapy in those aged 65–74 who have elevated diastolic blood pressure can be beneficial. Studies are also under way (Curb et al. 1985) to estimate the benefit of treating isolated high systolic blood pressure in older persons.

The Framingham Heart Study (Dawber and Kannel 1972) has been the foundation upon which many health policies for CHD have been built. It has provided evidence (Gordon et al. 1977) for the association of risk factors for CHD in healthy middle-aged whites as they move into the older age groups. Observations of the Framingham population show clearly that elevated blood pressure, high levels of serum cholesterol, increased relative weight, and cigarette smoking all exert a deleterious effect. In combination, the risk factor profile sharply differentiates various risk categories. Recently, a comparison of the major risk factors showed that the Framingham risk model fits the NHEFS data for CHD mortality remarkably well over a broad range of adult ages (Leaverton et al. 1987). The same risk factors were shown to be important to a similar degree when the same age groups (all white) were followed for a 10-year period.

In a 20-year study of the Framingham cohort members, Kannel and Gordon (Kannel and Gordon 1980) found differences in cardiovascular risk factors for the older cohort groups. In particular, they noted that the impact of the major risk factors was somewhat diminished by age but that systolic blood pressure became the most important single predictor of CHD for the oldest groups. However, the small sample size precluded analysis by precisely specified age subgroups.

In the Framingham cohort, it appears that the level of total cholesterol in serum and cigarette smoking lose their predictive power at older ages (Kannel and Gordon 1978). However, in other studies, either cholesterol or smoking has been shown to be associated with cardiovascular disease at older ages (Barrett-Conner et al. 1984; Jajich et al. 1984). Diabetes has been identified as a risk factor for mortality due to CHD in a broader age group, including the elderly, with the suggestion that the relative risk is higher in women (Kannel and Brand 1985).

In this chapter we report the relationship of the best-known cardiovascular risk factors to the incidence of coronary events in a population sample aged 55 years and older. Separate comparisons were executed for men and women, whites and blacks. The risk factors used were systolic blood pressure, total serum cholesterol, cigarette smoking, and history of diabetes. The importance of these factors in predicting CHD events during the 10 years of follow-up was evaluated.

Population and Methods

As described in Chapter 1, the National Health and Nutrition Examination Survey I (NHANES I, 1971–1975) surveyed individuals drawn from a clustered, multistage, stratified probability sample of 26,322 persons in the contiguous United States (Cornoni-Huntley et al. 1983). Among the major variables examined at baseline were age, race, gender, serum cholesterol, systolic blood pressure, cigarette smoking, history of diabetes, and body mass index. Information on some of these was collected only from a subsample. Those variables shown to be the most predictive of CHD in younger adults were selected for the present study. Age at baseline, race, and gender were recorded at follow-up and minor editorial corrections were incorporated into the data. The systolic blood pressure measurements at baseline are in millimeters of mercury (mmHg), and only the physician's measurement was used. Serum cholesterol was measured by a modification of the method of Abel and Kendall and is shown in milligrams per deciliter (mg/dl). At baseline only the subsample randomly selected for detailed examination was asked about cigarette smoking; responses are presented in a "current versus all others" format. However, when possible, a lifetime history of cigarette smoking was obtained at follow-up from both subjects and proxies. Therefore, for those with missing information at baseline, it was possible to reconstruct a "current versus all others" status at baseline from the follow-up history. History of diabetes consists of a positive response to either of two baseline questions: (1) "Has a doctor ever told you that you have . . . do you still have it?" from the medical history questionnaire; or (2) "Did a doctor ever tell you that you had . . . ?" from the detailed supplemental questionnaire. Body mass index was calculated from measured weight and height.

The follow-up end point of a CHD event was obtained as follows. A count of deaths due to CHD (ICD9 codes 410–414 inclusive) was obtained, as was the first record per subject of a hospital and/or nursing home discharge with a diagnosis of CHD (ICD9 codes 410–414 inclusive). These numbers were added to yield total number of incident CHD events during the follow-up period.

Several exclusionary criteria were used. From the ECG readings available at baseline on the subsample examined in detail, those identified as having had definite myocardial infarctions were excluded. Self-reported history of heart attack from either the medical history questionnaire or the supplemental cardiovascular questionnaire at baseline was also cause for exclusion. From the same supplemental cardiovascular questionnaire it was possible to construct a series of questions based on the questionnaire of Rose et al. (Rose et al. 1982; Rose 1965) for a diagnosis of angina pectoris on the subsample examined in detail. Analyses were done both with and without these individuals to determine whether angina pectoris should be considered as a preevent condition.

The logistic regression function was utilized for both univariate and multivariate analyses. Although there was some variation in the length of follow-up, the distribution of follow-up periods showed that most were in the range of 9.5–11 years. Proportional hazards modeling was also used but revealed little practical difference when compared with the multiple logistic model. The logistic model approach uses predicted probabilities of CHD death (holding age constant), sorts them into quintiles, and compares them to the observed rate for each quintile to assess how well the model fits. This model was constructed for three age categories at baseline: 55–64, 65–74, and these two groups combined, that is, 55–74 years. The relative odds were calculated from the logistic coefficients. The levels of risk factors chosen for estimation of the relative odds were approximately equal to two standard deviations of the variable for continuous measurements.

Results

Table 4–1 displays the sample sizes and summary statistics at baseline for all 5003 persons in the NHANES I sample who were free of CHD at baseline. The subsample available for blacks included only 806 persons, and the statistical power to detect true predictors was correspondingly reduced. The systolic blood pressure levels were about 10 mmHg higher in blacks, both men and women, than in whites.

Table 4–1 Means of Baseline (NHANES I) Measures of Persons Free of Coronary Heart Disease According to Race and Gender

Characteristic	White men (N = 1914)		White women (N = 2282)		Black men (N = 377)		Black women (N = 429)	
Age	66	(5.5)	66	(5.4)	65	(5.1)	66	(5.3)
Systolic blood pressure (mm/Hg)	144	(22.8)	148	(24.5)	153	(27.2)	159	(29.2)
Serum cholesterol (mg/dl)	226	(46.9)	248	(47.3)	225	(49.3)	247	(48.5)
Cigarette smoking (% current)	32	(47)	18	(38)	35	(48)	15	(36)
Diabetes (% ever)	6	(23)	7	(25)	7	(26)	12	(36)
Body mass index (kg/m²)	25.6	(4.0)	26.3	(5.1)	25.0	(4.6)	28.4	(6.5)
Alcohol (oz/week)	6	(13.3)	1.6	(5.0)	5.3	(14.7)	0.8	(3.1)
Education*	1.8	(1.0)	2.0	(1.0)	0.9	(1.0)	1.2	(1.0)

Note: Values given are reported or measured means (standard deviation).

*In computing mean years of education, the following scale was used: 0 = 0–4 years; 1 = 5–8 years; 2 = 9–11 years; 3 = ≥12 years.

Table 4–1a Means of Baseline (NHANES I) Measures of Persons Having Coronary Heart Disease According to Race and Gender*

Characteristic	White men (N = 327)		White women (N = 214)		Black men (N = 42)		Black women (N = 45)	
Age	67†	(5.3)‡	67†	(5.3)	67	(4.3)	66	(5.9)
Systolic blood pressure (mmHg)	143	(24.9)	154†	(26.7)	149	(28.7)	160	(30.8)
Serum cholesterol (mg/dl)	235†	(51.2)	250	(52.1)	226	(51.4)	256	(54.2)
Cigarette smoking (% current)	28	(45)	16	(37)	26	(45)	13	(34)
Diabetes (% ever)	14†	(35)	14†	(35)	12	(33)	22†	(42)
Body mass index (kg/m²)	25.8	(4.0)	27.5†	(5.6)	26.1	(4.7)	30.1	(7.9)
Alcohol (oz/week)	3.7†	(8.1)	1.5	(4.2)	1.5	(3.7)	0.3	(1.0)
Education 0 = 0–4 years	1.7	(1.0)	1.9	(1.0)	0.8	(1.0)	1.3	(0.9)
1 = 5–8 years								
2 = 9–11 years								
3 = ≥12‡ years								

*This group was excluded from subsequent analyses.
†Significantly different from analyzed sample $p < 0.05$.
‡Number in parentheses is standard deviation.

Otherwise there were no racial differences in the risk factors. The covariate education did differ among the groups. Women had higher cholesterol levels, and a higher proportion of them had diabetes; however, they smoked cigarettes at about half the rate reported by men.

Table 4–1a shows these same characteristics at baseline for the 628 sample persons who reported some form of CHD at their NHANES I interview. Statistical significance between the corresponding mean values for the two groups was analyzed by t-tests and χ^2 tests as appropriate. Those differences (Table 4–1 vs. Table 4–1a) that are statistically significant at the level of $p = 0.05$ are marked by a dagger in Table 4–1a. Several differences are apparent, and most were among whites, probably because of the much larger sample size. Those sample persons with CHD at baseline (Table 4–1a) were excluded from the predictive analyses. That is, only those free of CHD at baseline were included in the calculations of CHD incidence and the regression analyses.

Table 4–2 lists the incidences of CHD by hospitalizations (nonfatal), deaths, and combined (total) events for each of the four groups. Each race–gender group has been subdivided into two (baseline) age groups: 55–64 and 65–74 years as well as the combined group, 55–74 years. Differences in rates are roughly what one would expect. The results of univariate logistic regression analyses are summarized in Tables 4–3 and 4–3a. Table 4–3 shows the univariate regression coefficients for coronary heart disease (mortality plus hospitalizations) for white men and women in the groups aged 55–64 and 65–74 years and for the combined group aged 55–74 years. The sign of the coefficient indicates whether the estimate of the contribution of that risk factor to 10-year mortality due to CHD was positive (increasing the risk) or negative (decreasing the risk). Table 4–3a displays these same coefficients for blacks. Tables 4–4 and 4–4a show the coefficients derived from multiple logistic regression models that allow assessment of each variable while the others are held constant in the predic-

Table 4–2 Incidence of Coronary Heart Disease Events (Deaths and Hospitalizations) in 10 Years of Follow-up According to Race, Gender, and Age at Baseline (NHANES I)

Group	Sample size	Total events*	CHD deaths	CHD hospitalizations
Age 55–64				
White men	651	113 (17.4)	30 (4.6)	99 (15.2)
White women	763	61 (8.0)	10 (1.3)	58 (7.6)
Black men	95	11 (11.6)	6 (6.3)	6 (6.3)
Black women	129	13 (10.1)	4 (3.1)	9 (7.0)
Age 65–74				
White men	1263	355 (28.1)	161 (12.7)	259 (20.5)
White women	1520	345 (22.7)	108 (7.1)	292 (19.2)
Black men	282	66 (23.4)	33 (11.7)	45 (16.0)
Black women	300	65 (21.7)	25 (8.3)	46 (15.3)
Age 55–74				
White men	1914	468 (24.5)	142 (7.4)	358 (18.7)
White women	2283	406 (17.8)	98 (4.3)	350 (15.3)
Black men	377	77 (20.4)	26 (6.9)	51 (13.5)
Black women	429	78 (18.2)	21 (4.9)	55 (12.8)

*Single event per person. First recorded event only.

tion model. Tables 4–5 and 4–5a give the relative odds for development of CHD in relation to health characteristics at baseline.

Discussion

There are both similarities and differences in the risk factors for CHD for older Americans, as compared with their younger counterparts. All the risk factors exam-

Table 4–3 Relationship Between Baseline (NHANES I) Measures and Risk of a Coronary Heart Disease Event over a 10-year Interval for White Men and Women: Univariate Logistic Coefficients

Characteristic	Men			Women		
	55–64	65–74	55–74	55–64	65–74	55–74
Age	0.050	0.057*	0.061*	0.113*	0.045*	0.101*
Systolic blood pressure	0.009	0.008*	0.010*	0.012*	0.011*	0.014*
Serum cholesterol	0.001	0.002	0.001	−0.001	0	0
Cigarette smoking	0.426*	0.301*	0.264*	0.382	0.204	0.016
Diabetes	0.846	0.634*	0.734*	0.657	0.634*	0.730*
Body mass index	0.04	0.02	0.02	0.02	0.03*	0.03*
Alcohol	0.004	−0.01	−0.005	−0.02	−0.03	−0.04
Education†	−0.332*	−0.195*	−0.272*	−0.451*	−0.313*	−0.399*

*Significant at $p < 0.05$; t-test.

†In computing mean years of education, the following scale was used: 0 = 0–4 years; 1 = 5–8 years; 2 = 9–11 years; 3 = ≥12 years.

Table 4–3a Relationship Between Baseline (NHANES I) Measures and Risk of a Coronary Heart Disease Event over a 10-year Interval for Black Men and Women: Univariate Logistic Coefficients

| | Coefficient for indicated group | | | | | |
| | Men | | | Women | | |
Characteristic	55–64	65–74	55–74	55–64	65–74	55–74
Age	0.063	0.096*	0.088*	0.044	0.027	0.071*
Systolic blood pressure	0.022	0.013*	0.015*	0.009	0.002*	0.004
Serum cholesterol	−0.001	0.006*	0.005*	0.007	0	0.002
Cigarette smoking	−0.251	−0.399*	−0.473	—	0.357	−0.580
Diabetes	2.12	−0.273	−0.066*	1.05	1.07*	1.06*
Body mass index	0.04	−0.03	−0.02	0.006	−0.03	−0.02
Alcohol	0.02	0.01	0.01	−0.12	0.02	0.02
Education†	−0.58	0.03	−0.11	−0.40	−0.26	−0.33*

*Significant at $p < 0.05$; t-test.
†In computing mean years of education, the following scale was used: 0 = 0–4 years; 1 = 5–8 years; 2 = 9–11 years; 3 = ≥12 years.

ined here have often been shown to be predictors of CHD to a statistically significant degree in younger populations. Some of these variables were not statistically significant predictors in this study, as shown by the multivariate logistic regression models.

There are at least two possible explanations for such observations. First, the statistical power may simply have been too low because of the smaller size of the NHEFS sample (in the older age categories) as compared with the populations in Framingham and other studies. Second, for those who have survived free of heart disease to an older age, the risk factors may truly be different. Certainly, if the

Table 4–4 Relationship Between Baseline (NHANES I) Measures and Risk of a Coronary Heart Disease Event over a 10-year Interval for White Men and Women: Multivariate Logistic Coefficients

| | Coefficient for indicated group | | | | | |
| | Men | | | Women | | |
Characteristic	55–64	65–74	55–74	55–64	65–74	55–74
Age	0.032	0.035	0.044*	0.106*	0.055*	0.101*
Systolic blood pressure	0.013*	0.009*	0.010*	0.006	0.010*	0.010*
Serum cholesterol	0.001	0.002	0.002	−0.004	0	−0.001
Cigarette smoking	0.453	0.396*	0.408*	0.527	0.546*	0.538*
Diabetes	0.775	0.688*	0.719*	0.638	0.794*	0.794*
Body mass index	0.029	0.004	0.013	−0.016	0.018	0.013
Alcohol	0.004	−0.005	0	−0.013	−0.038	−0.029
Education†	−0.326*	−0.169*	−0.220*	−0.477*	−0.241*	−0.279*

*Significant at $p < 0.05$; t-test.
†In computing mean years of education, the following scale was used: 0 = 0–4 years; 1 = 5–8 years; 2 = 9–11 years; 3 = ≥12 years.

Table 4–4a Relationship Between Baseline (NHANES I) Measures and Risk of a Coronary Heart Disease Event over a 10-year Interval for Black Men and Women: Multivariate Logistic Coefficients

	Coefficient for indicated group					
	Men			Women		
Characteristic	55–64	65–74	55–74	55–64	65–74	55–74
Age	—	0.065	0.076*	—	0.009	0.070*
Systolic blood pressure	—	0.017*	0.016*	—	0.004	0.004
Serum cholesterol	—	0.007	0.005	—	0.003	0.003
Cigarette smoking	—	−0.729	−0.662	—	0.369	−0.605
Diabetes	—	−0.858	−0.944	—	1.518*	1.367*
Body mass index	—	−0.008	0.019	—	−0.068*	−0.048*
Alcohol	—	0.009	0.010	—	0.051	0.047
Education†	—	−0.041	−0.160	—	−0.403*	−0.448*

*Significant at $p < 0.05$; t-test.
†In computing mean years of education, the following scale was used: 0 = 0–4 years; 1 = 5–8 years; 2 = 9–11 years; 3 = ≥12 years.

regression coefficients are near zero, the latter explanation is more plausible. Because multivariate analysis is more appropriate than univariate analysis when there is correlation among the risk factors, we will restrict our comments about them to the results shown in Tables 4–4 and 4–4a.

We will first consider the analysis for the white population because it is a much larger sample. As might be expected, age was significant within the 20-year groups but not in the narrower 10-year groups. Diabetes and systolic blood pressure were the most consistently significant variables. Systolic blood pressure was a significant predictor in both genders for the combined ages as well as for each subgroup except women aged 55–64 years. Total serum cholesterol was not significant for any

Table 4–5 Relationship Between Baseline (NHANES I) Measures and Risk of a Coronary Heart Disease Event over a 10-year Interval for White Men and Women: Relative Odds Derived from Multiple Logistic Coefficients

	Difference in risk factor levels	Odds for indicated group					
		Men			Women		
Characteristic		55–64	65–74	55–74	55–64	65–74	55–74
Age	(4)	1.1	1.1	1.2	1.5	1.2	1.5
Systolic blood pressure	(50)	1.9	1.6	1.6	1.3	1.6	1.6
Serum cholesterol	(100)	1.1	1.2	1.2	(−)1.5	1.0	(−)1.1
Cigarette smoking	(Yes–no)	1.6	1.5	1.5	1.7	1.7	1.7
Diabetes	(Yes–no)	2.2	2.0	2.1	1.9	2.2	2.2
Body mass index	(10)	1.3	1.0	1.1	(−)1.2	1.2	1.1
Alcohol	(10)	1.0	(−)1.0	1.0	(−)1.1	(−)1.5	(−)1.3
Education*	(1)	(−)1.4	(−)1.2	(−)1.2	(−)1.6	(−)1.3	(−)1.3

*In computing mean years of education, the following scale was used: 0 = 0–4 years; 1 = 5–8 years; 2 = 9–11 years; 3 = ≥12 years.

Table 4–5a Relationship Between Baseline (NHANES I) Measures and Risk of a Coronary Heart Disease Event over a 10-year Interval for Black Men and Women: Relative Odds Derived from Multiple Logistic Coefficients

		Odds for indicated group					
	Difference in risk factor	Men			Women		
Characteristic	levels	55–64	65–74	55–74	55–64	65–74	55–74
Age	(4)	—	1.3	1.4	—	1.0	1.3
Systolic blood pressure	(50)	—	2.3	2.2	—	1.2	1.2
Serum cholesterol	(100)	—	2.0	1.6	—	1.3	1.3
Cigarette smoking	(Yes–no)	—	(−)2.1	(−)1.9	—	1.4	(−)1.8
Diabetes	(Yes–no)	—	(−)2.4	(−)2.6	—	4.6	3.9
Body mass index	(10)	—	(−)1.1	1.2	—	(−)2.0	(−)1.6
Alcohol	(10)	—	1.1	1.1	—	1.7	1.6
Education*	(1)	—	(−)1.0	(−)1.2	—	(−)1.5	(−)1.6

*In computing mean years of education, the following scale was used: 0 = 0–4 years; 1 = 5–8 years; 2 = 9–11 years; 3 = ≥12 years.

group. Since the coefficients are consistently near zero, it seems likely that cholesterol is of less importance for older persons who have remained free of CHD until age 55 than for those in younger age groups.

Cigarette smoking was a significant CHD risk factor for men and women aged 65–74 years and for the combined age groups of both genders. A history of diabetes was significantly related to risk of CHD for both combined age groups for men and women as well as for younger men and older women. Relative weight (or body mass index) and alcohol intake were not significant contributors to CHD. A higher level of education was associated with a reduced risk of CHD in all groups.

The sample of black persons had fewer significant predictors, a result undoubtedly influenced by the smaller numbers. Nevertheless, systolic blood pressure was significantly related to CHD for men, and diabetes was a predictor for women. Body mass index was significant for older black women. The negative coefficient implies a slight reduction in CHD risk for heavier weights at this age. Since this was the only such finding for body mass index in all the age, race, and gender groups, it is probably an artefact.

Although the logistic coefficients are comparable for the total sample and for the subgroups 65–74 years of age, when 5-year age subgroups are examined there is an apparent reduction in the magnitude of the coefficients from the youngest to the oldest subgroups. Also, when only CHD mortality was utilized as an end point, the coefficients changed very slightly. Thus, the prediction of coronary heart disease mortality or of morbidity plus mortality is virtually identical in this elderly population.

Methodologic issues that may affect the results need to be addressed, and the type of exclusions used merit comment. In general, the traditional risk factors have been less predictive in those with extant CHD (Kannel and Brand 1985). Electrocardiograms were available for only a subset of the population, therefore, some individuals with silent disease remain in the population. Furthermore, even a negative

ECG does not necessarily preclude the presence of CHD, and further tests are needed to provide a definitive diagnosis. The high prevalence of atherosclerosis in the elderly population may distort the usual chain of causation (risk factor leading to atherosclerosis, which in turn results in clinically manifest CHD) because of the lack of substantial variability between members of this older population. Whether NHEFS subjects whose responses to the Rose questionnaire (Rose et al. 1982) indicated the presence of angina were included in or excluded from the base population did not affect the results of the analysis. A history of heart attack was available for the entire population and was a reasonable exclusion, although the diagnoses were not independently verified.

The mortality end point represents the underlying cause of death (i.e., code 410–414, Ischemic Heart Disease) as shown on the death certificate. Similarly, hospitalizations with any mention of codes 410–414 were included in the CHD end point. Individuals with multiple admissions for CHD were counted only once.

The number of events in this study was modest. Because of small numbers, it was not possible to examine separately race subgrouping, hospitalizations alone, or sudden deaths in a reliable manner. Further follow-up of the cohort for events is under way, and subsequent analyses may be able to address these points more satisfactorily.

The confirmation of the finding that level of systolic blood pressure predicts CHD in this older, nationally representative population lends strong support to continued efforts in detection and control of hypertension. The coefficients for systolic blood pressure are similar for each 5-year subgroup and for both genders. The prevalence of those who had diastolic blood pressures of more than 90 mmHg or who were receiving antihypertensive treatment was similar to the 60–69-year-old group in the Hypertension Detection and Follow-up Program (HDFP) (Curb et al. 1985). There are slight methodologic differences between the two studies, however. HDFP used the average of the last two blood pressure measurements made in the subject's home while the NHANES I follow-up utilized a single blood pressure measured in the examination trailer.

In a population-based study in Puerto Rico (Kittner et al. 1983), where CHD mortality is lower than in the mainland United States, the adjusted relative odds for elevated systolic blood pressure as a risk factor for nonsudden CHD mortality among those aged 60 years and older was 3.7.

In the Framingham population aged 49–82 years, the multivariate logistic coefficients showed that systolic blood pressure was a significant predictor of CHD in men; for women a positive but nonsignificant relationship between systolic blood pressure and CHD was found. Left ventricular hypertrophy also was predictive of CHD in women. Thus, the evidence from NHEFS is consistent with the results of other studies (Sidney 1986).

Self-reported diabetes is also a significant predictor of CHD. Previous reports from Framingham (Dawber and Kannel 1972) and the Rancho Bernardo population, studied by the Lipid Research Clinic in La Jolla (Barrett-Conner and Wingard 1983), have suggested that the relationship between diabetes and CHD may be stronger in women than in men. In the 20-year follow-up of CHD in Framingham

(Kannel and McGee 1979), adjustment for other risk factors resulted in relative risks of 1.7 and 2.1 for men and women, respectively. In Rancho Bernardo the adjusted risk ratios were 2.4 and 3.5, respectively, for mortality due to ischemic heart disease (Barrett-Conner and Wingard 1983). Conversion of logistic coefficients to relative odds resulted in ratios of from 2.2 to 1.9, depending on the age and gender group (Table 4–5). Note that the relative odds estimates for black women were quite high (Table 4–5a).

Smoking was not a predictor of CHD among the elderly populations in Framingham (Kannel and Gordon 1980) or Rancho Bernardo (Barrett-Conner and Wingard 1983). In Puerto Rico (Kittner et al. 1983) as well, the adjusted relative odds for smoking and nonsudden CHD deaths among those 60 or older was not significant. However, a report (Jajich et al. 1984) from a Chicago population, aged 65–74 years, indicated that current smoking resulted in a mortality ratio of 1.52 for deaths due to CHD, but no breakdown by gender was presented. It also appeared that those who stopped smoking returned rather quickly to a lower-risk status. The NHEFS data indicate that white men and women who are smokers are at a higher risk for coronary heart disease at older ages. It was not possible to determine the effect of years stopped in this population. This report and the Chicago experience (Jajich et al. 1984) suggest the importance of encouraging those older than 55 who smoke to discontinue the use of cigarettes. There apparently is no age beyond which it is safe to smoke.

In this national sample, level of cholesterol in serum was not found to be a predictor of CHD. When total cholesterol was subdivided in Framingham into the major components of low-density lipoprotein (LDL) and high-density lipoprotein (HDL) cholesterol, both were significant. Unfortunately, HDL cholesterol determinations were not done at baseline in this investigation. Two other studies, Puerto Rico (Kittner et al. 1983) and Rancho Bernardo (Barrett-Conner and Wingard 1983), suggest that total concentration of cholesterol in serum can be a risk factor at older ages.

In summary, systolic blood pressure, cigarette smoking, and diabetes appear to be the major predictors of CHD in this older population. The fact that this NHEFS survey studied a national sample of the noninstitutionalized elderly persons adds credence and generalizability to these observations. With further follow-up of this population, recording of additional events will permit more detailed analysis.

Data from this study already provide information on which to base preventive and therapeutic strategies aimed at the aging population of the United States. Because the incidence of CHD and its sequelae is so high among the elderly, even modest changes can have a large impact.

HYPERTENSION

Most studies of the prevalence of hypertension in older persons have depended on statistics from single communities or other small areas (Cornoni-Huntley et al. 1989). Sometimes such studies have not documented important differences between the genders or major races. Only a few studies of nationwide populations have been able to examine the occurrence of new cases of hypertension over time or the prevalence of drug therapy (National Center for Health Statistics 1986). The availability of NHEFS enables us to examine these issues on a national sample of aging individuals. There is general acceptance that elevated diastolic blood pressure in older persons should be treated (HDFP Cooperative Group 1982), although treatment of the less common isolated systolic hypertension requires further study (Rowe 1983). Since a large proportion of the elderly is now receiving drug therapy, prevalence and incidence data should include treatment status as well as blood pressure level.

This section addresses the available NHEFS data on the prevalence of hypertension in the elderly at two points in time, compares the frequency of treatment at baseline with the frequency at follow-up, determines the incidence of new cases, highlights racial differences in incidence and prevalence, and discusses the methodologic issues important to the proper interpretation of these data.

Population and Method

The baseline NHEFS population included 14,407 participants, who at the time of characterization were 25 to 74 years when they were enrolled in NHANES I in 1971–1975. This analysis will be limited to the 5610 participants who were 55–74 years of age at baseline (NHANES I). Oversampling of some age, race, and gender groups occurred at baseline and resulted in nonrepresentative numbers in certain subgroups (Table 4–6). Also, the numbers will vary between the initial ascertainment and the follow-up because of mortality, aging of the population, losses to follow-up, and missing data (Table 4–7). For the incidence analysis (Table 4–8), persons with hypertension (definite, isolated systolic, or borderline) as defined later, and persons on treatment for hypertension were excluded.

In NHANES I blood pressure was measured at the time of NHANES I in the

Table 4–6 Rate of Hypertension by Traditional Categories According to Race, Gender, and Age at Baseline (NHANES I) (in percent)

Group	Sample size	Borderline	Isolated systolic	Definite by blood pressure	Treated	Total definite*
Ages 55–64						
White men	740	25.7	1.9	21.0	13.1	36.0
White women	816	23.9	3.2	16.9	18.3	38.4
Black men	106	21.7	2.8	33.0	16.0	51.8
Black women	138	16.7	4.4	29.7	29.0	63.1
Ages 65–74						
White men	1496	25.3	6.7	19.5	16.4	42.6
White women	1673	23.1	7.1	19.1	28.0	54.2
Black men	312	21.2	6.1	21.8	21.8	57.7
Black women	329	16.1	11.6	28.6	31.0	71.2

*Includes isolated systolic, definite by blood pressure, and treated categories.

Table 4–7 Rate of Hypertension by Traditional Categories According to Race, Gender, and Age at Follow-up (NHEFS) (in percent)

Group	Sample size	Borderline	Isolated systolic	Definite by blood pressure	Treated	Total definite*
Age 55–64						
White men	698	19.2	1.9	6.6	26.2	34.7
White women	879	12.6	2.1	3.5	32.1	37.7
Black men	95	13.7	5.3	11.6	34.7	51.6
Black women	136	11.0	3.7	8.1	44.9	56.7
Age 65–74						
White men	522	19.4	4.0	4.6	33.0	41.6
White women	632	14.6	4.8	3.0	42.6	50.4
Black men	67	14.9	7.5	9.0	43.3	59.8
Black women	109	16.5	2.8	3.7	58.7	65.2
Age 75–86						
White men	641	22.2	8.9	5.0	30.6	44.5
White women	963	17.3	7.3	2.2	49.1	58.6
Black men	107	18.7	7.5	5.6	44.9	58.0
Black women	161	14.3	9.9	4.4	59.0	73.3

*Includes isolated systolic, definite by blood pressure, and treated categories.

Mobile Examination Center. The physician measured blood pressure with a standard sphygmomanometer using the bell of the stethoscope on the right arm while the subject was seated. For NHEFS the blood pressure measurement was obtained at a home visit by a trained observer, who used the same techniques. For comparability between the time periods, only the single blood pressure is used as a criterion for hypertension.

Table 4–8 Category at Follow-up According to Race, Gender, and Age Among Subjects Normal at Baseline (NHANES I)

| Group | Sample size | No. of events (% of group) | | |
		Normal	Borderline	Definite
Age 55–64				
White men	206	136 (66.0)	33 (16.0)	37 (18.0)
White women	243	147 (60.5)	40 (16.5)	56 (23.1)
Black men	15	8 (53.3)	3 (20.0)	4 (26.7)
Black women	21	14 (66.7)	1 (4.8)	6 (28.6)
Age 65–74				
White men	236	121 (51.3)	63 (26.7)	52 (22.0)
White women	234	123 (52.6)	63 (26.9)	48 (20.5)
Black men	33	18 (54.6)	6 (18.2)	9 (27.3)
Black women	18	8 (44.4)	1 (5.6)	9 (50.0)
Age 55–74				
White men	442	257 (58.1)	96 (21.7)	89 (20.1)
White women	477	270 (56.6)	103 (21.6)	104 (21.8)
Black men	48	26 (54.2)	9 (18.8)	13 (27.1)
Black women	39	22 (56.4)	2 (5.1)	15 (38.5)

Definite hypertension has been defined as systolic blood pressure measurement of ≥160 mmHg and/or diastolic blood pressure of ≥95 mmHg. The group with isolated systolic hypertension includes persons with systolic blood pressure measurement of ≥160 mmHg but with diastolic blood pressure measure of <90 mmHg. Borderline is defined as systolic blood pressure measurement of ≥140 but <160 mmHg and/or a diastolic blood pressure measurement of >95 mmHg. Normal is defined as a systolic blood pressure of <140 and a diastolic blood pressure <90 mmHg.

Current reported usage of antihypertensive medications was the criterion for "treated" hypertension; usage was determined at interview. For a subset of the NHANES I population, current treatment included medication taken for hypertension during the previous six months (Cornoni-Huntley et al. 1989). The total number with definite hypertension includes three groups: those treated; definite hypertension, as defined earlier; and isolated systolic hypertension.

Standard descriptive and analytical statistical procedures were used for evaluation of the data.

Results

Prevalences of hypertension categories are presented by age, race, and gender at baseline (NHANES I) in Table 4–6 and at follow-up (NHEFS) in Table 4–7. Because of the aging of the cohort, substantial numbers of the population reached ages 75–86 in the period 1982–1984, and data from this older group are shown in Table 4–7. In both tables the numbers of black men and women in the sample are relatively small.

At ages 55–64 there are modest gender differences in total prevalence of definite hypertension at the two time points; however, at older ages there is an excess prevalence of this category in women at both examinations. In every race–gender subgroup, regardless of age, more women than men are being treated. At the follow-up visit the proportion of black women being treated is particularly noteworthy, being almost 60% of all those 65–86 years old. The percentage of those treated almost doubled in every subgroup, regardless of race, over the approximately 10-year follow-up period.

The frequencies of total definite hypertension are similar between the two time periods, even with the major increase in treatment. Almost in a corresponding manner, the percentage of those with definite hypertension by ascertained blood pressure measurement alone was lower. Besides better detection, some of this difference may have been due to the fact that at NHEFS blood pressures were measured at home rather than in the Mobile Examination Center. When blood pressures of those not receiving drug therapy at either examination are compared, the mean systolic and diastolic blood pressures for the various subgroups were approximately 8 mmHg lower at follow-up (Cornoni-Huntley et al. 1989).

Although isolated systolic hypertension is less common than other categories of hypertension, its frequency generally increases from ages 55–64 to ages 75–86 (Table 4–7).

Table 4–8 gives the numbers and percentages of individuals with various types of hypertension at follow-up among those with both systolic blood pressure of <140 mmHg and diastolic blood pressure of <90 mmHg at baseline. These data are indicators of the incidence over approximately 9.5 years of borderline and definite hypertension. Among white men and women, the percentage developing definite hypertension is about the same for the two older age groups. For the combined white group aged 55–74 years, those with hypertension represent about 20% of the surviving cohort. Comparison with younger age groups shows that there is an absolute rise in the proportion of persons with hypertension of 5% for each 10-year interval of age (Cornoni-Huntley et al. 1989). The population available for study of incidence among blacks was too small for evaluation (Table 4–8). Part of the reason for the small number of blacks is the fact that over 50% had definite hypertension and another 20% were in the borderline range at baseline and therefore were excluded from analysis of incidence.

As systolic blood pressure was a major risk factor for subsequent incidence of CHD (including CHD mortality), so definite hypertension at baseline predicted survival during follow-up (Cornoni-Huntley et al. 1989). Among white men and women aged 50 years or more, the proportion surviving was highest among the normotensives at baseline, intermediate among those with borderline elevated blood pressure, and lowest among those with definite hypertension. Overall, women were more likely than men to survive. The general findings were similar in blacks, but small numbers precluded definite conclusions. Elevated blood pressure at baseline, no matter what the treatment status, appeared to be an independent predictor of mortality (Havlik et al. 1989).

DISCUSSION

The striking observation in this analysis is the very high prevalence of hypertension among the elderly. In both Tables 4–6 and 4–7, which represent two periods of time, only about one third of older white men and women, one fifth of older black men, and one sixth of older black women could be considered to have normal blood pressure status. Although this finding has been noted previously (National Center for Health Statistics 1986), its repeated observation in a nationally representative population adds strength to the original report.

At every reported older age, blacks have a higher prevalence of total definite hypertension than whites, and this finding is consistent over the two time periods. The possible reasons for this racial difference have not been adequately explained; however, the observation has been almost universal in various populations in the United States (Gillum and Gillum 1984). It appears, however, that any gap in the receipt of therapy has been closed because treatment in blacks and whites has increased about twofold in the 10-year period of this study.

As is evident in Tables 4–6 and 4–7, women tend to have a higher frequency of hypertension than men, no matter which race or age subgroup is examined. Studies of incidence of new cases of hypertension can help in understanding the development of the observed differences in prevalence. However, Table 4–8 shows that for the combined age group 55–74 years, there is no observed gender difference in incidence of definite hypertension among whites. In addition, these incidence studies must be interpreted in the context of possible differential survival, since men are less likely than women to survive until very old age. In fact, this gender-related difference in survival was found in this population group. Thus, it suggests that any differences in hypertension prevalence between men and women are likely to be due to greater mortality among men with hypertension, rather than to gender differences in incidence.

As indicated in the first part of this chapter, systolic blood pressure continues to be a predictor of CHD at older ages. More generally, hypertension is negatively associated with survival in this population. The continuing importance of adequate detection and treatment of hypertension in the elderly is therefore evident. Some observers have suggested that treatment of elevated blood pressure, because of its wide use at all ages, is a likely reason for the decline in mortality due to cardiovascular diseases (Feinleib et al. 1982). A recent report of the Fourth Joint National Committee containing an increased variety of recommended treatments (Moser 1988) will promote more flexibility in customizing therapy for older patients. In the NHEFS population, diuretics and beta blockers were the most common drugs prescribed (Havlik et al. 1989). Evaluation of the results of the Systolic Hypertension in the Elderly Program will be necessary before widespread treatment of isolated elevated systolic blood pressure can be recommended (Rowe 1983).

The NHEFS provided an insight into a methodologic issue in the interpretation of prevalence of hypertension in a population. This opportunity evolved from the circumstances of NHEFS, with blood pressure being measured in an examination trailer at baseline and in the home at follow-up. Previous observers suggested that blood pressure could be expected to be lower at home than elsewhere (Kleinert et al. 1984). Even in subgroups of normotensive persons of similar ages, there was an approximate difference of 8 mmHg between the baseline and follow-up groups in this population (Cornoni-Huntley et al. 1989). It is unlikely that this difference was due entirely to a true decrease in mean blood pressure over time. It is more likely to be due to the different methodology. Also, because blood pressure was measured in the home, the estimates of definite hypertension at the follow-up in 1982–1984, as portrayed in Table 4–7, should be considered to be conservative. In the Third National Health and Nutrition Examination Survey, initiated in 1988, a new sample of the U.S. population will be surveyed. In this survey, a special effort to examine this methodologic question will be made by measurement of blood pressure in the home and by doing a separate measurement in the examination trailer.

Coronary heart disease and hypertension are interwoven manifestations of cardiovascular disease. NHEFS gives a 10-years view of the dynamics of risk factors for coronary heart disease and hypertension in the United States. The results of NHEFS provide further support for the notion that continued emphasis on detection and adequate treatment of hypertension should continue. However, further etiologic studies of CHD and risk factors for hypertension as well as development of potentially better preventive strategies at all ages are likely to have the greatest impact on the future cardiovascular status of the elderly.

REFERENCES

Barrett-Connor, E., L. Suarez, K. Khaw, M. H. Criqui, and D. L. Wingard. 1984. "Ischemic heart disease risk factors after age 50." *J Chron Dis* 37:903–908.

Barrett-Connor, E., and D. L. Wingard. 1983. "Sex differential in ischemic heart disease mortality in diabetics: A prospective population-based study." *Am J Epidemiol* 118:489–496.

Cornoni-Huntley, J., H. E. Barbano, J. A. Brody, B. Cohen, J. J. Feldman, J. C. Kleinman, and J. Madans. 1983. National Health and Nutrition Examination I—Epidemiologic Follow-up Survey. *Public Health Rep* 98:245–251.

Cornoni-Huntley, J., A. Z. LaCroix, R. J. Havlik. 1989. Race and Sex Differentials in the Impact of Hypertension in the United States: The NHANES I Epidemiologic Follow-up Study. *Arch Intern Med.* 149: 780–788.

Curb, J. D., N. O. Borhani, E. Schnaper, E. Karr, G. Entwistle, W. Williams, and R. Berman. 1985. "Detection and treatment of hypertension in older individuals." *Am J Epidemiol* 121:371–376.

Dawber, T. R., and W. B. Kannel. 1972. "Current status of coronary prevention; lessons from the Framingham Study." *Prevent Med* 1:499–512.

Eavenson, D., O. T. Grier, J. G. Cission, and R. F. Witter. 1966. "A semiautomated procedure for the determination of serum cholesterol using the Abel–Kendall method." *J Am Oil Chem Soc* 43:652–656.

Feinleib, M., R. J. Havlik, and T. J. Thom. 1982. "The changing pattern of ischemic heart disease." *Cardiov Med* 7:139–148.

Gillum, R. F., and B. S. Gillum. 1984. "Potential for control and prevention of essential hypertension in the black community." In *Behavioral Health,* J. D. Matarazzo, S. M. Weiss, J. A. Herd, N. E. Miller, and S. M. Weiss, eds. New York: John Wiley and Sons, pp. 825–835.

Gordon, T., W. B. Castelli, M. C. Hjortland, W. B. Kannel, and T. R. Dawber. 1977. "Predicting coronary heart disease in middle-aged and older persons: The Framingham Study." *JAMA* 238:497–499.

Harris, T. B., E. F. Cook, A. Schatzkin, W. B. Kannel, and L. Goldman. 1985. "Blood pressure experience and risk of cardiovascular disease in the elderly." *Hypertension* 7:118–124.

Havlik, R. J., A. Z. LaCroix, J. C. Kleinman, D. D. Ingram, T. Harris, and J. Cornoni-Huntley. 1989. "Antihypertensive drug therapy and survival by treatment status in national survey. *Hypertension* 13 (suppl. I): I-25–I-32.

Hypertension Detection and Follow-up Program Cooperative Group. 1982. "Five-Year findings of the Hypertension Detection and Follow-up Program: III. Reduction in stroke incidence among persons with high blood pressure." *JAMA* 247:633–638.

Jajich, C. L., A. M. Ostfeld, and D. H. Freeman, Jr. 1984. "Smoking and coronary heart disease mortality in the elderly." *JAMA* 252:2831–2834.

Kannel, W. B. 1985. "Hypertension and aging." In *Handbook on the Biology of Aging,* 2nd ed. E. C. Finch and E. L. Schiedner, eds. New York: Van Nostrand Reinhold Co., pp. 859–877.

Kannel, W. B., and F. N. Brand. 1985. "Cardiovascular risk factors in the elderly." In *Principles of Geriatric Medicine*. R. Andrew, F. L. Bierman, and W. R. Hazzard, eds. New York: McGraw-Hill Book Co., pp. 104–119.

Kannel, W. B., and T. Gordon. 1978. "Evaluation of cardiovascular risk in the elderly: The Framingham Study." *Bull NY Acad Med*. 54(6):573–591.

Kannel, W. B., and T. Gordon. 1980. "Cardiovascular risk factors in the aged: The Framingham Study." In *Second Conference on the Epidemiology of Aging*. S. G. Haynes and M. F. Feinleib, eds. NIH Publication No. 80-969, pp. 65–89.

Kannel, W. B., and D. L. McGee. 1979. "Diabetes and glucose tolerance as risk factors for cardiovascular disease: The Framingham Study 1979." *Diabetes Care* 2:120–126.

Kittner, S., M. R. Garcia-Palmieri, R. Costas Jr., M. Cruz-Vidal, R. D. Abbott, and R. J. Havlik. 1983. "Alcohol and coronary heart disease in Puerto Rico." *Am J Epidemiol* 17:538–550.

Kleinert, H. D., G. A. Harshfield, T. G. Pickering, R. B. Devereau, P. A. Sullivan, R. M. Marion, W. K. Mallory, and J. H. Laragh. 1984. "What is the value of home blood pressure measurement in patients with mild hypertension?" *Hypertension* 6:574–578.

Leaverton, P. E., P. O. Sorlie, J. C. Kleinman et al. 1987. "Representativeness of the Framingham risk model for coronary heart disease mortality: A comparison with a national cohort study." *J Chron Dis* 40:775–784.

Moser, M. 1988. "Some highlights of the fourth Joint National Committee Report on the Detection, Evaluation, and Treatment of High Blood Pressure." *Hypertension* 11:560–562.

National Center for Health Statistics. 1985. *Health, United States, 1985*. Health Statistics, DHHS Pub. No. (PHS) 86-1232. Washington, DC: U.S. Government Printing Office, pp. 8–10.

National Center for Health Statistics. 1986. T. Drizd, A. L. Dannenberg, and A. Engel, Blood Pressure Levels in Persons 18–74 Years of Age in 1976–80, and Trends in Blood Pressure from 1960 to 1980 in the United States. *Vital and Health Statistics*. Series 11, No. 234. DHHS Publication No. (PHS) 86-1684. Hyattsville, MD.

National Center for Health Statistics. 1987. R. J. Havlik, B. M. Liu, M. G. Kovar et al., Health Statistics on Older Persons, United States, 1986. *Vital and Health Statistics*. Series 3, No. 25. DHHS Pub. No. (PHS) 87-1409. Washington, DC: U.S. Government Printing Office.

Rose, G. A. 1965. "Chest pain questionnaire." *Milbank Mem Fund Q* 43(2):32–39.

Rose, G. A., H. Blackburn, R. F. Gillum, and R. J. Prineas. 1982. *Cardiovascular Survey Methods*. Geneva: World Health Organization, pp. 162–165.

Rosenberg, H. M., and A. J. Klebba. 1979. "Trends in cardiovascular mortality with a focus on cardiovascular disease: United States, 1950–76." In *Proceedings of the Conference on the Decline in Coronary Heart Disease Mortality*, R. J. Havlik and M. Feinleib, eds. NIH publication no. 79-1610, pp. 11–41.

Rowe, J. W. 1983. "Systolic hypertension in the elderly." *N Engl J Med* 309:1246–1247.

Sidney, S. 1986. "Risk factors for coronary heart disease in the elderly." CVD Epidemiology Newsletter 39:30.

World Health Organization. 1977. Manual of International Statistical Classification of Diseases, Injuries, and Cause of Death. Based on recommendations of 9th Revision Conference. Geneva: World Health Organization.

5

Cancer

ARTHUR SCHATZKIN, D. YVONNE JONES,
TAMARA B. HARRIS, PHILIP R. TAYLOR,
ROBERT N. HOOVER, CHRISTINE L. CARTER,
REGINA G. ZIEGLER, AND LOUISE A. BRINTON

EPIDEMIOLOGIC INVESTIGATIONS OF CANCER IN NHEFS

At least three features make the data set from the NHANES I (National Health and Nutrition Examination Survey-I) Epidemiologic Follow-up Study, or NHEFS, particularly useful for researchers in cancer epidemiology. First, since the study was based on a probability sample of the population of the United States, the NHEFS cohort has greater heterogeneity in educational background, occupation, and geographic residence than one traditionally finds in cohorts. Second, information on characteristics and exposures of subjects was gathered before diagnosis. Cancer is known to affect many systems within the body and may certainly affect constituents of the blood and other biologic end points, as well as various aspects of life-style, including diet and exercise. Moreover, the diagnosis of cancer may influence a person's recall and reporting of information. These potential problems of reverse causation and recall bias are obviated in large part by the prospective cohort design of NHEFS. Third, relatively "hard" data on cancer end points are available from both hospital records and death certificates.

We have previously used the NHEFS data set to examine three hypotheses of considerable public health importance: (1) Alcohol consumption is positively associated with breast cancer; (2) dietary fat consumption is positively associated with breast cancer; and (3) serum cholesterol is inversely associated with cancer (at all sites combined and at certain specific sites, especially the colorectum). In this chapter we present a review of our earlier analyses (Jones et al. 1987; Schatzkin, Jones et al. 1987; Schatzkin, Taylor et al. 1987; Schatzkin et al. 1988). In addition, we present results of a study of the relation between socioeconomic status and cancer. These studies reflect a common premise that the identification of socioenvironmental factors involved in the etiology of cancer is a critical step in the prevention of malignant disease.

71

IDENTIFICATION OF CASES: GENERAL CONSIDERATIONS

For our analyses involving the incidence of "all cancers," a study participant was classified as an incident case if there was any diagnosis of cancer (International Classification of Diseases codes 140 through 208, excluding nonmelanoma skin cancer, ICD code 173) on a hospital record or death certificate. (With incident cases identified from death certificates, both the underlying and contributing causes of death were relevant.) Cancer cases at specific sites were similarly identified from the hospital records and/or death certificates. A few cases listed as primary lung cancer were found on review of the hospital records to be secondary cancers (metastatic from some other site). An individual could have had an incident cancer at more than one site.

For cases identified through hospital records, the date of first admission for a specific cancer listed in the discharge diagnosis was regarded as the date of incidence for that site. The date of death was considered to be the incidence date for cancers for which the only data available were those on the death certificate.

In analyses of mortality, only cancer listed as the underlying cause of death was considered to be a case.

We excluded persons with prevalent cancer at baseline from all our analyses. A person was considered to be a prevalent case if, at the first hospitalization, one of the ICD V-codes indicating a "history" of cancer at a specific site was listed. A person with a history of cancer at one site, however, was still at risk for cancer at another site and would not have been excluded from some of the site-specific investigations.

ALCOHOL AND BREAST CANCER

Evidence that alcohol consumption increases the risk of breast cancer in women appeared over a decade ago (Williams and Horm 1977). Since that time, a number of epidemiologic studies have shown this association. Although not all case-control investigations of the relation between alcohol consumption and breast cancer showed the positive association (Begg et al. 1983; Byers and Funch 1982; Paganini-Hill and Ross 1983; Webster at al. 1983, Wynder et al. 1960), the majority of them indicated that the risk of breast cancer increased with moderate alcohol consumption (Harvey et al. 1987; La Vecchia et al. 1985; Le et al. 1984; O'Connell et al. 1987; Rosenberg et al. 1982; Talamini et al. 1984). Three cohort studies observed an elevation in risk of 50–100% in relation to drinking. Hiatt and Bawol reported a 40% excess risk among women consuming three or more drinks per day (Hiatt and Bawol 1984). Willet et al. showed a 60% increase in risk for women drinking a little more than a drink per day, with a dose–response relation being evident (Willet et al. 1987). Hiatt et al. recently showed that women consuming one or two drinks per day had a 50% elevation in risk, with "past drinkers" being at more than twice the risk of nondrinkers (Hiatt et al. 1988).

Analytic Methodology

The original NHEFS cohort consisted of 8596 women, of whom 83% were white. We initially identified 131 incident breast cancers in NHEFS, 111 from hospital records and 20 from death certificates.

In this study (Schatzkin et al. 1987), women were excluded from the original cohort as follows: 30 women were excluded because baseline information on drinking was missing; 281 women who were pregnant or breast-feeding at the time of the NHANES I interview were excluded, since alcohol consumption was likely to have been affected by these conditions; 675 of the eligible women could not be traced; 483 women were found to be alive but did not have a follow-up interview, either because they refused to participate or could not be contacted; 12 women were considered to be prevalent cases at baseline. A small number of women fell into more than one of these exclusion categories.

After these exclusions the population available for analysis consisted of 7188 women, of whom 121 developed breast cancer. The median follow-up time for the cohort was 10 years.

We were concerned that the breast cancer rate in this cohort should be at least roughly comparable to that in other U.S. populations. Therefore, we applied the age- and race-specific incidences derived from the Connecticut Cancer Registry to our cohort. The ratio of observed to expected cases was 1.07 (95% confidence interval, 0.89–1.28).

Questions on frequency and quantity of alcohol consumption were asked during the baseline interview. Each woman was asked if she had at least one drink of beer, wine, or liquor during the previous year. If she had, she was then asked how often she drank (the possible responses being every day, just about every day, about two or three times per week, about one to four times per month, more than three but less than 12 times per year, or no more than two or three times per year). Those women reporting having had at least one drink in the previous year were also asked how much they usually drank per 24-hour period (in glasses or drinks). We calculated the average number of ounces of ethanol consumed per day by the formula (number of drinks per day) × (a drinking frequency factor) × (0.5 oz). The factor 0.5 oz was an estimate of the amount of ethanol in a "shot" of liquor, a 5-oz glass of wine, or a 12-oz glass of beer. The frequency factors were as follows: 1 for drinking every day, 5/7 for just about every day, 5/14 for two to three times per week, 5/60 for one to four times per month, 15/730 for 3 to 12 times per year, and 5/730 for two to three times per year. Ounces of ethanol were converted into grams, with one ounce being approximately equal to 25 grams (or roughly two drinks).

Unfortunately, information on quantity of the specific type of alcoholic beverage consumed was not available. Since questions on drinking at earlier ages were asked in the follow-up interview, we attempted a case-control analysis of the relation of drinking at various ages to risk of breast cancer. However, the number of women with breast cancer who provided this information in the follow-up survey was too small for stable analysis.

Information on most of the important covariates, including age, education, poverty index ratio, body mass index, parity, age at menarche, age at menopause, and diet, was provided in the baseline interview. The dietary data came from a 24-hour recall interview conducted by a trained nutritionist using three-dimensional graduated food portion models (National Center for Health Statistics 1972). Standard data on food composition were used for calculation of nutrient intake (Watt and Merrill 1963). Information on family history of breast cancer (in mother or sister) and age at birth of first child was available only from the follow-up interview. Information was collected on smoking at baseline from only 43% of women in the original NHEFS cohort. For those women lacking smoking data at baseline, we inferred smoking status at baseline from the follow-up information. A woman without baseline smoking data who reported at follow-up, for example, that she was a current smoker and that she began smoking 20 years before her baseline examination would have been classified as a current smoker at baseline, with a 20-year duration of smoking.

We found that the distributions of alcohol consumption and most risk factors for breast cancer were virtually identical in the NHEFS cohort used in our analyses and the total NHEFS cohort. The analytic cohort was slightly older than the total cohort (26% vs. 23% $\geq$ 65 years of age) and had a slightly greater proportion of postmenopausal women (52% vs. 47%).

Observed Correlations between Alcohol Use and Breast Cancer

The mean age at baseline of women in our analytic cohort was 49 years. Fifty-five percent were under 50, and 25% were over 65 years of age. Women who developed breast cancer were older than those who did not; mean baseline ages were 56 years for cases and 49 years for noncases. Of the 7188 women in the analytic cohort, 42% had not graduated from high school at baseline, whereas 21% had completed more than 12 years of education.

We examined the relation of alcohol consumption to a number of risk factors for breast cancer (Table 5–1). Younger women reported more drinking than older women. The age-adjusted proportions of women reporting drinking were higher among women with more education, lower body mass index, older age at first birth, and lower parity; those who smoked and had a higher fat intake also reported more alcohol use. There was little difference in reported frequency of drinking according to menopausal status, family history of breast cancer, or age at menarche.

Crude incidences of breast cancer according to category of drinking were calculated by the formula (number of cases of breast cancer among women in the category)/(total number of person-years contributed by women in that category). The number of person-years contributed by an individual woman was calculated from baseline to the time of diagnosis of breast cancer, death, or the follow-up interview, whichever came first.

Age-adjusted incidences are shown in Fig. 5–1. The incidence was higher among drinkers than among nondrinkers, and it increased moderately with amount of alcohol consumed.

Table 5–1 Relationship Between Levels of Alcohol Intake and Risk of Breast Cancer

Relative risk estimates	Alcohol intake level (grams per day)				
	None	Any	>0–1.2	1.3–4.9	>5
Age-adjusted*	1.0	1.5	1.4	1.5	1.6
(95% Confidence interval)		(1.1–2.2)	(0.9–2.3)	(0.9–2.6)	(1.0–2.7)
Multivariate†	1.0	1.6	1.4	1.6	2.0
(95% Confidence interval)		(1.0–2.5)	(0.8–2.5)	(0.9–3.1)	(1.1–3.7)

Source: This table is reprinted with permission of *The New England Journal of Medicine*.

*Based on age-adjusted regression coefficients from the proportional-hazards models (121 cases).

†Based on 88 cases with complete covariate informatics, including age (years); education (>12 years); body mass index (combined second through fourth quintiles 21–29; fifth quintile, >30); total dietary fat (grams per day) (separate second through fifth quintiles; 34.2–47.5; 47.6–61.4; 61.5–80.6; ≥80.7); age at first parturition (19–20, 21–22, 23–24, and ≥25), age of menarche (≤12), parity (nulliparity, one or two births), positive family history; and premenopausal status.

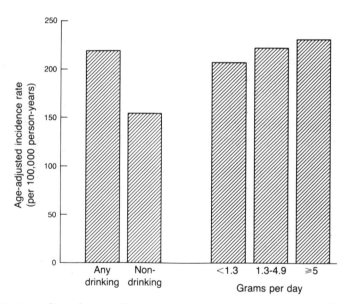

Fig. 5–1. Age-adjusted rates of breast cancer according to level of alcohol consumption. These rates have been age-adjusted by the indirect method (Fleiss 1981), on the basis of the crude and age-specific incidence rates for breast cancer among women 25 to 74 years of age from the Connecticut Cancer Registry. Age-adjusted rates calculated by the direct method (Fleiss 1981) (on the basis of the analytic cohort) were 150 and 218, respectively, for no drinking and any drinking, and 206, 204, 271 for the lowest through the highest levels of drinking. Five grams of ethanol per day is roughly equivalent to three drinks per week. (Figure modified from Schatzkin, Jones, Hoover, et al., 1987.)

To analyze the simultaneous relation of alcohol, age, and other variables to incidence of breast cancer in the cohort, we used Cox's proportional hazards regression technique (Cox and Oakes 1984). The analyses were performed with the PROC PHGLM procedure available in the SAS statistical package (SAS Institute, Inc. 1983). Estimates of relative risk (and 95% confidence intervals) were derived from the regression coefficients (and standard errors of the coefficients) yielded by the regression models.

Table 5–1 depicts the results of proportional-hazards models comprising variables for age and alcohol use only. The estimated relative risk (95% confidence interval) for any drinking compared to nondrinking was 1.5 (1.1–2.2); the estimates for the three tertiles of drinking, from lowest to highest, were 1.4 (0.9–2.3), 1.5 (0.9–2.6), and 1.6 (1.0–2.7), respectively.

We next performed a series of analyses based on various "trivariate" models that included variables for age, alcohol consumption, and one of several potential confounders, including education (<12, 12, >12 years), total dietary fat in grams per day (quintiles), age at first birth (<19, 19–20, 21–22, 23–25, ≥26), age at onset of menarche (≤11, 12, 13, 14, ≥15), parity (nulliparity, one, two, three, or more than four live births), family history of breast cancer, menopausal status, body mass index (quintiles), or cigarette smoking (never, former, current smoker; or, 0, 1–13, or >13 pack-years). These analyses yielded relative risks for the highest tertile of drinking in the range of 1.4 to 2.0. Estimates were largely unchanged when quintile indicators for saturated fat, or fat as a percentage of total calories, were substituted for total fat, nor were they altered in separate analyses that included quintile indicators for protein, dietary cholesterol, or total calories.

Models that simultaneously included a variety of potential confounders generated relative risk estimates (95% confidence intervals) of 1.6 (1.0–2.5) for any drinking compared to nondrinking. For the three textiles of drinking (relative to nondrinking), the estimates from lowest to highest were 1.4 (0.8–2.5), 1.6 (0.9–3.1), and 2.0 (1.1–3.7) (Table 5–2). (Because of missing information on covariates, especially smoking and dietary variables, the number of cases analyzed in the multivariate regressions was somewhat lower.)

We used the multivariate proportional hazards analysis to examine a linear trend variable for alcohol consumption (with four values: nondrinking and three tertiles of alcohol use). The p-value for trend was 0.020 for that variable. In a similar analysis of a linear trend variable limited to the three tertiles of drinking, the p-value was 0.50.

Finally, we performed stratum-specific analyses for a number of risk factors to examine the possibility that the relation between alcohol and breast cancer differed across risk factor subgroups. The relative risk estimates for any drinking (relative to nondrinking) were greatest for women under 50, premenopausal women, and women with the lowest body mass index. These three groups had relative risks (95% confidence intervals) of 2.1 (1.1–4.1), 2.0 (1.0–3.8), and 3.5 (1.6–7.9), respectively. Relative risk estimates for any drinking were not materially changed in analyses carried out within categories of age at first birth, parity, age at menarche,

Table 5–2 Percentage Distribution by Fat Intake According to Risk Factors for Breast Cancer

Risk factor	Fat (g/day) for indicated quartiles				Fat (% of kcal/day) for indicated quartiles			
	<38	38–53.9	54–73.9	>74	<30	30–35.9	36–41.9	>42
Age (years)								
25–34	19	23	25	33	23	26	27	24
35–54	21	22	26	31	21	25	28	26
55–64	30	26	24	20	26	28	23	23
≥65	33	28	24	15	28	27	24	21
Poverty index ratio* (≥3.75 top quartile)	20	26	25	29	23	29	26	22
Body mass index* (≥30.0 top quartile)	32	26	21	21	26	25	24	25
Age at menarche* (<12 years)	24	25	27	24	24	27	25	24
Premenopausal*	18	23	29	30	24	22	32	22
Family history of breast cancer (first degree relative)*	22	26	27	25	26	27	25	22

*Age-adjusted.

family history of breast cancer, fat consumed (grams per day or percentage of total calories), or smoking.

Discussion

This investigation using the NHEFS data set showed a 50–100% elevation in risk of breast cancer for women who reported any drinking. The data were consistent with a modest dose–response relation across the levels of alcohol consumption (Schatzkin et al. 1987).

It is noteworthy that women in the NHEFS cohort were relatively light drinkers; only 9% consumed one or more drinks per day. Too few women in the NHEFS cohort reported heavy drinking for us to determine whether heavier drinking conferred an even greater excess risk of breast cancer.

Controlling for a number of potentially confounding covariates did not eliminate the association between alcohol and breast cancer. However, controlling for dietary factors in NHEFS is problematic. This limitation is of some importance because dietary factors have been implicated in the etiology of breast cancer and dietary intake is correlated with alcohol consumption. The assessment of a woman's "usual" intake by the 24-hour recall method is limited by the substantial day-to-day variation in what is eaten (Block 1982). Considerable misclassification can occur when this method is used for assignment of individuals to quintiles of nutrient intake (Freudenheim et al. 1987). Although it has become generally accepted that random misclassification in the exposure variable (alcohol in this case) results in dilution of the relative risk toward no association (Rothman 1986), the less extensive literature on misclassification of a confounder indicates that the effect on the relative risk can be in either direction (Greenland and Robins 1985). Since the number of cases in this study was relatively small, we cannot rule out the possibility that misclassification of dietary intake could have resulted in inadequate control of confounding.

Adequate information on a history of benign breast disease was not available from the NHEFS data set. However, there is little evidence for an association between alcohol use and benign breast disease, and in other cohort studies a history of benign breast disease did not confound the positive relation between alcohol and breast cancer (Hiatt and Bawol 1984; Willett et al. 1987; Hiatt et al. 1988). Therefore, it is unlikely that confounding by a history of benign breast disease could account for our findings.

With regard to our findings of a stronger association between alcohol and breast cancer in younger, leaner, and premenopausal women, it is of interest that the risk of breast cancer associated with drinking was greater in those women with the least risk at baseline (i.e., younger and possibly leaner women). Alternatively, the higher risk in younger women might simply reflect a harmful effect of drinking at earlier, as opposed to later, ages, as has been suggested by a recent case-control study (Harvey et al. 1987). This latter hypothesis can be tested later with the NHEFS data set, since questions on the amount of drinking at various ages were asked in the follow-up interview. In the future, when the number of cases with information on early drinking becomes larger, a case-control analysis of the relationship between breast cancer and drinking at earlier versus later ages can be carried out.

DIETARY FAT AND BREAST CANCER

Laboratory (Tannenbaum 1942; Carroll and Khor 1970; Carroll 1980) and human correlation (Armstrong and Doll 1975; Carroll and Khor 1975; Drasar and Irving 1973; Enig, Munn, and Keeney 1978; Gaskill et al. 1979; Gray, Pike, and Henderson 1979; Hirayama 1978; Ingram 1981; Lea 1965; Miller et al. 1978) studies have suggested that consumption of large amounts of fat predisposes women to breast cancer, but the evidence is far from conclusive. Some recent experimental work suggests that when both fat and total energy intake are considered, total energy intake contributes to incidence of mammary cancer (Kritchevsky et al. 1984; Kritchevsky et al. 1986). Inter- and intranational ecologic studies provide some of the strongest support for the hypothesis linking dietary fat to breast cancer, but again it is difficult to disentangle total energy intake (and intake of other nutrients) from fat intake. Some case-control studies have estimated dietary fat (Graham et al. 1982; Hirohata et al. 1985; Miller et al. 1978; Nomura et al. 1985); others have provided information on consumption of certain foods or food groups high in fat (Hislop et al. 1986; Katsouyanni et al. 1986; Kinlen 1982; Le et al. 1986; Lubin et al. 1981; Lubin 1986; Phillips 1975; Talamini et al. 1984) and have produced inconsistent results. A study of a Japanese cohort found that meat consumption was associated with an increased risk of breast cancer (Hirayama 1978), but another study among Seventh Day Adventists in the United States did not find this association (Phillips and Snowdon 1983). A recent large cohort study of over 600 cases of breast cancer showed no positive association between dietary fat (as assessed by a food frequency questionnaire) and subsequent breast cancer (Willett et al. 1987).

Analytic Methodology

The criteria for exclusion of women from this study were somewhat different from those used in the study of the relation between alcohol and breast cancer that was described earlier. Initially excluded were 1727 women from whom no dietary data were obtained at baseline, 205 whose dietary data were obtained from a proxy, 35 whose dietary information was considered "unsatisfactory" by the nutritionist collecting the data, and 117 with imputed data. Also excluded were 244 women who were pregnant or breast feeding, seven with prevalent breast cancer at baseline, and 776 who were lost to follow-up either because they could not be traced or because they refused to participate. The final analytic cohort consisted of 5485 women.

Breast cancer was identified by the same procedures as those used in the study of the effects of alcohol use. (All hospital records indicating breast cancer were reviewed in detail.) Ninety-nine cases were identified: 84 from hospital records and

15 from death certificates. The ratio of observed to expected cases, again based on the age- and race-specific incidences of breast cancer from the Connecticut Tumor Registry, was 0.93 (0.75–1.13). Thirty-four cases were premenopausal, and 65 were postmenopausal at baseline.

Dietary exposure data were the same as those described in the preceding section of this chapter. The key variables in the study of the link between fat intake and breast cancer were intakes of total fat, percent of energy intake derived from fat, and intakes of monounsaturated fat and of cholesterol. Ten persons for whom we had no data on fatty acid and cholesterol intake were excluded from all analyses of these dietary variables. Information on other covariates was obtained as described in the study of alcohol consumption.

Observed Correlations between Fat Intake and Breast Cancer

In Table 5–2 we present data on the distribution of age groups and age-adjusted distribution of several risk factors for cancer across categories of dietary fat. Younger women tended to report total fat intakes in the upper quartiles and older women in the lower quartiles. This pattern reflected, in part, the fact that younger women reported larger energy intakes than did older women, since the trend was weakened considerably when fat intake as a percentage of energy was examined. Women with higher relative income and premenopausal women were found disproportionately in the higher quartiles of fat intake. Relatively overweight women, however, had total fat intakes concentrated in the two lower quartiles. Little association was seen between fat intake and either age at menarche or family history of breast cancer. For fat as a percentage of total caloric intake, no association was seen for these two risk factors for breast cancer.

Mean intakes of fat for cases and noncases are presented in Table 5–3. These mean values were adjusted for age and other risk factors for breast cancer risk by

Table 5–3 Comparison of Mean Daily Nutrient Intakes Between Cases and Noncases of Breast Cancer*

	Age-adjusted		Full model†	
Nutrients (units)	Cases (n = 99)	Noncases (n = 5386)	Cases (n = 86)	Noncases (n = 4912)
Fat (g)	57.0 (3.2)	59.9 (0.4)	55.0 (3.4)	60.3 (0.5)
Fat (% of energy)	34.6 (0.9)	36.0 (0.1)	34.6 (0.9)	36.0 (0.1)
Energy (kcal)	1441 (61)	1465 (8)	1404 (65)	1475 (9)
Saturated fat (g)	20.0 (1.3)	21.4 (0.2)	19.4 (1.4)	21.5 (0.2)
Polyunsaturated fat (g)	6.6 (0.6)	6.6 (0.1)	6.1 (0.6)	6.7 (0.1)
Monounsaturated fat (g)	21.8 (1.3)	22.9 (0.2)	21.0 (1.4)	23.1 (0.2)
Cholesterol (mg)	282 (24)	305 (3)	268 (26)	305 (3)

Note: No statistically significant differences were found in any of these nutrient comparisons.

*Standard error of the mean in parentheses.

†Model includes age, poverty index ratio, body mass index, age at menarche, menopausal status/age at menopause, and family history of breast cancer. Analyses were done on a subset of women with complete information.

means of general linear regression, with the dietary variables as the dependent variable, with age and the other risk factors as covariates, and with case status as an indicator variable. (Because all the dietary variables except percentage of energy from fat were skewed to the right, the regression analyses were repeated with use of logarithmic transformed values. The results of both analyses were similar; therefore, the untransformed results are presented here.) Although the mean intake for cases was less than that for noncases for each of the dietary variables, these differences were not statistically significant.

Estimates of relative risk (and 95% confidence intervals) derived from proportional hazards regression models are presented in Table 5–4. Women in the upper quartiles for fat intake and for saturated fat intake had a lower risk of breast cancer than those in the lowest quartile. The multivariate relative risks (95% confidence intervals) for women in the upper quartiles were 0.34 (0.16–0.73) and 0.29 (0.12–0.67), respectively, for intakes of total and saturated fat. The multivariate trend tests (for a protective association) were significant ($p = 0.03$ for fat, $p = 0.04$ for saturated fat). The trend test for fat as a percentage of total energy yielded a marginally significant (protective) result ($p = 0.06$). None of the other dietary fat and energy variables showed an association with incidence of breast cancer.

Analyses according to baseline menopausal status demonstrated that the protective effect of high fat intake was strongest in premenopausal women (relative risk, 0.08; 95% confidence interval, 0.01–0.61). In postmenopausal women, the protective effect was still apparent (relative risk, 0.63, 95% confidence interval, 0.30–1.54), but the confidence interval now included 1.0.

When the relation between fat intake was examined within tertiles of body mass index, nonsignificant protective associations were observed for the highest quartile of fat intake: For body mass index of 22.0 or less, the relative risk (95% confidence interval) values were 0.65 (0.17–2.52); for body mass index of 22.1–28.0, the values were 0.08 (0.01–0.65); and for body mass index of 28.1 or more, 0.41 (0.11–1.47).

Discussion

We found no positive association between dietary fat intake and risk of breast cancer in the NHEFS data set. If anything, the data are consistent with a slight inverse relation. These findings are qualitatively similar to those of Willett et al. (Willett et al. 1987).

Again, the potential misclassification of dietary intake resulting from the 24-hour recall must be considered. In this study dietary variables were the exposure of interest. Since random misclassification would tend to reduce a positive association toward a relative risk of 1.0, it is plausible that the lack of association between breast cancer and several of the dietary variables could have resulted from such misclassification.

The NHANES I data seem to indicate a slight negative association between obesity and energy intake in women (Braitman et al. 1985). One explanation for this finding is differential underreporting of intake by the obese who might be at in-

Table 5–4 Relationship Between Dietary Fat and Energy Intake and the Occurrence of Breast Cancer

Variable	Age-adjusted			Full model*		
	No. of cases ($n = 99$)	No. of noncases ($n = 5386$)	Relative risk (95% confidence interval)†	No. of cases ($n = 86$)	No. of noncases ($n = 4912$)	Relative risk (95% confidence interval)†
Fat (g)‡						
≤38	33	1337	1.00	29	1198	1.00
38–53.9	24	1313	0.78 (0.46–1.33)	21	1194	0.73 (0.42–1.29)
54–73.9	29	1350	0.95 (0.58–1.58)	27	1234	0.96 (0.57–1.63)
≥74	13	1386	0.47 (0.25–0.91)	9	1286	0.34 (0.16–0.73)
			p for trend = 0.07			p for trend = 0.03
Fat (% of energy)‡						
<30	26	1277	1.00	22	1157	1.00
30–35.9	38	1397	1.38 (0.84–2.27)	35	1279	1.50 (0.88–2.56)
36–41.9	20	1403	0.77 (0.43–1.38)	16	1292	0.73 (0.38–1.38)
≥42	15	1309	0.62 (0.33–1.19)	13	1184	0.66 (0.33–1.31)
			p for trend = 0.05			p for trend = 0.06
Energy (kcal)‡						
<1030	26	1338	1.00	23	1193	1.00
1030–1378.9	31	1337	1.23 (0.73–2.08)	28	1209	1.23 (0.71–2.13)
1379–1775.9	24	1349	0.99 (0.57–1.71)	21	1260	0.89 (0.49–1.63)
≥1776	18	1362	0.87 (0.47–1.61)	14	1250	0.70 (0.36–1.40)
			p for trend = 0.54			p for trend = 0.22

Saturated fat (g)[‡]						
<13	34	1431	1.00	29	1282	1.00
13–18.9	23	1275	0.81 (0.47–1.37)	21	1176	0.83 (0.47–1.45)
19–26.9	30	1287	1.07 (0.65–1.76)	29	1172	1.18 (0.70–1.98)
≥27	12	1383	0.44 (0.23–0.86)	7	1272	0.29 (0.12–0.67)
			p for trend = 0.07			p for trend = 0.04
Polyunsaturated fat (g)[‡]						
<3	31	1398	1.00	27	1229	1.00
3–4.9	19	1144	0.78 (0.44–1.37)	17	1065	0.75 (0.41–1.38)
5–8.9	28	1555	0.90 (0.54–1.50)	26	1423	0.93 (0.54–1.59)
≥9	21	1279	0.93 (0.53–1.63)	16	1185	0.73 (0.39–1.36)
			p for trend = 0.85			p for trend = 0.45
Monounsaturated fat (g)[‡]						
<14	31	1365	1.00	28	1225	1.00
14–19.9	24	1222	0.90 (0.53–1.53)	20	1124	0.82 (0.46–1.45)
20–28.9	25	1415	0.81 (0.48–1.38)	24	1318	0.83 (0.48–1.43)
≥29	19	1338	0.74 (0.41–1.34)	14	1235	0.59 (0.30–1.13)
			p for trend = 0.28			p for trend = 0.14
Cholesterol (mg/dl)[‡]						
<130	25	1333	1.00	11	1197	1.00
130–232.9	31	1321	1.29 (0.76–2.18)	30	1221	1.33 (0.76–2.31)
233–414.9	24	1370	0.95 (0.54–1.66)	19	1261	0.79 (0.43–1.46)
≥415	19	1352	0.80 (0.44–1.47)	15	1223	0.70 (0.36–1.37)
			p for trend = 0.32			p for trend = 0.12

*Full model includes age, poverty index ratio, body mass index, age at menarche, menopausal status/age at menopause, and family history of breast cancer. Analyses were done on subset of women with complete information.

[†]Relative risks (95% confidence intervals) for the proportional hazards model.

[‡]Age-adjusted.

creased risk of breast cancer. This underreporting is considered unlikely because of the careful and standardized dietary assessment techniques used in that survey (Braitman et al. 1985). Furthermore, if underreporting by more overweight women were the explanation for the overall findings regarding any relation between fat and breast cancer, then one would except no association between dietary fat and breast cancer to be evident in the leaner tertiles. The fact that the point estimates for fat intake were substantially less than 1.0 for each of the tertiles of body mass index argues against this underreporting explanation.

In addition to expressing fat intake as a percentage of calories, other means of adjusting fat intake for body size and energy intake include examining fat intake per kilogram body weight and examining residuals of fat after regressing calories (on fat). We found that both of these approaches yielded results similar to those obtained when fat was assessed as a percentage of caloric intake, with multivariate relative risk estimates for the upper quartile, relative to the lowest quartile, of 0.66 for fat/kg of body weight and of 0.68 for fat residuals. The confidence intervals for both point estimates included 1.0.

We should note, especially given the results of the analysis of the relationship between alcohol consumption and breast cancer in the NHEFS data set as well as the findings from other studies (Harvey et al. 1987; Hiatt and Bawol 1984; Hiatt et al. 1987; La Vecchia et al. 1985; Le et al. 1984; O'Connell et al. 1987; Rosenberg et al. 1982; Talamini et al. 1984; Willett et al. 1987), that controlling for alcohol consumption did not materially affect the association between fat intake and breast cancer.

Since it is conceivable that different effects of dietary fat on incidence and on survival could have influenced our results, we performed similar analyses after exclusion of the 15 cases identified from death certificates only, with date of death used as date of incidence. Although the numbers were obviously much smaller, the same inverse association between breast cancer and high intake of fat was seen in cases determined by death certificates as in those identified through hospital records.

Two additional limitations merit discussion. First, the women in this study are generally consumers of a large amount of fat, certainly in relation to the levels consumed in some other countries (e.g., Japan). Therefore, if there were a substantially reduced risk of breast cancer at lower levels of dietary fat intake (e.g., 20% of energy), one would not be able to observe this protective effect in the NHEFS data set. Second, data on exposure in early life to dietary fat and other nutrients were not available.

SERUM CHOLESTEROL AND CANCER

In this third investigation in the epidemiology of cancer done with the NHEFS data set, we consider men as well as women, incidence at sites other than the breast, incidence at all sites combined, and total mortality attributable to cancer (Schatzkin et al. 1987).

The relation between serum cholesterol and cancer has long been a controversial topic. A number of cohort studies have found that among men, serum cholesterol and cancer, particularly cancer of the colon, are inversely related (Beaglehole et al. 1980; Cambien et al. 1980; Feinleib 1981; Garcia-Palmieri et al. 1981; International Collaborative Group 1982; Kagan et al. 1981; Kark, Smith, and Hames 1980; Kozarevic et al. 1981; Morris et al. 1983; Peterson and Trell 1983; Rose et al. 1974; Rose and Shipley 1980; Sherwin et al. 1987; Stemmerman et al. 1981; Wallace et al. 1982; Williams et al. 1981). A number of other cohort studies, though, found no such inverse relation, either for all cancer or for cancer of the colon (Dyer et al. 1981; Hiatt et al. 1982; Hiatt and Fireman 1986; Keys et al. 1985; Morris et al. 1983; Salonen 1982; Sorlie and Feinleib 1982; Thomas et al. 1982; Westlund and Nicolaysen 1972; Wingard et al. 1984; Yaari et al. 1981). Most studies of cholesterol and cancer in women have reported no significant association (Dyer et al. 1981; Hiatt and Fireman 1986; Kark et al. 1980; Morris et al. 1983; Sorlie and Feinleib 1982; Wallace et al. 1982; Wingard et al. 1984), although a few studies have shown a nonsignificant inverse (Kark, Smith, and Hames 1980; Morris et al. 1983; Sorlie and Feinleib 1982) or direct (Wallace et al. 1982) association. A positive association between level of cholesterol in serum and colorectal cancer has recently been described (Tornberg et al. 1986).

Since a few studies have found that the inverse relation between serum cholesterol and cancer was confined to the first few years of follow-up (Cambien, Ducimitiere, and Richard 1980; International Collaborative Group 1982; Rose and Shipley 1980; Sherwin et al. 1987; Wallace et al. 1982), some investigators suggested a "preclinical cancer effect" (i.e., the metabolic depression of serum cholesterol by undiagnosed cancers) as an explanation for the finding (Rose and Shipley 1980; McMichael et al. 1984). Again, the data on this particular hypothesis are inconsistent. Some studies found that the inverse relation did not disappear for malignancies diagnosed 2–15 or more years after measurement of the concentration of cholesterol in serum (Beaglehole et al. 1980; Garcia-Palmieri et al. 1981; Kark, Smith, and Hames 1980; Peterson and Trell 1983; Sorlie and Feinleib 1982).

Analytic Methodology

The procedure for identifying incident cases and deaths due to cancer in NHEFS was described earlier. The ratio and 95% confidence interval of observed to expected number of cases (based on age-, gender-, and race-specific incidence rates from the Connecticut Tumor Registry) for all incidence of cancer in men was 1.04 (0.95–1.14). The comparable ratio of observed to expected number of cases among women was 1.01 (0.91–1.11).

Criteria for exclusion of subjects were slightly different for the analyses of incidence and mortality. At the time of NHEFS, 351 eligible men and 675 eligible women could not be traced; 309 men and 483 women were traced and found to be alive but did not have a follow-up interview, either because they could not be contacted or because they refused to participate; and 20 men and 61 women had no baseline data on serum cholesterol. Ten men and 25 women with cancer at any site (except nonmelanoma skin cancer) at baseline were excluded from the analyses of all cancer. A smaller number of prevalent cases were excluded from the site-specific analyses; the precise number varied from site to site. A few men and women fell into more than one of these exclusion categories. For the analyses of mortality, only those missing baseline data on serum cholesterol and/or those identified as prevalent cases were excluded.

Overall, 5125 men and 7363 women were included in the analysis of incidence with cancers developing in 459 men and 398 women. The analyses of mortality comprised 5791 men and 8535 women, including 258 men and 186 women dying with cancer as the underlying cause.

Concentration of cholesterol in serum was determined from blood specimens obtained from nonfasting subjects; a semiautomated modified ferric chloride–sulfuric acid method was used. Measurements were done in the lipid laboratory of the Centers for Disease Control, Atlanta, Georgia (National Center for Health Statistics 1980; Eavenson et al. 1966); other covariate data were obtained as described in the two preceding sections.

Observed Correlations between Serum Cholesterol and Cancer

The mean age at baseline of men in our study population was 52 years; that of women, 48 years. (These simple descriptive data for women are nearly identical to those presented in the section on alcohol consumption and breast cancer, but they are repeated here for comparison with the findings for men and because the cohorts analyzed were slightly different.) Of the 5125 men, 48% did not graduate from high school, whereas 25% had more than 12 years of education; the analogous figures for women were 42% and 21%. Eighty-six percent of the men and 84% of the women were white.

The mean serum cholesterol levels for the entire group ($\pm$standard deviation) were 221 ($\pm$47) mg/100 ml for men and 222 ($\pm$50) mg/100 ml for women.

We examined the interrelation of serum cholesterol level with various risk factors for cancer. Among both men and women, high levels of cholesterol in serum at baseline were associated with older age, poverty index ratio, body mass index, cigarette smoking, alcohol assumption, and lower consumption of fiber. There was little difference across levels of serum cholesterol in years of education, race, and, for women, age at first birth, age at menarche, and parity. Intake of fat was directly related to cholesterol in women but essentially unrelated in men.

Age-related incidence and mortality rates (computed by the method described in the study of alcohol consumption–breast cancer) are shown in Fig. 5–2. Among men there was an inverse relation between cholesterol and both incidence of cancer and mortality due to cancer. Among women the inverse relation for mortality was stronger than that for incidence, with elevations in cancer rates being largely confined to those in the lowest quintile of serum cholesterol.

In Fig. 5–3 we present data for those specific sites with at least ten cases in both sexes (except for cancers of the prostate, cervix, endometrium, and ovaries, for which ten cases were required in the appropriate gender group). In men an inverse

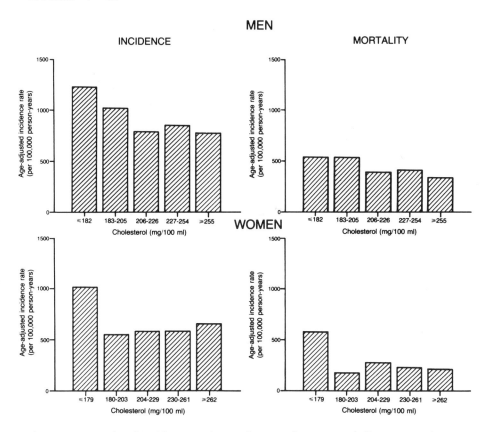

Fig. 5–2. Age-related incidence and mortality rates for cancer of all sites according to levels of serum cholesterol and gender. Rates were age-related by the direct method (Fleiss 1981) according to the age distribution of the cohort.

relation can be seen for all cancers as well as for lung, colorectal, pancreas, and bladder cancers and for leukemia. There was little association between cholesterol and prostate cancer or lymphoma. Among women, inverse associations were apparent for cancers of the lung, pancreas, bladder, and cervix and for leukemia. Little relation between cholesterol level and cancer was evident for breast, colorectal, ovarian, and uterine corpus cancers. (Note, however, that the incidence rates for some sites were based on a small number of cases within cholesterol levels.)

Age-adjusted and multivariate estimates of relative risk from proportional hazards regression models are presented in Table 5–5. There was an inverse association between cholesterol and incidence of cancer in men; the multivariate relative risk estimates (95% confidence intervals) for the first through fourth quintiles of cholesterol (in comparison to the highest quintile) were, respectively, 1.7 (1.2–2.6), 1.5 (1.0–2.2), 1.0 (0.7–1.5), and 1.2 (0.8–1.8). The multivariate trend test for incidence was significant ($p = 0.003$). Similar results were obtained when mortality

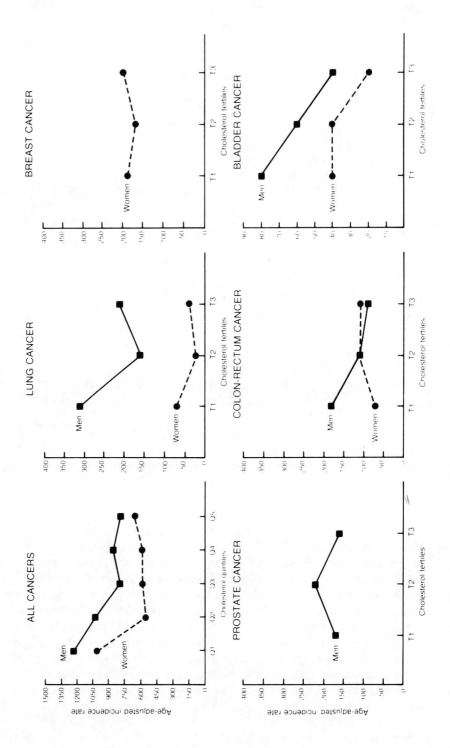

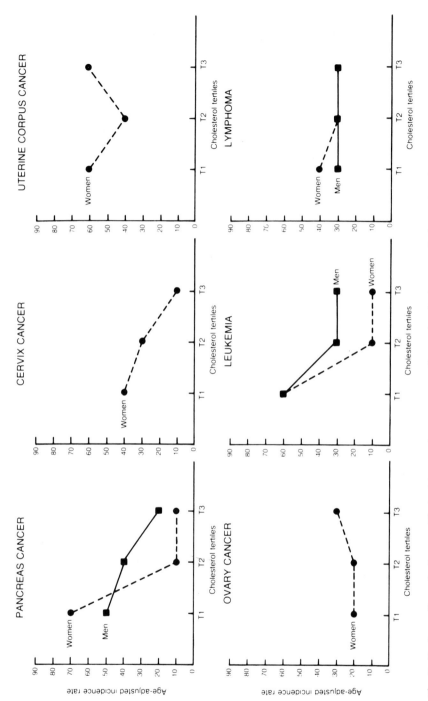

Fig. 5-3. Age-adjusted, site-specific incidence of cancer according to level of serum cholesterol and gender. The first through third tertiles of cholesterol (mg/100 ml) are defined as follows: for men, ≤200, 201–235, ≥236; for women, ≤196, 197–239, ≥240.

Table 5-5 Relationship Between Level of Serum Cholesterol and Cancer in All Sites According to Gender

Incidence

Men

	Cholesterol (mg/100ml)				
	≤182	183–205	206–226	227–254	≥255
Relative risk*	1.6	1.3	1.0	1.1	(1.0)
(95% confidence interval)	(1.2–2.1)	(1.0–1.9)	(0.7–1.3)	(1.8–1.4)	—
Multivariate relative risk†	1.7	1.5	1.0	1.2	(1.0)
(95% confidence interval)	(1.2–2.6)	(1.0–2.2)	(0.7–1.5)	(0.8–1.8)	—

Women

	Cholesterol (mg/100ml)				
	≤179	180–203	204–229	230–261	≥262
Relative risk*	1.4	1.0	1.0	1.0	(1.0)
(95% confidence interval)	(1.0–2.0)	(0.7–1.4)	(0.7–1.3)	(0.8–1.3)	—
Multivariate relative risk‡	1.2	1.0	0.8	0.9	(1.0)
(95% confidence interval)	(0.8–1.9)	(0.7–1.5)	(0.6–1.2)	(0.6–1.2)	—

Mortality

Men

	Cholesterol (mg/100ml)				
	≤182	183–205	206–226	227–254	≥255
Relative risk*	1.6	1.6	1.1	1.2	(1.0)
(95% confidence interval)	(1.0–2.3)	(1.1–2.3)	(0.7–1.7)	(0.6–1.7)	—
Multivariate relative risk†	1.9	1.9	1.4	1.4	(1.0)
(95% confidence interval)	(1.0–3.4)	(1.1–3.4)	(0.8–2.5)	(0.8–2.5)	—

Women

	Cholesterol (mg/100ml)				
	≤179	180–203	204–229	230–261	≥262
Relative risk*	2.6	1.0	1.5	1.2	(1.0)
(95% confidence interval)	(1.6–4.1)	(0.6–4.1)	(1.0–2.3)	(0.8–1.9)	—
Multivariate relative risk‡	2.0	1.0	1.2	1.2	(1.0)
(95% confidence interval)	(1.0–3.8)	(0.5–2.1)	(0.7–2.2)	(0.7–2.0)	—

*Aged-adjusted in proportional hazards model that included variables for age and cholesterol.

†Model includes variables for age, education, body mass index, smoking (pack-years), alcohol, dietary fat as a percentage of total calories, dietary fiber, and cholesterol. Because some subjects lacked information on smoking (even when follow-up data were used) and/or diet, the number of cases in the multivariate models for incidence and mortality was reduced to 257 and 127, respectively.

‡Model includes variables for age, education, body mass index, smoking (pack-years), alcohol, dietary fat as a percentage of total calories, age at first birth, age at menarche, parity, and cholesterol. Because some subjects lacked information on smoking (even when follow-up data were used) and/or diet, the number of cases in the multivariate models for incidence and mortality was reduced to 268 and 107, respectively.

was analyzed and when incident cases reported by death certificate only were eliminated.

For incidence of cancer in women, there was a small, nonsignificant increase in risk confined to the lowest quintile of cholesterol (Table 5–5). The multivariate relative risk estimates for incidence in women were 1.2 (0.8–1.9), 1.0 (0.7–1.5), 0.8 (0.6–1.2), and 0.9 (0.6–1.2). The multivariate trend test for incidence was not significant ($\chi^2 = 2.34; p = 0.13$). Negligible differences resulted from the elimination of those incident cases identified from death certificate only. In the analysis of mortality, the risk was higher for women in the lowest quintile for cholesterol (relative risk, 1.9; 95% confidence interval, 1.0–3.4).

In Table 5–6 we show more detailed data on the association between serum cholesterol and colorectal cancer. Although there was a suggestion of an inverse relation between cholesterol and colorectal cancer among men, none of the relative risk estimates were statistically significant. No association was seen in women.

Because the curves depicting incidence and the results of regression analyses suggested an inverse relation between concentration of cholesterol in serum and several site-specific cancers known to be related to cigarette smoking, we aggregated sites a posteriori to form categories of smoking-related and non-smoking-related cancers. The smoking-related cancers in men were those of the lung, mouth, larynx, esophagus, pancreas, and bladder and leukemia (Wynder and Hoffman 1982; Austin and Cole 1986). In women the smoking-related cancers were at the same sites as those in men, plus the additional site of the cervix (Wynder and Hoffman 1982; Austin and Cole 1986). Age-adjusted incidence rates for the smok-

Table 5–6 Relationship Between Level of Serum Cholesterol and Colorectal Cancer According to Gender

	Cholesterol Quartiles			
	<198	190–216	217–246	>247
Men				
No. of cases	16	18	10	18
Relative risk*	1.3	1.2	0.6	(1.0)
(95% confidence interval)	(0.6–2.5)	(0.6–2.4)	(0.3–1.3)	—
Multivariate relative risk†	1.7	1.2	0.5	(1.0)
(95% confidence interval)	(0.8–3.7)	(0.5–2.6)	(0.2–1.4)	—
	<186	187–217	218–251	>252
Women				
No. of cases	6	13	23	26
Relative risk‡	0.9	1.1	1.2	(1.0)
(95% confidence interval)	(0.4–2.2)	(0.6–2.2)	(0.7–2.2)	—
Multivariate relative risk‡	1.0	0.9	1.3	(1.0)
(95% confidence interval)	(0.3–2.7)	(0.4–2.1)	(0.6–2.4)	—

*Based on proportional hazards models including variables for age and cholesterol.

†Model includes variables for age, education, body mass index, smoking (pack-years), alcohol, fat as a percentage of calories, dietary fiber, and cholesterol. Forty-five cases were analyzed in the multivariate model.

‡Model includes variables for age, education, body mass index, smoking (pack-years), alcohol, fat as a percentage of calories, age at first birth, age at menarche, parity, and cholesterol. Forty-eight cases were analyzed in the multivariate model.

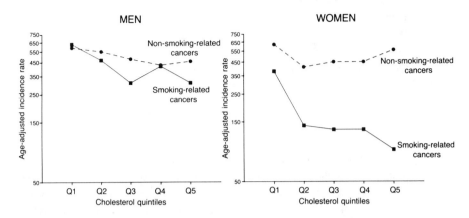

Fig. 5–4. Age-adjusted incidence of smoking- and non-smoking related cancers according to level of serum cholesterol and gender. The first through fifth quintiles of cholesterol (mg/100 ml) were as follows: for men, ≤182, 183–205, 206–226, 227–254, ≥255; for women, ≤179, 180–203, 204–229, 230–261, ≥262.

ing-related and non-smoking-related cancers by quintiles of cholesterol are displayed in Fig. 5–4.

A definite inverse relation between cholesterol and cancer similar to that seen for all cancer was found for smoking-related cancers, whereas only a weak inverse relation was noted for non-smoking-related cancers. Among women only, an inverse relation was also apparent for smoking-related cancers, but not for non-smoking-related cancers.

Table 5–7 gives the relative risk estimates for smoking-related and non--smoking-related cancers in men in each of the serum cholesterol quintiles. A clear inverse relation was present for smoking-related cancers in men (Table 5–7), with multivariate relative risk estimates of 2.1 (1.1–3.8), 1.6 (0.8–2.9), 1.1 (0.6–2.2), and 1.4 (0.7–2.5) for the first to fourth quintiles. (The highest quintile is the reference group.) The multivariate test for trend was significant ($p = 0.02$). Since the etiologic link between smoking and leukemia is not as well established as that for the other smoking-related cancers mentioned, we performed separate analyses without leukemia in the smoking-related cancers group. The multivariate risk estimates for smoking-related cancers minus leukemia (101 cases) were 2.1 (1.1–4.0), 1.8 (0.9–3.3), 1.1 (0.6–2.2), and 1.3 (0.7–2.4). (Again, the reference group was the highest cholesterol quintile.) The trend test showed a p-value of $= 0.01$. In addition, since the ascertainment of cancer solely by death certificate might have been less accurate than ascertainment by hospital records, we examined the relation between cholesterol and cancer for smoking-related cancers confirmed by hospital records. Estimates of relative risk were not substantially altered. For the non-smoking-related cancers, there was a weak inverse relation, with $\chi^2 = 3.35$ ($p = 0.07$) for the multivariate trend test.

For women an inverse relation, considerably stronger than the one for all

Table 5–7 Relationship Between Levels of Serum Cholesterol and the Occurrence of Smoking-related and Nonsmoking-related Cancers for Men

Men	Serum cholesterol level (mg/100ml)				
	<182 (n = 1008)	183–205 (n = 1000)	206–226 (n = 1023)	227–254 (n = 1065)	>255 (n = 1029)
Smoking-related cancers					
No. of cases	49	44	32	48	38
Relative risk*	2.0	1.4	0.9	1.3	(1.0)
(95% Confidence interval)	(1.3–3.0)	(0.9–2.2)	(0.6–1.5)	(0.8–2.0)	—
Multivariate relative risk†	2.1	1.6	1.1	1.4	(1.0)
(95% Confidence interval)	(1.1–3.8)	(0.8–2.9)	(0.6–2.2)	(0.7–2.5)	—
Non-smoking-related cancers					
No. of cases	45	51	49	49	54
Relative risk*	1.3	1.2	1.0	0.9	(1.0)
(95% Confidence interval)	(0.8–1.9)	(0.8–1.7)	(0.7–1.5)	(0.7–1.4)	—
Multivariate relative risk†	1.6	1.4	0.9	1.2	(1.0)
(95% Confidence interval)	(0.9–2.7)	(0.9–2.4)	(0.5–1.6)	(0.7–2.0)	—

*Based on proportional hazards model including variables for age and cholesterol.

†Model includes variables for age, education, body mass index, smoking (pack-years), alcohol, fat as a percentage of calories, dietary fiber, and cholesterol. The total number of cases in the multivariate models for all cancers, smoking-related cancers, and non-smoking-related cancers were, respectively, 261, 112, 149. Multivariate trend tests for the relation of cholesterol to all cancer, smoking-related cancers, and non-smoking-related cancers in men yielded, respectively, $\chi^2 = 8.83$ ($p = 0.003$), $\chi^2 = 5.48$ ($p = 0.02$), $\chi^2 = 3.35$ ($p = 0.07$).

cancer, was evident for the smoking-related cancers, with a multivariate relative risk estimate of 3.3 (1.4–7.8) for the lowest compared to the highest quintile (Table 5–8). The test for trend for smoking-related cancers yielded $p = 0.02$. The estimates of relative risk for smoking-related cancers minus leukemia (only 45 cases) were 2.2 (0.8–5.7), 1.2 (0.5–3.2), 0.7 (0.3–1.8), and 0.9 (0.4–2.0) (highest cholesterol quintile as reference), with a multivariate trend test yielding $\chi^2 = 1.44$ ($p = 0.23$). Relative risk estimates for smoking-related cancers did not differ materially, whether based on hospital records alone or on hospital records combined with death certificates. No association was evident between cholesterol and non-smoking-related cancers in women.

The relation of cholesterol to incidence of all cancers, incidence of smoking-related and non-smoking-related cancer, and mortality due to cancer was similar across subgroups of various risk factors for cancer, including age, education, body mass index, smoking, alcohol consumption, and fat consumption. Among women the inverse relation observed between cholesterol and cancer for incidence of all cancers was restricted to women under the age of 50 years.

Because of concern for residual confounding by smoking, we focused on the relation between cholesterol and smoking-related cancers (not exclusively attributable to smoking) among nonsmokers. For male nonsmokers the relative risk estimates and 95% confidence intervals from the first to the fourth cholesterol quintiles for smoking-related cancers (25 cases) were 4.7 (1.3–17), 2.0 (0.5–8.4), 1.2 (0.2–5.8), and 1.0 (0.2–4.9) (reference was highest cholesterol quintile). The analogous estimates for smoking-related cancers (40 cases) among nonsmoking women were 2.5 (0.8–8.1), 2.2 (0.8–6.3), 2.0 (0.8–5.0), and 1.8 (0.8–4.3).

Finally, to explore the possibility that preclinical cancer was depressing cholesterol levels (the "preclinical cancer effect" hypothesis), we analyzed the relation between cholesterol and cancer within three distinct follow-up periods: 0 to 1.9, 2 to 5.9, and 6 or more years from the measurement of cholesterol measurement to the diagnosis of cancer. For incidence of all cancer, we analyzed only those cases confirmed by hospital records, since the time of cancer diagnosis was thought to be less reliable for cases identified by death certificate only. As Table 5–9 demonstrates, the inverse relation among men was strongest for cases diagnosed 6 or more years after serum cholesterol was determined. For women there was a statistically significant excess risk only among women in the lowest cholesterol quintile in whom cancer was diagnosed within two years of measurement of cholesterol.

As the data in Table 5–10 show, the inverse relation between cholesterol and smoking-related cancers persisted in both men and women for cases that were diagnosed more than 6 years or more than 8 years after measurement of cholesterol. Results were not altered in the analyses of smoking-related cancers confirmed by hospital records or in multivariate models including variables for cholesterol, age, education or poverty index ratio, race, body mass index, smoking, alcohol consumption, dietary fat intake, dietary fiber intake, and, for women, age at first birth, age at menarche, parity, and menopausal status. For the 41 smoking-related cancers in men diagnosed 8 or more years after measurement of cholesterol, the age-adjusted relative risk estimates for the first through fourth quintiles, relative to the

Table 5–8 Relationship Between Levels of Serum Cholesterol and the Occurrence of Smoking-related and Nonsmoking-related Cancers for Women

Women	Serum cholesterol level (mg/100ml)				
	<179 (n = 1409)	180–203 (n = 1502)	204–229 (n = 1489)	230–261 (n = 1484)	>262 (n = 1479)
Smoking-related cancers					
No. of cases	19	12	16	21	18
Relative risk*	4.1	1.7	1.5	1.4	(1.0)
(95% Confidence interval)	(2.1–8.0)	(0.8–3.6)	(0.8–3.0)	(0.8–2.8)	—
Multivariate relative risk†	3.3	1.7	0.7	1.1	(1.0)
(95% Confidence interval)	(1.4–7.8)	(0.7–4.1)	(0.3–1.9)	(0.5–2.4)	—
Non-smoking-related cancers					
No. of cases	37	44	59	74	98
Relative risk*	1.0	0.9	0.9	0.9	(1.0)
(95% Confidence interval)	(0.7–1.6)	(0.6–1.3)	(0.6–1.2)	(0.7–1.2)	—
Multivariate relative risk†	0.9	0.9	0.8	0.8	(1.0)
(95% Confidence interval)	(0.6–1.5)	(0.6–1.3)	(0.6–1.2)	(0.5–1.2)	—

*Based on proportional hazards model including variables for age and cholesterol.

†Model includes variables for age, education, body mass index, smoking (pack-years), alcohol, fat as a percentage of calories, dietary fiber, age at first birth, age at menarche, parity, and cholesterol. The total number of cases in the multivariate models for all cancer, smoking-related cancers, and non-smoking-related cancers were 268, 52, 261, respectively. Multivariate trend tests for the relation of cholesterol to all cancer and smoking-related cancers in women yielded $\chi^2 = 0.34$ ($p = 0.5$), and $\chi^2 = 5.42$ ($p = 0.02$), respectively.

Table 5–9 Relationship of Levels of Serum Cholesterol and Relative Risk of Cancer as Confirmed by Hospital Records According to Years of Follow-up and Gender

Serum cholesterol level (mg/100ml)	Relative risk (95% confidence interval) after indicated years of follow-up		
	Zero–1.9	2–5.9	≥6
Men (no. of cases)	56	134	168
≤182	0.8 (0.3–1.9)	1.5 (0.9–2.5)	2.2 (1.3–3.7)
183–205	1.3 (0.6–2.6)	1.0 (0.6–1.7)	1.8 (1.1–3.1)
206–226	0.6 (0.2–1.4)	0.9 (0.6–1.6)	1.7 (1.0–2.9)
227–254	0.8 (0.4–1.7)	0.8 (0.7–2.0)	1.8 (1.1–3.0)
≥255	(1.0) —	(1.0) —	(1.0) —
Women (no. of cases)	58	125	153
≤179	3.3 (1.3–8.2)	0.6 (0.3–1.3)	1.0 (0.6–1.8)
180–203	1.3 (0.4–3.8)	1.0 (0.6–1.8)	0.8 (0.5–1.4)
204–229	2.8 (1.5–5.9)	0.8 (0.5–1.3)	0.7 (0.4–1.2)
230–261	1.9 (0.9–4.0)	0.6 (0.4–1.0)	1.0 (0.7–1.5)
≥262	(1.0) —	(1.0) —	(1.0) —

Note: Age-adjusted relative risks and 95% confidence intervals were derived from follow-up time-specific proportional hazards models that included variables for age and cholesterol. Estimates were only minimally altered in multivariate models that included variables for age, cholesterol, education, body mass index, smoking (pack-years), alcohol, dietary fat as a percentage of total calories, dietary fiber, and, for women, age at first birth, age at menarche, and parity.

highest quintile, were 5.9 (2.0–18), 1.5 (0.4–5.5), 2.2 (0.7–7.2), and 2.2 (0.7–7.2). (There were only 17 such cases in women.)

Discussion

Our analysis of the relation between serum cholesterol level and cancer in men confirmed the inverse association that has been reported in numerous cohort studies. There was at most, however, a small, nonsignificant inverse relation for colorectal cancer. The inverse relation was somewhat stronger for smoking-related as opposed to non-smoking-related cancers, with a doubling in risk of smoking-related cancer among men in the lowest cholesterol quintile. The inverse relation for incidence of all cancer and of smoking-related cancers persisted for several years after cholesterol was measured (Schatzkin et al. 1987, 1988).

Among women we found a nonsignificant inverse relation between serum cholesterol level and incidence of cancer that was restricted to women in the lowest cholesterol quintile. For mortality attributable to cancer, however, the inverse relation (again confined to the lowest quintile) was considerably stronger. There was also a strong inverse association of cholesterol level with smoking-related cancers in women but no association with the non-smoking-related cancers. The findings for smoking-related and non-smoking-related cancers are compatible with results of the analysis of mortality, in that the mortality experience associated with smoking-related cancers in women tends to be less favorable than that associated with non-smoking-related cancers (e.g., cancer of the breast and uterine corpus) (Sondik et al. 1986). The inverse relation seen for all cancer in women was confined largely to

Table 5–10 Relationship of Levels of Serum Cholesterol and Relative Risk of Smoking-related Cancers According to Years of Follow-up and Gender

Serum cholesterol level (mg/100ml)	Relative risk (95% confidence interval) after indicated years of follow-up		
	0–1.9	2–5.9	≥6
Men (no. of cases)	32	90	80
≤182	1.3 (0.4–4.2)	1.7 (0.9–5.1)	2.5 (1.3–4.9)
183–205	1.9 (0.7–2.5)	1.3 (0.7–2.5)	1.4 (0.7–2.8)
206–226	0.4 (0.1–2.0)	0.9 (0.5–1.9)	1.2 (0.6–2.4)
227–254	1.7 (0.6–4.8)	1.0 (0.5–1.9)	1.5 (0.7–2.9)
≥255	(1.0) —	(1.0) —	(1.0) —
Women (no. of cases)	15	38	33
≤179	8.8 (1.5–49)	1.8 (0.6–5.6)	6.2 (2.1–18)
180–203	3.0 (0.4–22)	1.7 (0.6–4.6)	1.3 (0.3–5.3)
204–229	1.8 (0.3–13)	1.1 (0.4–3.0)	2.0 (0.7–6.1)
230–261	3.2 (0.6–17)	1.1 (0.5–2.8)	1.5 (0.5–4.5)
≥262	(1.0) —	(1.0) —	(1.0) —

Note: Relative risks (95% confidence intervals) were derived from proportional hazards models that included variables for age and cholesterol. Although the multivariate models were relatively unstable due to the small number of cases, estimates were only minimally altered in models that included variables for age, cholesterol, education, body mass index, smoking (pack-years), alcohol, dietary fat as a percentage of total calories, dietary fiber, and, for women, age at first birth, age at menarche, and parity.

the first 2 years of follow-up, but for the smoking-related cancers the inverse relation persisted over a longer period of follow-up.

The "preclinical cancer effect" hypothesis for the observed inverse relation between cholesterol and cancer is an attractive explanation given the protean physiologic manifestations of malignant disease, which could well include depression of serum cholesterol levels. In that regard, it has long been known that patients with leukemia have reduced cholesterol levels (Muller 1930), and it has recently been shown that leukemic cells have an elevated low-density lipoprotein receptor activity that is inversely correlated with plasma cholesterol levels (Vitols et al. 1985). We found, however, that the inverse relation between cholesterol and all incident cancer in men held for several years after cholesterol was measured. For smoking-related cancers this relation held for women as well as for men. Although one cannot totally exclude the possibility that nascent neoplasms could alter cholesterol metabolism several years prior to clinical diagnosis, our findings and those from a few other studies (Beaglehole et al. 1980; Garcia-Palmieri et al. 1981; Kark, Smith, and Hames 1980; Peterson and Trell 1983; Sorlie and Feinleib 1982) suggest that there is more to the inverse relation between cholesterol and cancer than a short-term effect of preclinical cancer. We note also that the inverse relation between cholesterol and leukemia obtained even after exclusion of cases diagnosed within the first 2 years after determinations of cholesterol levels.

Finally, if smoking-related cancers stemmed from pathologic processes common to those anatomic sites most susceptible to the carcinogenic effects of tobacco smoke, and if these processes were linked with depression of the serum cholesterol level, then the inverse relation between cholesterol and smoking-related cancers would be found. However, it is unclear whether a low level of cholesterol is a necessary precondition for such processes or merely an incidental effect. If the latter were true, then the explicit reduction of serum cholesterol for prevention of coronary disease would not in itself increase the risk of cancer. We emphasize that our aggregation of cancer sites into smoking-related and non-smoking-related cancers was not driven by a prior hypothesis. Inferences drawn from this kind of post hoc grouping must be considered cautiously, and our finding for smoking-related cancers needs to be examined with other sets of data.

Although we cannot now offer more than a very general explanation for the observed inverse relation between cholesterol and cancer, we conclude that the findings are strong enough to merit continued epidemiologic investigation.

SOCIOECONOMIC STATUS AND CANCER

The relation between two sociodemographic variables, education and income, and cancer (incidence and mortality for cancer at all sites, and incidence at major sites) is the subject of our fourth investigation of the epidemiology of cancer, utilizing the NHEFS data set. Since the NHEFS cohort was derived from a probability sample of the U.S. population, accompanied by oversampling of groups hypothesized to be at increased risk of nutritional deprivation, there is a considerable spread of educational achievement and income across the cohort.

Previous studies have shown higher rates of total malignant disease among those at the lower end of the socioeconomic scale (American Cancer Society 1986; Kitagawa and Hauser 1973; Logan 1982). For several cancer sites, including lung (Devesa and Diamond 1983), cervix (Brinton and Fraumeni 1986), esophagus (Day 1975), and stomach (Haenszel and Correa 1975), inverse relations with socioeconomic status have generally been reported. However, consistent trends across social classes have not been demonstrated for colorectal (Schottenfeld and Winawer 1982) or prostate (Mandel and Schuman 1979) cancer. Although a positive association between socioeconomic status and breast cancer has been found (Kelsey 1979), the magnitude of this relation is not great and may be diminishing over time (Logan 1982).

Analytic Methodology

The cohorts used in the analyses of education and income in relation to cancer were similar to those analyzed in the study of the cholesterol-cancer association. Baseline data on education were missing for 54 men and 51 women, whereas baseline data on income were missing for 225 men and 322 women.

The analyses of education and incident cancer included 5100 men and 7374 women; those for income and cancer included 4952 men and 7146 women. The comparable analyses for mortality due to cancer involved 5757 men and 8545 women for education, 5586 men and 8274 women for income.

Smoking-related and non-smoking-related cancers were defined in the same manner as in the study of the association between cholesterol and cancer.

Observed Correlations between Socioeconomic Status and Cancer

Classification of the cohorts studied by broad education and income groups indicated that a substantial proportion of subjects had relatively little formal education, with 33% of the men and 23% of the women completing no more than elementary school. Only 21% of the men and 17% of the women had any education beyond high school. At least some schooling in grades 9 through 12 was reported by 46% of the men and 60% of the women. With regard to income, 20% of the men and 24% of the women reported less than $4000 per year, whereas only about 22% of the men and 19% of the women received $10,000 or more annually. Similar proportions of men and women (58% and 57%, respectively) had annual incomes in the mid-range $4000–9999).

Data reflecting the relations between the two socioeconomic status variables and other potential risk factors for cancer can be summarized as follows. In most instances, the associations with other risk factors were similar for education and income. Low socioeconomic status and educational achievement tended to be associated with being older and nonwhite, consuming more fat (as a percentage of total energy) and less fiber, and, in women, having an earlier age at first birth, later age at menarche, and greater parity. Among women, obesity, as reflected by body mass index, was inversely related to both education and income and, to a lesser degree, to education in men, but there was a slight positive association of obesity with income among men. A greater proportion of men with lower, as opposed to higher, socioeconomic status reported being current smokers, but among men there was little association between total pack-years of smoking and socioeconomic status. Smoking levels for women were generally lower than those for men, and they were largely unrelated to education and slightly inversely related to income. (More men and women in higher, as compared with lower, education and income brackets reported being former smokers.) Among men there was no association between serum cholesterol and education, but there was a small inverse association between income and cholesterol level. Data for women showed a positive relation for cholesterol level and education, with little apparent relation between cholesterol level and income. The proportion of menopausal women was slightly higher among those with more education and income. Among both men and women, alcohol consumption was positively associated with socioeconomic status. As one would expect, there was a strong direct association between educational achievement and income.

Figures 5–5 and 5–6 depict age-adjusted incidence and mortality rates for all cancer by level of education and income. Figures 5–7 through 5–10 display the socioeconomic status level-specific rates for major cancer sites and for the smoking- and non-smoking-related cancers.

Men of lower socioeconomic status had higher overall rates of cancer, with the inverse trend being somewhat stronger for mortality than for incidence. This inverse association appeared largely among the smoking-related, as opposed to non--

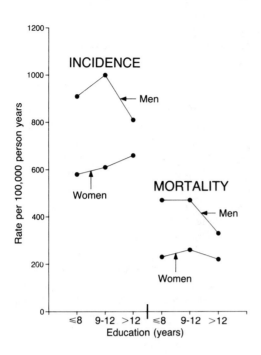

Fig. 5–5. Age-adjusted cancer incidence and mortality rates (per 100,000 persons-years) according to education and gender.

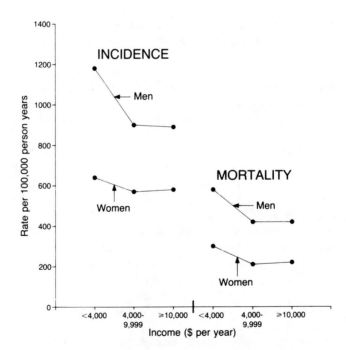

Fig. 5–6. Age-adjusted cancer incidence and mortality rates (per 100,000 person-years) according to income and gender.

Fig. 5–7. Age-adjusted incidence (per 100,000 person-years) of lung, prostate, colorectal, and smoking- and non-smoking-related cancers according to level of education for men.

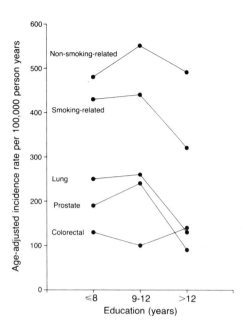

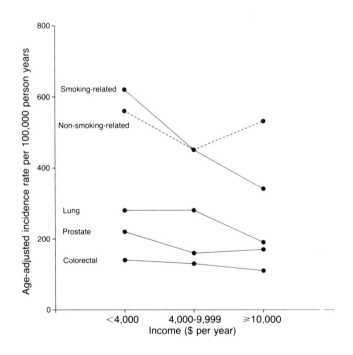

Fig. 5–8. Age-adjusted incidence (per 100,000 person-years) of lung, prostate, colorectal, and smoking- and non-smoking-related cancers according to level of income for men.

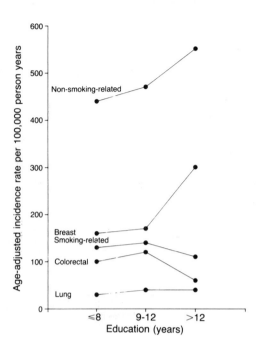

Fig. 5–9. Age-adjusted incidence (per 100,000 person-years) of lung, breast, colorectal, and smoking- and non-smoking-related cancers according to level of education for women.

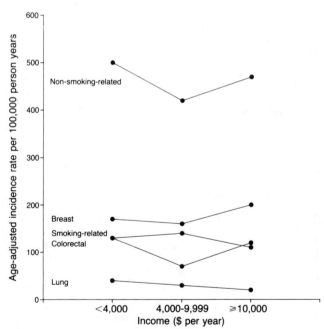

Fig. 5–10. Age-adjusted incidence (per 100,000 person-years) of lung, breast, colorectal, and smoking- and non-smoking-related cancers according to level of income for women.

Table 5–11 Rates of Cancer (per 10,000 person years) According to Years of Education, Gender and Age at Baseline (NHANES I)

| | Indicated age groups and years of education | | | | | | | | |
| | <55 Years of age | | | 55–64 Years of age | | | >65 Years of age | | |
	<8	9–12	>12	<8	9–12	>12	<8	9–12	>12
Men									
All cancer incidence	530	280	210	1210	1320	1220	2280	2550	2060
All cancer mortality	350	140	70	680	610	680	1080	1250	800
Smoking cancer incidence	280	150	70	600	440	600	1030	1180	800
Nonsmoking cancer incidence	250	130	140	610	870	610	1230	1350	1250
Women									
All cancer incidence	300	260	250	560	760	1400	1340	1420	1260
All cancer mortality	850	840	600	240	400	540	620	650	440
Smoking cancer incidence	70	50	40	130	100	280	270	410	200
Nonsmoking cancer incidence	240	210	230	480	600	960	990	1080	1100

smoking-related, cancers. Men with lower educational achievement and income had higher rates of lung cancer than their male counterparts with higher socioeconomic status. There was at most a small inverse relation between prostate cancer and socioeconomic status, whereas for colorectal cancer there was no association for education and a slight inverse relation for income.

Since a deterioration in health status before diagnosis of cancer might lower income (Luft 1978), we examined the relation between income and cancer after elimination of the first two person-years of follow-up. The income–cancer relations were not materially different from those described earlier.

The relation between socioeconomic status and cancer among women was different. Incidence of cancer showed a small positive relation to education, whereas there was no consistent trend for income. For mortality due to cancer, there was a small inverse trend for income and an even smaller inverse association for education. Smoking-related cancers, which made up a considerably smaller proportion of all cancers in women than in men, demonstrated only a small inverse association with socioeconomic status. There was no trend for lung cancer in relation to socioeconomic status, but the number of cases in women was quite small. A positive association was observed between both socioeconomic status variables and breast cancer. As among men, there was no clear relation among women between education or income and colorectal cancer.

Age-specific cancer rates are presented in Tables 5–11 and 5–12. Among men the inverse relations appeared to be more prominent for younger subjects. Among women, inverse socioeconomic status–cancer relations were evident for groups aged under 55 and 65 years and older groups; however, the associations were positive for women aged 55–64 years. These age-specific patterns need to be

Table 5–12 Rates of Cancer (per 10,000 person years) According to Income, Gender, and Age at Baseline (NHANES I)

	Cancer rates for indicated age groups and income level								
	<55 Years of age			55–64 Years of age			>65 Years of age		
	<$4000	4–9999	>10,000	<4,000	4–9999	>10,000	<4000	4–9999	>10,000
Men									
All cancer incidence	780	310	280	1740	1190	1240	2330	2250	2480
All cancer mortality	470	140	100	1070	470	670	1020	1120	1170
Smoking cancer incidence	600	140	70	960	500	490	860	1200	1040
Nonsmoking cancer incidence	200	170	146	780	670	740	1440	1030	1410
Women									
All cancer incidence	280	270	250	760	500	1130	1460	1320	1180
All cancer mortality	1230	890	630	440	240	470	720	520	490
Smoking cancer incidence	70	50	40	130	100	280	270	410	200
Nonsmoking cancer incidence	200	230	210	620	400	850	1190	910	980

viewed cautiously, however, because the numbers of cases within each of the age-specific and socioeconomic status–specific categories were rather small.

In Tables 5–13 and 5–14 we present results from proportional hazards regression analyses of the relation between the two socioeconomic status variables and all cancer incidence and mortality. The relative risk estimates for education and income from models that also include only age paralleled the age-adjusted incidences discussed earlier. Men who had 12 or fewer years of schooling, as compared with those who had some education past high school, had approximately a 10–20% greater risk of cancer. In comparison with those who had incomes of $10,000 or more, the relative risk estimate for incidence was 1.3 (95% confidence interval 1.0–1.6) for men with incomes of less than $4000. The excess risk of mortality among men was somewhat greater, with marginally significant point estimates of 1.4 (1.0–2.1) for the least versus the most educated, and 1.6 (1.0–2.3) for an income of less than $3000 as compared with $10,000 or more.

Inclusion of smoking as well as age in the models for men lowered these point estimates considerably. Inclusion of multiple risk factors in the regression models reduced these estimates to or very near 1.0.

For women the age-adjusted point estimates of cancer incidence for the lowest category of education and income, relative to the highest, were negligibly different from 1.0 and did not change with adjustment for smoking and other risk factors. For mortality due to cancer, risk was at most minimally increased with education. There was, however, a marginally significant excess risk for those with incomes of less than $4000, compared with $10,000 or more. This effect did not diminish after adjustment for smoking and other risk factors.

Discussion

Our analyses have shown that the inverse relation between socioeconomic status, as reflected by educational achievement or income, and cancer was of modest dimension, with at most a 50% excess risk. Overall the inverse association was somewhat greater for men than for women, for younger than for older subjects, and for cancer mortality as compared with cancer incidence. The increased risk of death due to cancer among those in the lowest, as opposed to highest, brackets of both education and income for men and of income for women was approximately 50%. The excess risks observed in relation to socioeconomic status, with the exception of a persistent association between income and mortality due to cancer in women, largely disappeared after adjustment for smoking and other risk factors for cancer.

Studies of socioeconomic status and cancer (or any disease, for that matter) tend to lack specificity in the sense that particular (and potentially modifiable) "biologic" exposures are not investigated. Education and income are considered to be surrogates for elements of the sociophysical environment that have a causal relation to disease. That is, it is not the differences in income itself that account for the variation in cancer rates, but the differences in smoking, diet, or some unmeasured factors across the different income groups that govern the corresponding income-related differences in frequency of cancer.

Table 5–13 Relationship Between Education and Income and Cancer Incidence and Mortality for Men

Variable	Age-adjusted		Age-smoking-adjusted		Multiple risk factor adjusted*	
	Relative risk	95% Confidence interval	Relative risk	95% Confidence interval	Relative risk	95% Confidence interval
All cancer incidence						
Education						
≤8	1.1	(0.6–1.5)	1.0	(0.7–1.4)	1.0	(0.7–1.4)
9–12	1.2	(0.9–1.6)	1.0	(0.7–1.4)	1.0	(0.7–1.4)
≥12	(1.0)	—	(1.0)	—	(1.0)	—
Income						
<$4000	1.3	(1.0–1.6)	1.1	(0.8–1.5)	1.1	(0.8–1.6)
4001–9999	1.1	(0.8–1.4)	1.0	(0.8–1.3)	1.0	(0.8–1.3)
≥10,000	(1.0)	—	(1.0)	—	(1.0)	—
All cancer mortality						
Education						
≤8	1.4	(1.0–2.1)	1.2	(0.8–1.8)	1.0	(0.7–1.4)
9–12	1.4	(1.0–2.1)	1.1	(0.7–1.6)	1.0	(0.7–1.4)
≥12	(1.0)	—	(1.0)	—	(1.0)	—
Income						
<$4000	1.6	(1.0–2.3)	1.2	(0.8–1.8)	1.1	(0.8–1.6)
4001–9999	1.1	(0.7–1.6)	1.0	(0.7–1.4)	1.0	(0.8–1.3)
≥10,000	(1.0)	—	(1.0)	—	(1.0)	—
Incidence of smoking-related cancers						
Education						
≤8	1.4	(0.9–2.1)	1.1	(0.7–1.8)	1.2	(0.7–1.9)
9–12	1.3	(0.9–2.1)	1.0	(0.6–1.6)	1.0	(0.6–1.6)
≥12	(1.0)	—	(1.0)	—	(1.0)	—
Income						
<$4000	1.5	(1.0–2.3)	1.4	(0.9–2.3)	1.4	(0.9–2.3)
4001–9999	1.5	(1.0–2.1)	1.4	(0.9–2.1)	1.4	(1.0–2.2)
≥10,000	(1.0)	—	(1.0)	—	(1.0)	—

*Model includes age, race, smoking (pack-years), body mass index, and alcohol along with education or income (all entered as indicators).

Table 5-14 Relationship Between Education and Income and Cancer Incidence and Mortality for Women

Variable	Age-adjusted		Age-smoking-adjusted		Multiple risk factor adjusted*	
	Relative risk	95% Confidence interval	Relative risk	95% Confidence interval	Relative risk	95% Confidence interval
All cancer incidence						
Education						
≤8	0.9	(0.7–1.2)	0.8	(0.6–1.1)	0.9	(0.6–1.2)
9–12	0.9	(0.7–1.2)	0.9	(0.9–1.2)	0.8	(0.9–1.1)
≥12	(1.0)	—	(1.0)	—	(1.0)	—
Income						
<$4000	1.1	(0.8–1.4)	1.1	(0.8–1.5)	1.3	(0.9–1.8)
4001–9999	0.9	(0.8–1.2)	0.9	(0.7–1.2)	1.0	(0.7–1.3)
≥10,000	(1.0)	—	(1.0)	—	(1.0)	—
All cancer mortality						
Education						
≤8	1.1	(0.7–1.7)	1.1	(0.7–1.8)	1.0	(0.6–1.8)
9–12	1.2	(0.8–1.9)	1.3	(0.8–2.0)	1.1	(0.7–1.9)
≥12	(1.0)	—	(1.0)	—	(1.0)	—
Income						
<$4000	1.6	(1.0–2.3)	1.6	(1.0–2.4)	1.7	(1.0–3.0)
4001–9999	1.1	(0.7–1.6)	1.1	(0.7–1.7)	1.2	(0.7–1.9)
≥10,000	(1.0)	—	(1.0)	—	(1.0)	—
Incidence of smoking-related cancers						
Education						
≤8	1.3	(0.7–2.5)	1.3	(0.6–2.6)	1.4	(0.6–3.2)
9–12	1.3	(0.7–2.5)	1.1	(0.6–2.3)	0.9	(0.4–1.9)
≥12	(1.0)	—	(1.0)	—	(1.0)	—
Income						
<$4000	1.0	(0.6–1.9)	1.1	(0.6–2.2)	0.9	(0.4–2.0)
4001–9999	1.2	(0.7–2.2)	1.2	(0.7–2.3)	1.0	(0.5–2.0)
≥10,000	(1.0)	—	(1.0)	—	(1.0)	—

*Model includes age, race, smoking (pack-years), body mass index, alcohol, age at first birth, parity, age at menarche and age at menopause (all entered as indicators).

Our results clearly show that risk factors for cancer vary markedly with both education and income. Moreover, the results of the multiple regression analyses suggest that known risk factors for cancer, especially smoking, are largely responsible for the inverse relations between socioeconomic status and cancer. In other words, the data suggest that much of the excess cancer observed among men in the lower education and income groups would be eliminated if those men did not smoke more than men in the highest socioeconomic status groups.

Except for the link between income and cancer mortality, there was little relation between socioeconomic status and cancer in women. This finding may reflect the facts that breast cancer, the leading incident cancer in women, had a positive relation with both education and income and that smoking-related cancers (which showed an inverse relation between socioeconomic status and cancer in men) accounted for a substantially smaller proportion of the total cases of cancers in women than in men. The inverse association between income and mortality due to cancer among women that persisted even after adjustment for multiple risk factors suggests that the income variable in women actually may have been a surrogate for other risk factors not included in the regression models. Since mortality reflects survival as well as incidence, it is conceivable that income-related differences in cancer mortality reflect differences in some factors related to survival of women who have cancer.

Although the elevation in cancer risk among those of lower socioeconomic status was small, even a 20–30% increase in risk would have etiologic and public health importance. Where known risk factors can account for socioeconomic differences in cancer rates, it follows that elimination or modification of these factors, such as smoking, could go a long way toward eliminating those differences. It is plausible, although by no means assured, that a reduction in socioeconomic status disparities would be accompanied by a comparable reduction in differential exposure to cancer risk factor across socioeconomic status groups. Finally, the existence of socioeconomic differences in cancer rates not adequately explained by known risk factors suggests the need for discovering other cancer-related factors that vary across categories of socioeconomic status.

POSSIBILITIES FOR FUTURE RESEARCH

Some of the cancer studies using the NHEFS data that are presently under way at the National Cancer Institute illustrate additional possibilities for research offered by this data set. Again, it is important to note that NHEFS is an ongoing study. Although the number of cases of cancer at certain sites is rather small for detailed analysis, more cases will accrue in the coming years. Therefore, certain studies of site-specific cancer that are not now possible will become so over the next decade. Moreover, particular hypotheses, such as those relating consumption of alcohol and fat to breast cancer, can be reexamined as additional cases develop in the original NHANES I cohort.

There is considerable interest in the relation of various indexes of body size and growth to cancer at different sites. The extensive anthropometric data gathered as part of NHANES I have permitted current evaluations of the relation between obesity and measures of frame size to breast cancer. Questions from the NHEFS interview, including those relating to body weight at different ages, may be valuable when examined in a case-control context, especially as the number of available cases increases.

Many research questions remain to be explored with data on dietary factors, from both the baseline and follow-up examinations. Investigators are now examining cancer in relation to reported patterns of consumption of the various food groups. These data were compiled from 24-hour diet recall queries included in the baseline survey.

Information on dietary calcium is being examined in relation to cancer of the large bowel and other sites. Since it is likely that nutrient interactions are important in carcinogenesis, we have begun to look at various combinations of dietary lipids and fiber in relation to breast cancer. In addition to serum cholesterol, other biochemical factors (serum retinol, for example) can be investigated in terms of their correlation with the incidence of cancer.

These samples of ongoing studies illustrate the potential role of the NHEFS data in epidemiologic investigations of the etiology of malignant disease.

REFERENCES

American Cancer Society. 1986. *Cancer in the Economically Disadvantaged*. New York: The American Cancer Society.

Armstrong, B., and R. Doll. 1975. "Environmental factors and cancer incidence and mortality in different countries, with special reference to dietary practices." *Int J Cancer* 15:617–631.

Austin, H., and P. Cole. 1986. "Cigarette smoking and leukemia." *J Chronic Dis* 39:417–421.

Begg, C. B., A. M. Walker, B. Wessen, and M. Zelen. 1983. "Alcohol consumption and breast cancer" (letter). *Lancet* 1:293–294.

Beaglehole, R., M. A. Foulkes, I. A. M. Prior et al. 1980. "Cholesterol and mortality in New Zealand Maoris." *Br Med J* 1:285–287.

Block, G. 1982. "A review of validations of dietary assessment methods." *Am J Epidemiol* 115:492–505.

Braitman, L. E., E. V. Adlin, and J. L. Stanton, Jr. 1985. "Obesity and caloric intake: The National Health and Nutrition Examination Survey of 1971–1975 (HANES I)." *J Chronic Dis* 38:727–732.

Brinton, L. A., and J. F. Fraumeni, Jr. 1986. "Epidemiology of uterine cervical cancer." *J Chronic Dis* 39:1051–1065.

Byers, T., and D. P. Funch 1982. "Alcohol and breast cancer" (letter). *Lancet* 1:799–800.

Cambien, F., P. Ducimitiere, and J. Richard. 1980. "Total serum cholesterol and cancer mortality in a middle-aged population." *Am J Epidemiol* 112:388–394.

Carroll, K. K. 1980. "Lipids and carcinogenesis." *J Environ Pathol Toxicol* 3:253–271.

Carroll, K. K., and H. T. Khor. 1970. "Effects of dietary fat and dose level of 7,12-dimethylbenz(a)anthracene on mammary tumor incidence in rats." *Cancer Res* 30:2226–2264.

Carroll, K. K., and H. T. Khor. 1975. "Dietary fat in relation to tumorigenesis." *Prog Biochem Pharmacol* 10:308–353.

Cox, D. R., and D. Oakes. 1984. *Analysis of Survival Data*. London: Chapman and Hall.

Day, N. E. 1975. "Some aspects of the epidemiology of esophageal cancer." *Cancer Res* 35:3304–3307.

Devesa, S. S., and E. L. Diamond. 1983. "Socioeconomic and racial differences in lung cancer incidence." *Am J Epidemiol* 118:818–831.

Drasar, B. S., and D. Irving. 1973. "Environmental factors and cancer of the colon and breast." *Br J Cancer* 27:167–172.

Dyer, A. R., J. Stamler, O. Paul et al. 1981. "Serum cholesterol and risk of death from cancer and other causes in three Chicago epidemiological studies. *J Chronic Dis* 34:249–260.

Eavenson, D., O. T. Grier, J. G. Cision, and R. F. Witter. 1966. "A semiautomated procedure for the determination of serum cholesterol using the Abell–Kendall method." *J Am Oil Chem Soc* 43:652–656.

Enig, M. G., R. J. Munn, and M. Keeney. 1978. "Dietary fat and cancer trends—a critique." *Fed Proc* 37:2215–2220.

Feinleib, M. 1981. "On a possible inverse relationship between serum cholesterol and cancer mortality." *Am J Epidemiol* 114:5–10.

Fleiss, J. L. 1981. *Statistical Methods for Rates and Proportions*. New York: Wiley.

Freudenheim, J. L., N. E. Johnson, and R. L. Wardrop. 1987. "Misclassification of nutrient intake of individuals and groups using one-, two-, three-, and seven-day food records." *Am J Epidemiol* 126:703–713.

Garcia-Palmieri, M. R., P. D. Sorlie, R. Costas et al. 1981. "An apparent inverse relationship between serum cholesterol and cancer mortality in Puerto Rico." *Am J Epidemiol* 114:29–40.

Gaskill, S. P., W. L. McGuire, C. K. Osborne et al. 1979. "Breast cancer mortality and diet in the United States." *Cancer Res* 39:3628–3637.

Graham, S., J. Marshall, C. Mettlin et al. 1982. "Diet in the epidemiology of breast cancer." *Am J Epidemiol* 116:68–75.

Gray, G. E., M. C. Pike, and B. E. Henderson. 1979. "Breast cancer incidence and mortality rates in different countries in relation to known risk factors and dietary practices." *Br J Cancer* 39:1–7.

Greenland, S., and J. M. Robins. 1985. "Confounding and misclassification." *Am J Epidemiol* 122:495–506.

Haenszel, W., and P. Correa. 1975. "Developments in the epidemiology of stomach cancer over the past decade." *Cancer Res* 35:3452–3459.

Harvey, E. B., C. Schairer, L. A. Brinton, R. N. Hoover, and J. F. Fraumeni, Jr. 1987. "Alcohol consumption and breast cancer." *Natl Cancer Inst* 78:657–661.

Hiatt, R. A., and R. O. Bawol. 1984. "Alcoholic beverage consumption and breast cancer incidence." *Am J Epidemiol* 12:676–683.

Hiatt, R. A., and B. H. Fireman. 1986. "Serum cholesterol and the incidence of cancer in a large cohort." *J Chronic Dis* 39:861–870.

Hiatt, R. A., G. D. Friedman, R. D. Bawol et al. 1982. "Breast cancer and serum cholesterol." *JNCI* 68:885–889.

Hiatt, R. A., A. Klatsky, and M. A. Armstrong. 1988. "Alcohol consumption and the risk of breast cancer in a prepaid health plan." *Cancer Res* 48:2284–2287.

Hirayama, T. 1978. "Epidemiology of breast cancer with special reference to the role of diet." *Prev Med* 7:173–195.

Hirohata, T., T. Shigematsu, A. M. Nomura et al. 1985. "Occurrence of breast cancer in relation to diet and reproductive history: A case-control study in Fukuoka, Japan." *Natl Cancer Inst Monogr* 69:187–190.

Hislop, T. G., A. J. Coldman, J. M. Elwood et al. 1986. "Childhood and recent eating patterns and risk of breast cancer." *Cancer Detect Prev* 9:47–58.

Ingram, D. M. 1981. "Trends in diet and breast cancer mortality in England and Wales 1928–1977." *Nutr Cancer* 3:75–80.

International Collaborative Group. 1982. "Circulating cholesterol level and risk of death from cancer in men aged 40–69 years: experience of an international collaborative group." *JAMA* 248:2853–2859.

Jones, D. Y., A. Schatzkin, S. B. Green et al. 1987. "Dietary fat and breast cancer in the National Health and Nutrition Examination Survey I Epidemiologic Follow-up Study." *J Natl Cancer Inst* 79:465–471.

Kagan, A., D. L. McGee, K. Yano et al. 1981. "Serum cholesterol and mortality in a Japanese-American population: The Honolulu Heart Program." *Am J Epidemiol* 114:11–20.

Kark, J. D., A. H. Smith, and C. G. Hames. 1980. "The relationship of serum cholesterol to the incidence of cancer in Evans County, Georgia." *J Chronic Dis* 33:311–322.

Katsouyanni, K., D. Trichopoulos, P. Boyle et al. 1986. "Diet and breast cancer: A case-control study in Greece." *Int J Cancer* 38:815–820.

Kelsey, J. L. 1979. "A review of the epidemiology of human breast cancer." *Epidemiol Rev* 1:74–109.

Keys, A., C. Aravanis, H. Blackburn et al. 1985. "Serum cholesterol and cancer mortality in the Seven Countries Study." *Am J Epidemiol* 121:870–883.

Kinlen, L. J. 1982. "Meat and fat consumption and cancer mortality: A study of strict religious orders in Britain." *Lancet* 1:946–949.

Kitagawa, E. M., and P. M. Hauser. 1973. *Differential Mortality in the United States: A Study in Socioeconomic Epidemiology.* Cambridge, MA: Harvard University Press.

Kozarevic, D. J., D. McGee, N. Vojvodic et al. 1981. "Serum cholesterol and mortality: The Yugoslavia Cardiovascular Disease Study." *Am J Epidemiol* 114:21–28.

Kritchevsky, D., M. M. Weber, C. L. Buck et al. 1986. "Calories, fat and cancer." *Lipids* 21:272–274.

Kritchevsky, D., M. M. Weber, and D. M. Klurfeld. 1984. "Dietary fat versus caloric content in initiation and promotion of 7,12-dimethylbenz(*a*)anthracene-induced mammary tumorigenesis in rats." *Cancer Res* 44:3174–3177.

La Vecchia, C., A. Decarli, S. Franceschi et al. 1985. "Alcohol consumption and the risk of breast cancer in women." *JNCI* 75:61–65.

Le, M. G., C. Hill, A. Kramer, and R. Flamant. 1984. "Alcoholic beverage consumption and breast cancer in a French case-control study." *Am J Epidemiol* 120:350–357.

Le, M. G., L. H. Moulton, C. Hill, and A. Kramer. 1986. "Consumption of dairy produce and alcohol in a case-control study of breast cancer." *JNCI* 77:633–636.

Lea, A. J. 1965. "New observations on distribution of neoplasms of female breast in certain European countries." *Br Med J* 1:488–490.

Logan, W. P. 1982. *Cancer mortality by occupation and social class 1851–1971.* London:

Her Majesty's Stationary Office (Studies on Medical and Population Subjects No. 44) (also IARC Scientific Publication No. 36).

Lubin, J. H., P. E. Burns, W. J. Blot et al. 1981. "Dietary factors and breast cancer risk." *Int J Cancer* 28:685–689.

Lubin, F., Y. Wax, and B. Modan. 1986. "Role of fat, animal protein, and dietary fiber in breast cancer etiology: A case-control study." *JNCI* 77:605–612.

Luft, H. S. 1978. *Poverty and Health*. Cambridge, MA: Ballinger.

Mandel, J. S., and L. M. Schuman. 1979. "Epidemiology of cancer of the prostate." *Epidemiol Rev* 1:1–73.

McMichael, A. J., O. M. Jensen, D. M. Parkin, and D. G. Zaridze. 1984. "Dietary and endogenous cholesterol and human cancer." *Epidemiol Rev* 6:192–216.

Miller, A. B., A. Kelly, N. W. Choi et al. 1978. "A study of diet and breast cancer." *Am J Epidemiol* 107:499–509.

Morris, D. L., N. O. Borhani, E. Fitzsimons et al. 1983. "Serum cholesterol and cancer in the Hypertension Detection and Follow-up Program." *Cancer* 52:1754–1759.

Muller, H. G. 1930. "The cholesterol metabolism in health and anemia." *Medicine* 9:119–174.

National Center for Health Statistics. 1972. *Instruction Manual. Data Collection. Part 15a.* NHANES Examination Staff Procedures Manual for the Health and Nutrition Examination Survey, 1971–1973. Washington, DC: U.S. Government Printing Office 722-554/89.

National Center for Health Statistics. 1980. Serum cholesterol levels by persons 4–74 years of age by socioeconomic characteristics. *Vital and Health Statistics*. Series 11, No. 217. DHEW Pub. No. (PHS) 80-1667. Washington, DC: U.S. Government Printing Office.

Nomura, A. M., T. Hirohata, L. N. Kolonel et al. 1985. "Breast cancer in Caucasian and Japanese women in Hawaii." *Natl Cancer Inst Monogr* 69:191–196.

O'Connell, D. L., B. S. Hulka, L. E. Chambless et al. 1987. "Cigarette smoking, alcohol consumption, and breast cancer risk." *JNCI* 78:229–234.

Paganini-Hill, A., and R. K. Ross. 1983. "Breast cancer and alcohol consumption." *Lancet* 2:626–627.

Peterson, B., and E. Trell. 1983. "Premature mortality in middle-aged men: Serum cholesterol as risk factor." *Klin Wochenschr* 63:795–801.

Phillips, R. L. 1975. "Role of life-style and dietary habits in risk of cancer among Seventh-Day Adventists." *Cancer Res* 35:3513–3522.

Phillips, R. L., and D. A. Snowdon. 1983. "Association of meat and coffee use with cancers of the large bowel, breast, and prostate among Seventh-Day Adventists: Preliminary results." *Cancer Res* 43(suppl 5):2403a–2408s.

Rose, G., H. Blackburn, A. Keys et al. 1974. "Colon cancer and blood cholesterol." *Lancet* 1:181–183.

Rose, G., and M. J. Shipley, 1980. "Plasma lipids and mortality, a source of error." *Lancet* 1:523–526.

Rosenberg, L., D. Stone, S. Shapiro et al. 1982. "Breast cancer and alcoholic-beverage consumption." *Lancet* 1:267–271.

Rosner, B., W. C. Willett, and D. Spiegelman. In press. "Correction of logistic regression relative risk estimates and confidence intervals for systematic within-person measurement error." *Stat Med*.

Rothman, K. J. 1986. *Modern Epidemiology*. Boston: Little, Brown.

Salonen, J. T. 1982. "Risk of cancer and death in relation to serum cholesterol: a longitudinal study in an Eastern Finnish population with high overall cholesterol level." *Am J Epidemiol* 116:622–630.

SAS Institute, Inc. 1983. *SUGI Supplemental Library User's Guide, 1983.* Cary, NC.

Schatzkin, A., R. N. Hoover, P. R. Taylor et al. 1988. "A site-specific analysis of total serum cholesterol and incident cancer results from the NHANES I Epidemiologic Follow-up Study." *Cancer Res* 48:452–458.

Schatzkin, A., D. Y. Jones, R. N. Hoover et al. 1987. "Alcohol consumption and breast cancer in the epidemiologic follow-up study of the first National Health and Nutrition Examination Survey." *N Engl J Med* 316:1169–1173.

Schatzkin, A., P. R. Taylor, C. L. Carter et al. 1987. "Serum cholesterol and cancer in the NHANES I epidemiologic follow-up study." *Lancet* 2:298–301.

Schottenfeld, D., and S. J. Winawar. 1982. Large intestine. In *Cancer Epidemiology and Prevention.* D. Schottenfeld and J. F. Fraumeni, Jr., eds. Philadelphia: W. B. Saunders Company, pp. 703–727.

Sherwin, R. W., D. N. Wentworth, J. A. Cutler et al. 1987. "Serum cholesterol levels and cancer mortality in 361,662 men screened for the Multiple Risk Factor Intervention Trial." *JAMA* 257:943–948.

Sondik, E. J., J. L. Young, J. W. Horm, and L. A. G. Riles. 1986. *1986 Annual Cancer Statistics Review.* DHHS, Public Health Service, National Institutes of Health, National Cancer Institute, Bethesda, MD.

Sorlie, P. D., and M. Feinleib. 1982. "The serum cholesterol–cancer relationship: An analysis of time trends in the Framingham Study." *JNCI* 69:989–996.

Stemmerman, G. N., A. Nomura, L. K. Heilbrun et al. 1981. "Serum cholesterol and colon cancer incidence in Hawaiian Japanese men." *JNCI* 67:1179–1182.

Talamini, R., C. La Vecchia, A. Decarli et al. 1984. "Social factors, diet and breast cancer in a northern Italian population." *Br J Cancer* 49:723–729.

Tannenbaum, A. 1942. "The genesis and growth of tumors. III. Effects of high-fat diet." *Cancer Res* 2:468–475.

Thomas, C. B., K. R. Duszynski, and J. W. Schaffer. 1982. "Cholesterol levels in young adulthood and subsequent cancer: A preliminary note." *Johns Hopkins Med J* 150:89–94.

Tornberg, S. A., L. E. Holm, J. M. Carstensen, and G. A. Eklund. 1986. "Risks of cancer of the colon and rectum in relation to serum cholesterol and beta-lipoprotein." *New Engl J Med* 315:1629–1633.

Vitols, S., M. Bjorkkolm, G. Gahrton, and C. Peterson. 1985. "Hypocholesterolaemia in malignancy due to elevated low-density-lipoprotein-receptor activity in tumour cells: Evidence from studies in patients with leukemia." *Lancet* 2:1150–1154.

Wallace, R. B., C. Rost, L. F. Burmeister et al. 1982. "Cancer incidence in humans: relationship to plasma lipids and relative weight." *J Natl Cancer Inst* 68:915–918.

Watt, B. K., and A. L. Merrill. 1963. *Composition of Foods: Raw, Processed, Prepared. Agriculture Handbook. 8th ed. (rev.).* Washington, DC: U.S. Department of Agriculture.

Webster, L. A., P. M. Layde, P. A. Wingo et al. 1983. "Alcohol consumption and risk of breast cancer." *Lancet* 2:724–726.

Westlund, K., and Nicolaysen, R. 1972. "Ten-year mortality and morbidity related to serum cholesterol." *Scand J Clin Lab Invest* 30(suppl 127):3–24.

Willett, W. C., G. A. Colditz, M. J. Stampfer et al. 1986. "A prospective study of alcohol intake and risk of breast cancer (abstract)." *Am J Epidemiol* 124:540–541.

Willett, W. C., M. J. Stampfer, G. A. Colditz et al. 1987. "Dietary fat and the risk of breast cancer." *N Engl J Med* 316:22–28.

Williams, R. R., and J. W. Horm. 1977. "Association of cancer sites with tobacco and alcohol consumption and socioeconomic status of patients: Interview study from the Third National Cancer Survey." *J Natl Cancer Inst* 58:525–547.

Williams, R. R., P. D. Sorlie, M. Feinleib et al. 1981. "Cancer incidence by levels of cholesterol." *JAMA* 245:247–252.

Wingard, D. L., M. H. Criqui, M. J. Holdbrook, and E. Barrett-Connor. 1984. "Plasma cholesterol and cancer morbidity and mortality in an adult community." *J Chronic Dis* 37:401–406.

Wynder, E. L., I. J. Bross, and T. Hirayama. 1960. "A study of the epidemiology of cancer of the breast." *Cancer* 13:559–601.

Wynder, E. L., and D. Hoffman. 1982. Tobacco. In *Cancer Epidemiology and Prevention.* D. Schottenfeld and J. F. Fraumeni, J., eds. Philadelphia: W. B. Saunders Company, pp. 277–292.

Yaari, S., U. Goldbourt, S. Evan-Zohar et al. 1981. "Associations of serum high density lipoprotein and total cholesterol with total, cardiovascular, and cancer mortality in a 7-year prospective study of 10,000 men." *Lancet* 1:1011–1014.

6

Cerebrovascular Disease

LON R. WHITE, KATALIN G. LOSONCZY,
AND PHILIP A. WOLF

In most developed countries, cerebrovascular disease is the most common neurologic cause of mortality and physical disability in later life. Stroke, the most dramatic manifestation of cerebrovascular disease, is a sudden and often catastrophic event whose complex pathogenesis usually involves slowly progressive vascular disease processes begun decades earlier and culminating in an abrupt failure of perfusion of some part of the brain. The final event of the pathogenic chain may be precipitated by changes in physical or chemical factors such as those that alter local laminar blood flow or that encourage clot formation and propagation at the site of a disrupted atheromatous plaque (Toole 1983). Factors influencing development of the underlying cardiovascular disease usually act over a time course of decades, whereas those that directly influence the final precipitous event are likely to express their influence at or shortly before a stroke. Strategies for the prevention of strokes may be effectively directed at any or all of these components of the total pathogenic chain. Some strategies aim to delay the onset or progression of the underlying vascular process, whereas others aim to prevent the final precipitous event.

Although we know that atherosclerosis is an important component of the vascular process leading to cardiovascular disease (including stroke) and that clotting at the time of the stroke is involved in a high proportion of cases, our understanding of the pathogenesis of stroke is far from complete. This situation is underscored by certain paradoxical relationships observed in epidemiologic studies. First, although both obesity and serum cholesterol level have been identified consistently as predictors of heart disease, neither has been identified as an important risk factor for stroke in most studies (Wolf 1985). Second, stroke was the leading cause of death in Japan for many years, and heart disease was of lesser importance; however, in recent years there has been a reversal in Japan, with stroke becoming less important and heart disease increasing, whereas the rates of both have decreased in the United States (Takeya et al. 1984).

Over the past two to three decades mortality attributed to stroke has fallen dramatically in this country (Takeya et al. 1984). The improvement seems to be due mainly to decreasing incidence in both genders and all age groups, rather than to lessening of case-fatality rates (Takeya et al. 1984; Kurtzke 1985). The factors that brought about this decline, although not thoroughly understood, may well include control of hypertension, diminishing smoking, and dietary changes. Of these three candidate factors, only hypertension has been unambiguously associated with strokes in older persons (Wolf 1985). A full explanation for these dramatic decreases in incidence of and mortality from stroke and for the paradoxical phenomena mentioned earlier remains a challenge to epidemiologists, clinical scientists, and basic scientists alike.

The central objective of this chapter is to present an overview of available information related to incident cerebrovascular disease among participants in the National Health and Nutrition Examination Survey (NHANES I) during the interval between initial contact (1971–1975) and the follow-up a decade later (NHEFS 1982–1984). Special emphasis is given to methodologic issues concerning mechanisms and validity of ascertainment of cerebrovascular disease, the spectrum and total burden of different types of cerebrovascular disease, its prognostic significance, and factors that influence the development of cerebrovascular disease.

METHODOLOGY AND STUDY DESIGN

A description of the overall study design is provided in Chapter 1. The analyses to be described employed the following variables:

Baseline history of stroke: affirmative response to baseline query, "Has a doctor ever told you that you had a stroke?

History of incident stroke: affirmative response to follow-up interview query, "Did a doctor ever tell you that you had any of the following conditions: . . . small stroke, sometimes known as TIA . . . stroke, sometimes called a CVA . . . ?"

Medical record documentation of cerebrovascular disease: data from NHEFS hospitalization and death files (for codes included, see later).

Physical disability index: described in detail in Chapter 12; summary score of 1.0 or greater to indicate the presence of physical disability.

Cognitive disability: created by an algorithm that identified a person as disabled if the follow-up interview was conducted with a proxy for reasons of cognitive impairment (not stringently defined), and/or if the subject correctly answered five or fewer items on the mental status examination (MSQ score recalculated and not used on the NHEFS data tape from the National Center for Health Statistics; MSQ administered only to persons aged 60 and older at follow-up interview) (Pfeiffer 1975).

Blood pressure: sitting pressures taken by the physician at baseline examination.

Diabetes: A physician coding of the diagnosis of the baseline examination, or affirmative response to either: (1) "Has a doctor ever told you that you have diabetes? . . . Do you still have it?" or (2) "Did a doctor tell you that you had sugar diabetes?"

Heart disease at baseline: either (1) an affirmative response to the baseline query, "Has a doctor ever told you that you have had a heart attack?" or (2) affirmative responses to the question, "Have you seen a doctor . . . about the chest or lung conditions you mentioned? . . . What did he say it was?" (ischemic heart disease), (3) baseline physician coding of ICD9 412 (old myocardial infarct) or ICD9 413 (angina pectoris), or (4) identification of angina based on a standard algorithm and interview items developed by Dr. Geoffrey Rose of the University of London (Rose et al. 1982).

Alcohol consumption: an estimate of the usual daily consumption of ethanol calculated from responses to three baseline questions (generating an estimate of the number of drinks per day), with the assumption that an average drink contained 0.5 oz of ethanol (Chapter 9).

Smoking: a composite variable generated from baseline data when available, augmented with follow-up information designed to estimate what the responses to the baseline questions would have been had they been asked. Categories of baseline exposure: current smoker, ex-smoker, or never smoked cigarettes; and number of years smoked.

Body mass index: calculated as weight (kilograms) divided by height (meters squared) as measured at baseline examination (NHANES I).

Dietary intakes of fat, potassium, sodium, and calcium: calculated from the 24-hour food recall questionnaire at baseline (NHANES I).

Hemoglobin, cholesterol, and uric acid levels in blood: determined by standard methods on blood samples drawn at baseline (NHANES I).

ANALYSIS RELATED TO CEREBROVASCULAR DISEASE

Among 10,896 participants aged 35–74 years at the baseline contact, 135 men and 148 women reported that they had experienced a stroke. The gender- and age-specific prevalences of history of stroke are shown in Table 6–1. Participants who

Table 6–1 Prevalence of History of Prior Stroke Reported at Baseline (NHANES I)

Age	No. with stroke/No. examined (%)	
	Men	Women
35–44	5/928 (0.5%)	17/2013 (0.8%)
45–54	14/1058 (1.3%)	8/1220 (0.6%)
55–64	24/861 (2.8%)	28/962 (2.9%)
65–69	48/1067 (4.5%)	47/1148 (4.1%)
70	44/769 (5.7%)	48/870 (5.5%)

Table 6–2 Distribution of Number of Persons for the Analysis of Incidence of Cerebrovascular Disease According to Gender and Age at Baseline (NHANES I)

Age	No. of men	No. of women	Total no.
35–49	1226	2265	3491
50–54	462	533	995
55–59	424	439	863
60–64	328	403	731
65–69	874	959	1833
70+	618	704	1322
Total	3932	5303	9235

gave a history of stroke when initially examined were excluded from the remainder of this analysis. An additional 496 persons were lost to follow-up, whereas for 882 only vital status was ascertained. The age and gender distributions of the remaining 9235 subjects, comprising the base population for the analyses to be described, are presented in Table 6–2. The analysis focused mainly on the 4749 persons who were aged 55–74 years at their baseline examinations. For intracranial hemorrhagic events it was decided to utilize data from the entire 35–74-year age range, partly because the number of cases with this type of stroke was small and partly because the pathogenesis of hemorrhagic stroke may involve factors not as clearly related to aging as are other types of cerebrovascular disease.

Identification and Definition of Cases of Cerebrovascular Disease

Subjects developing cerebrovascular disease during the course of the surveillance were identified by a hospital, nursing home, or death certificate diagnosis in the ICD9 430–437.1 group of codes and/or by an affirmative response to the follow-up interview query concerning occurrence of stroke since baseline. Overlap between these ascertainment methods was incomplete, partly because available data were incomplete and partly as a reflection of the inadequacy of ascertainment by any single mechanism. Figure 6–1 illustrates that overlapping sources of information for the total group of 923 persons reported to have developed some sort of cerebrovascular disease according to one, two, or all three of the information sources. The sources of the information providing this evidence according to the individual categories of cerebrovascular disease are shown in Table 6–3.

During the follow-up interval there were a total of 14,694 hospitalizations and nursing home admissions among subjects aged 55 and older in the base population for this analysis. Of these institutional admissions, 5.5% were associated with one or more diagnoses of the cerebrovascular disease ICD9 code series 430–437.1.

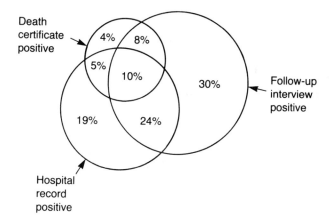

Fig. 6–1. Sources used to identify and classify incident cases of cerebrovascular disease.

Concordance of Historical and Medical Record Evidence of Cerebrovascular Disease

Among the 645 study participants for whom a history of stroke was obtained at follow-up interview, there were 594 for whom a death certificate, hospital, and/or nursing home record was available. In this group the occurrence of interim cerebrovascular disease was confirmed by concordance with medical record information for 62% of cases (370/594).

A cerebrovascular disease code was identified in a hospital–nursing home file and/or on a death certificate for 648 study participants. Concordance by an affirmative answer to the question (asked at follow-up of either the respondent or a proxy) concerning occurrence of a stroke was 58% (370/648). When the calculation was limited to persons with ICD9 diagnostic codes of 430–434 (hemorrhagic and thromboembolic stroke groups, excluding other types of cerebrovascular diseases), concordance was 60% (155/258).

Classification of Subjects According to Type of Cerebrovascular Disease

For simplication of the analysis, each of the 9235 subjects was assigned to one of seven cerebrovascular disease categories; one of the seven was for persons with no evidence of cerebrovascular disease. Because it was common for individuals to have been assigned more than one diagnosis in the ICD9 430–437.1 code series, a hierarchy of codes was established so that the classification system was exhaustive and categories were mutually exclusive. The category definitions are given in Table 6–4.

Each of the cerebrovascular disease categories represented an aggregate of

Table 6–3 Sources of Information for Identification and Categorization of New Cases of Cerebrovascular Disease

Hosp or NH record*	Death certificate*	History of stroke*	Stroke categories					
			Hem stroke	TE stroke	Mixed Hem + TE stroke	TIA only	ILL DEF CbVD	Stroke by history only
+	Alive	+	7	61	1	42	55	0
+	Alive	−	5	28	0	48	36	0
−	Alive	+	0	0	0	0	0	116
+	+	+	10	12	4	0	39	0
+	+	−	9	9	2	1	12	0
+	−	+	5	28	1	16	34	0
+	−	−	4	16	0	13	34	0
−	−	+	0	0	0	0	0	66
−	+	+	2	7	0	0	0	0
−	+	−	1	2	0	0	0	0
NA	+	+	4	13	0	0	29	0
NA	−	−	13	14	0	0	31	0
NA	Alive	+	0	0	0	0	0	51
NA	−	+	0	0	0	0	0	42
Total			60	190	8	120	270	275

Note: Abbreviations: HEM = hemorrhagic; TE = thromboembolic; TIA = transient ischemic attack.

*The first three columns define the sources of information: Hospital (Hosp) or nursing home (NH) record, death certificate, or as indicated by history of stroke, response to a question concerning stroke asked at the follow-up interview. Symbols indicate positive, negative, or not available (NA).

Table 6–4 Cerebrovascular Disease Categories: Definitions and ICD9 Codes

Category	Definition
Hemorrhagic stroke	Includes ICD codes 430–432.9; excludes thromboembolic stroke (433–434.9); ignores other codes
Thromboembolic stroke	Includes ICD codes 433–434.9; excludes persons with hemorrhagic stroke (430–432.9); ignores other codes
Thromboembolic and hemorrhagic stroke (in combination)	Includes ICD codes 430–432.9 and 433–434.9; ignores other codes
Transient ischemic attack without diagnosed hemorrhagic or thromboembolic stroke	Includes ICD codes 435.0–435.9; excludes ICD codes 430–434.9; ignores other codes. (Note: codes 436–437.1 may be in this category.)
Ill-defined cerebrovascular disease without either stroke or transient ischemic attack	Includes 436.0–437.1; excludes persons with ICD codes 430–435.9; ignores other codes
History of stroke given at follow-up interview, no other evidence of cerebrovascular disease	Affirmative answer to interview query regarding stroke, but not records and/or death certificate available, or no cerebrovascular disease codes recorded

more specific categories. In the group referred to as hemorrhagic stroke, 25% of the cases had a diagnosis of subarachnoid hemorrhage; 67%, a diagnosis of intracerebral hemorrhage; and the remaining 8%, some other type of nontraumatic intracranial bleeding, such as subdural hematoma. These are shown with finer breakdowns by age and gender in Table 6–5.

The thromboembolic stroke group represents the aggregation of diagnoses involving occlusion by embolism or thrombosis of intracranial or extracranial vessels. The breakdown by age, gender, and ICD9 code is shown in Table 6–6. Eight subjects whose records included diagnostic codes in both the ICD9 430–432.9 and the ICD9 433–434.9 series, that is, those persons designated by the category "mixed hemorrhagic and thromboembolic stroke" in Table 6-3, were excluded from the data in Tables 6-5 and 6-6.

Table 6–5 Cases of Hemorrhagic Stroke According to Gender and Age at Baseline (NHANES I) by Assigned Diagnostic ICD9 Codes

Age at baseline	Subarachnoid ICD 430		Intracerebral ICD 431		Other, ICD ICD 432–432.9		Total
	Women	Men	Women	Men	Women	Men	
35–49	3	2	2*	1	1	2	11
50–54	2	1	0	2	0	0	5
55–59	2	0	3	1	0	0	6
60–64	1	0	2†	1	0	0	4
65–69	0	1	5	8*	1	0	15
70–74	1	2	7†	8	0	1	19
Total	9	6	19	21	2	4	60

*One person in this cell also had a code of 430.

†One person in this cell also had a code of 432.1.

Table 6–6 Cases of Thromboembolic Stroke According to Gender and Age at Baseline (NHANES I) by Assigned Diagnostic ICD9 Codes

Age at baseline	Precerebral Artery Occlusion/Stenosis ICD 433–433.9		Cerebral Artery Occlusion/Thromb ICD 434–434.0		Cerebral Embolism ICD 434.1		Total
	Women	Men	Women	Men	Women	Men	
35–49	3	3	0	2	2	3	13
50–54	1	2	2	0	2	3	10
55–59	1	4	2	1	1	2	11
60–64	0	1	0	3	5	3	12
65–69	4	11	11	14	9	16	65
70–74	5	10	22	16	12	14	79
Total	14	31	37	36	31	41	190

The ill-defined cerebrovascular disease group was composed of two diagnostic codes, ICD9 436 and ICD9 437–437.1. The ICD9 436 category, acute but ill-defined cerebrovascular disease, included the following diagnostic terms: apoplexy not otherwise stated, cerebral apoplexy, apoplectic attack, apoplectic seizure, cerebral seizure, cerebrovascular accident not otherwise stated, and stroke not otherwise stated. The ICD9 437 code group, described as "Other and ill-defined cerebrovascular disease," included ICD9 code 437.0 (cerebral atherosclerosis, atheroma of cerebral arteries) and ICD9 437.1 codes (other generalized ischemic cerebrovascular disease, acute cerebrovascular insufficiency not otherwise stated, and chronic cerebral ischemia). As shown in Table 6–7, the preponderance of persons assigned to the ill-defined cerebrovascular disease group had codes in the ICD9 436 series, with only 21 individuals having codes in both the ICD9 436 and the ICD9 437–437.1 series. Although we have no means for verification, it is our impression that the ill-defined group, and especially the ICD9 436 code group, contained many

Table 6–7 Cases of Ill-defined Cerebrovascular Disease According to Gender and Age at Baseline (NHANES I) by Assigned Diagnostic ICD9 Codes

Age at baseline	Acute ill-defined stroke or CVA NOS; apoplexy ICD9 436		Chronic ill-defined cerebral arteriosclerosis ICD9 437–437.1		Both acute and chronic ill-defined ICD9 436 + 437–437.1		Total
	Women	Men	Women	Men	Women	Men	
34–49	8	6	0	0	0	0	14
50–54	4	4	0	0	0	0	8
55–59	3	7	1	0	0	1	12
60–64	6	9	3	3	1	0	22
65–69	26	37	17	14	7	4	105
70–74	36	37	14	14	5	3	109
Total	83	100	35	31	13	8	270

cases that might have been more precisely coded as hemorrhagic or thromboembolic strokes, had more specific information been available to the coder.

The Hierarchical Nature of the Cerebrovascular Disease Classification System

The cerebrovascular disease classification system that we have used allows individuals to be categorized in the hemorrhagic and the thromboembolic stroke groups even though they received other cerebrovascular disease diagnoses in the series ICD9 435–437.1. Because transient cerebral ischemia (codes ICD9 435–435.9) is above ill-defined cerebrovascular disease in the hierarchy, persons with conditions coded in both the ICD 435–435.9 and the ICD9 436–437.1 series were categorized only as cases of transient cerebral ischemia. Also, because of the hierarchical categorization, none of the persons classified as having transient cerebral ischemia had diagnoses of hemorrhagic or thromboembolic stroke. In contrast (but also because of the classification hierarchy), none of those in the ill-defined group had other cerebrovascular disease diagnoses. Our classification scheme reflected a decision to focus most of the analyses on clinically identified hemorrhagic and thromboembolic stroke, with less attention devoted to the other cerebrovascular disease diagnoses.

Occurrence of Strokes by Age and Time

The interval between initial contact and the first identified diagnosis of cerebrovascular disease was quite evenly distributed over the period of surveillance, a fact suggesting that ascertainment was probably not badly biased relative to timing of the initial event. The expected increasing frequency of clinical expression of cerebrovascular disease with advancing age is apparent in Fig. 6–2, illustrating the 10-year (approximately) incidence of cerebrovascular disease according to gender and age at baseline examination. When all six cerebrovascular disease categories were considered collectively, approximately 21% of participants aged 65–74 years at baseline developed some evidence of cerebrovascular disease in the decade of surveillance.

Prognosis and Outcome Associated with Cerebrovascular Disease

To examine the range of outcome associated with the different cerebrovascular disease categories defined earlier, we defined participant status at the time of follow-up by vital status and functioning. Physically disabled persons were identified by responses to questions on physical functioning (Chapter 12), with disability defined on the basis of a physical disability index equal to or greater than 1.0. Cognitively disabled persons were identified by their performance on a mental status questionnaire (MSQ; five or more errors on ten items) and/or the need for a proxy respondent for the follow-up interview (when this need was attributed to cognitive impairment). The "disabled" segments of the histograms shown in Fig.

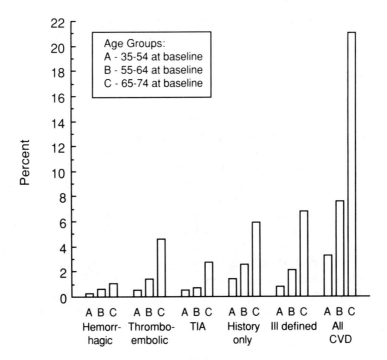

Fig. 6–2. Incidence of cerebrovascular disease over a 10-year follow-up period according to category and age at baseline (NHANES I).

6–3 represent the proportions of persons in the groups with cerebrovascular disease who were physically and/or cognitively disabled at follow-up. By this definition, the prevalence of disability (physical and/or cognitive) was approximately 20% among surviving participants who were aged 65–74 years at initial contact and who had no evidence of cerebrovascular disease over the decade of surveillance. The prevalence of physical or cognitive disability among persons in the transient ischemic attack group was in the same range, whereas approximately half of the surviving participants in the other cerebrovascular disease categories were disabled at follow-up.

The occurrence of death or survival with disability among the different categories of cerebrovascular disease is shown in Fig. 6–3. These are compared with outcomes among participants aged 65–74 years without evidence of cerebrovascular disease during the follow-up interval. As these data demonstrate, the most common outcome associated with hemorrhagic stroke was death. Thromboembolic strokes were less lethal but more disabling. As noted earlier, persons were categorized as having ill-defined cerebrovascular disease only if their records contained no diagnostic codes of thromboembolic or hemorrhagic stroke (ICD9 430–434.9) or transient ischemic attack (ICD9 code 435). Of the persons in this category, 204 of the 270 had one or more diagnoses of acute (rather than chronic), ill-defined cere-

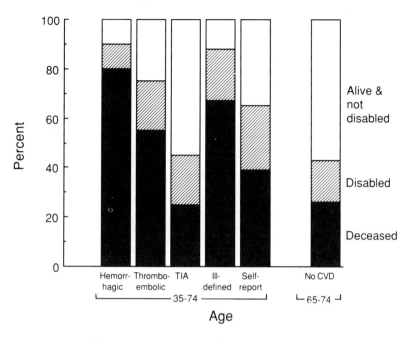

Fig. 6–3. Vital and functional status at follow-up according to category of cerebrovascular disease, compared with persons aged 65–74 years at baseline (NHANES I) who remained free of cerebrovascular disease during the follow-up period.

brovascular disease, and the group of 204 consisted largely of cases of "stroke, not otherwise defined" (ICD 436). The proportion of persons in the total group with ill-defined cerebrovascular disease who were alive and not disabled at follow-up was midway between the corresponding proportions for the hemorrhagic and thromboembolic stroke groups. This result is consistent with the interpretation that many of these individuals, particularly those with diagnoses in the ICD 436 series, had actually suffered a stroke that would have been categorized as either hemorrhagic or thromboembolic had supplementary information been available.

Individuals for whom a history of stroke was ascertained at follow-up but for whom no documentation was available had outcomes only slightly less dismal than those observed for persons with thromboembolic strokes. This group (stroke by history only) is almost certainly comprised of a mixture of types of cases: (1) those who actually had no cerebrovascular disease (having misunderstood a medical diagnosis or having some other condition, such as Alzheimer's disease or Parkinsonism mistakenly attributed to cerebrovascular disease), (2) those whose manifestations of cerebrovascular disease were not severe enough to require hospitalization, and (3) those for whom the pertinent hospital records were unavailable or incorrectly coded. Because they represent such a mixture of clinical types, the interpretation of information for this group is difficult.

The apparently innocuous nature of transient ischemic attacks as shown here is

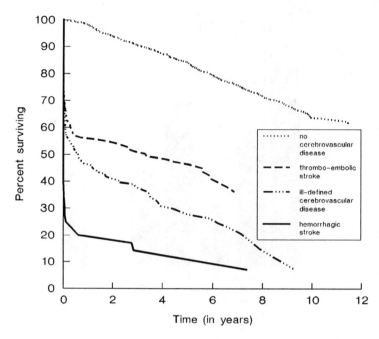

Fig. 6–4. Survival following initial stroke compared with survival from baseline for persons aged 65–74 years with incident st

partly an artifact of the category definitions. Individuals could be in this category only if they had no diagnoses in the ICD9 430–434.9 series in the entire period of surveillance. Cases in the group with transient ischemic attacks shown here were thereby selected not only for their expressed evidence of cerebrovascular disease, but also for the absence of diagnosed hemorrhagic or thromboembolic stroke. On the other hand, the hierarchical categorization allowed persons with ICD codes in both the ICD9 435 and 436–437.1 (ill-defined cerebrovascular disease) series to be identified only as cases of transient ischemic attack.

In Fig. 6–4 Kaplan–Meier curves depict survival after the first diagnosis of hemorrhagic stroke, thromboembolic stroke, or ill-defined cerebrovascular disease (Kaplan and Meier 1958). Data shown for cerebrovascular disease cases aged 55–74 at baseline. A comparison curve depicting survival after the baseline contact is presented for persons aged 65–74 without evidence of cerebrovascular disease during the follow-up interval. These curves demonstrate an immediate mortality of 35–40% following the first diagnosis of thromboembolic stroke and of 75–80% following a hemorrhagic stroke. Immediate mortality for the ill-defined cerebrovascular disease group was similar to that for thromboembolic stroke. Mortality in the years following the first stroke was much lower than that in the first few weeks but was greater than that among persons without diagnosed cerebrovascular disease. The worst prognosis for long-term survival was associated with ill-defined cerebrovascular disease (ICD codes 436–437.1).

Risk Factors

The risk factor analyses contained in this section include only factors previously implicated as influencing the risk for stroke. In addition to age, race, and gender, they include systolic blood pressure, diastolic blood pressure, pulse pressure, body mass index, diabetes, heart disease, smoking, dietary fat, dietary potassium, dietary sodium, dietary calcium, alcohol intake, serum cholesterol and uric acid, and hemoglobin levels. Usable information on atrial fibrillation or other electrocardiographic indicators of heart disease were unavailable at the time of these analyses.

An initial examination of these potential risk factors was based on univariate associations with hemorrhagic stroke and thromboembolic stroke; sets of univariate association indicators were calculated separately for these two cerebrovascular diagnostic categories. Associations with hemorrhagic stroke were calculated in a manner such that persons were considered negative for that outcome (hemorrhagic stroke not having been diagnosed) even if other types of cerebrovascular disease were present, that is, persons with thromboembolic stroke, transient ischemic attacks, ill-defined cerebrovascular disease, or stroke by history only were considered negative for hemorrhagic stroke. The inverse situation held for thromboembolic stroke; that is, persons with cerebrovascular disease other than thromboembolic stroke were grouped with persons who had no cerebrovascular disease. These preliminary analyses support possible associations of risk for thromboembolic stroke with age, elevated blood pressure, male gender, diabetes, dietary fat, elevated hemoglobin, and alcohol intake (slightly elevated risk associated with intake of more than 0.1 oz daily). Patterns of univariate relative risk (for thromboembolic stroke) across strata were variable for dietary sodium and fat as well as for serum cholesterol and uric acid levels.

Statistically significant univariate associations with hemorrhagic stroke were noted for age, black race, elevated blood pressure, obesity (elevated body mass index), diabetes, hemoglobin (both high and low levels suspect), alcohol (no alcohol intake associated with higher risk), and smoking (past smokers at lower risk). Although high univariate relative risks were associated with some strata of serum cholesterol and uric acid levels, the pattern across strata allowed no conclusions.

Multivariate analyses and significance testing were done with use of Cox proportional hazards methods to avoid distortions due to variable lengths of follow-up and variable intervals between initial contact and the cerebrovascular disease event (Cox 1972). As with other methods, this multivariate technique generates estimates of the influence of each variable controlling or adjusting for the simultaneous influences of the other independent variables whenever possible in the model. Factors identified as independently associated with stroke in such preliminary models were then analyzed in parsimonious proportional hazards models, with most continuous variables presented in quintile strata to better define patterns of association with level.

For thromboembolic stroke, the following eight factors were found to be significantly associated with risk:

1. Age was strongly associated in all models; older persons were at greater risk of developing strokes. In a single parsimonious model containing all the other major factors and limited to subjects aged 55–74 at baseline, the association of risk with advancing age was highly significant ($p < 0.0001$).
2. Gender was strongly associated in all models; the incidence of stroke was higher among men ($p < 0.01$).
3. Race was not significantly associated when analyzed for both genders combined. However, whereas analysis with stratification by gender showed no significant association between race and thromboembolic stroke among women, there was a substantially increased risk among black men as compared with white men ($p < 0.05$).
4. Elevated blood pressure was strongly and consistently associated with stroke. The association was stronger for systolic than for diastolic blood pressure. When risk was examined by quintile of systolic blood pressure, the association was statistically significant only for the highest quintile among both men and women. Comparison of persons having systolic blood pressure of ≥166 with persons having systolic blood pressure of less than 127 mmHg values gave p values of <0.01 for men and of <0.05 for women.
5. Diabetes was significantly associated with an increased risk of thromboembolic stroke for women ($p <0.05$) but not for men.
6. Heart disease was strongly associated with risk of stroke in models in which men and women were considered collectively. When the analysis was stratified by gender, the association among men weakened so that statistical significance was lost, whereas among women the association became more apparent ($p < 0.05$).
7. Hemoglobin levels, both elevated and low, were associated with an increased risk of thromboembolic stroke in men. In comparisons of the lowest quintile (<13.3 g/dl) with the middle quintile (14.2–14.9 g/dl) and of the highest (>15.7 g/dl) with the middle quintile, both p values for men were < 0.05. Among women, increased risk was associated only with elevated hemoglobin; risk for the highest quintile was significantly greater than that for the middle quintile ($p < 0.05$). Because the quintile strata were defined on the basis of combined-gender distributions of hemoglobin levels, approximately 35% of men but only about 5% of women had hemoglobin values in the highest quintile.
8. Cholesterol level was not associated with thromboembolic stroke in women. Among men, those in the second quintile (201–223 mg/dl) had a significantly lower risk than men with higher levels. However, no clear and consistent pattern of increasing risk with increasing cholesterol level was apparent.

These results are summarized in Table 6–8. Factors not found to be significantly associated with thromboembolic stroke after taking into account the effects of

Table 6–8 Relationship Between Baseline (NHANES I) Measures and Risk of Thromboembolic Stroke Over a 10-year Interval for Men and Women

Factor	Relative risk for T-E stroke		
	Men only	Women only	All
Age (10-year increment)	2.5*	3.8*	3.0*
Gender			
Female	—	—	(1.0)
Male	—	—	1.6*
Race			
White	(1.0)	(1.0)	(1.0)
Black	2.7†	0.9	1.4
Systolic BP, mmHg			
<127	(1.0)	(1.0)	(1.0)
127–139	1.7	1.5	1.5
140–148	1.4	1.1	1.3
149–166	1.3	2.2	1.6
>166	3.0*	2.8†	2.8*
Hemoglobin, g/dl			
<13.4	2.4†	1.3	1.6
13.4–14.1	1.3	1.1	1.2
14.2–14.9	(1.0)	(1.0)	(1.0)
15.0–15.7	1.4	1.1	1.3
>15.7	2.3†	3.0†	2.4*
Diabetes			
No	(1.0)	(1.0)	(1.0)
Yes	1.2	2.0†	1.7†
Heart disease			
No	(1.0)	(1.0)	(1.0)
Yes	1.6	2.0†	1.7*
Cholesterol, mg/dl			
<201	1.4	0.8	1.1
201–223	(1.0)	(1.0)	(1.0)
224–246	2.7*	1.0	1.7†
247–275	2.1†	0.8	1.4
>275	2.5†	0.9	1.5

Note: (1.0) indicates the reference category for each variable, relative to which the other categories are compared.

*Statistically significant at $p < 0.01$.

†Statistically significant at $p < 0.05$, > 0.01.

the main factors included uric acid level; dietary intake of fat, potassium, calcium, and sodium; smoking; alcohol consumption; and body mass index.

For multivariate analysis of factors associated with hemorrhagic stroke, the population was extended to include persons aged 35 and older, because the number of cases was relatively small. Analyses were carried out as described for thromboembolic stroke, except that no models were developed with stratification by gender because of small numbers. Five factors were found to be significantly associated with hemorrhagic stroke.

1. Older age was strongly associated with risk ($p < 0.01$).
2. Blood pressure was strongly associated with risk. Although a trend of increasing risk was seen for the three highest quintiles of systolic blood pressure, the association was statistically significant only for the highest quintile (>166 mmHg) as compared with the lowest quintile (<127 mmHg) ($p < 0.05$).
3. Elevated hemoglobin level was strongly associated with risk. The association was statistically significant in a comparison of the highest quintile (>15.7 g/dl) with the third quintile (14.2–14.9) ($p < 0.01$).
4. Diabetes was strongly associated with risk ($p < 0.01$).
5. Black race was strongly associated with increased risk ($p < 0.01$).

After the strong associations of the main factors were accounted for, the strengths of association of hemorrhagic stroke with the following characteristics fell below the threshold of statistical significance: gender; uric acid level; dietary intake of fat, potassium, and calcium; smoking; alcohol consumption; body mass index; and heart disease at baseline. In a preliminary parsimonious model with factors entered as continuous variables, serum cholesterol showed a statistically significant inverse relationship with hemorrhagic stroke. As shown in Table 6–9 this significance was lost in models in which quintile strata of serum cholesterol were examined.

Results of multivariate analyses are summarized in Tables 6–8 and 6–9 with estimate of relative risk as the index of association. Strengths of association with both hemorrhagic and thromboembolic stroke were compared among systolic blood pressure, diastolic blood pressure, and pulse pressure in preliminary models containing only one of these (either continuous or as quintile strata) together with the other main factors. In such models, diastolic blood pressure was found to be least strongly associated with the stroke end points, whereas systolic blood pressure and pulse pressure showed nearly identical strengths of association. Common convention led us to identify systolic blood pressure rather than pulse pressure as a main factor.

Excess Risk Attributable to Recognized Risk Factors

The comparison of the incidence of cerebrovascular disease in the general population with that in a subset of persons exposed to none of the major recognized risk factors allows one to gain some appreciation of the excess risk possibly due to these factors, i.e., the population-attributable proportion. We estimated the population attributable proportion for four major risk factors among the participants in two age strata, 55–64 and 65–74 years at the baseline examination. Participants were considered risk factor negative if none of the following characteristics were identified at baseline: diabetes, systolic blood pressure greater than 149 mmHg, hemoglobin level above 15.7 g/dl, or evidence of prior heart disease. As shown in Table 6-10, the crude incidence of cerebrovascular disease (all types combined; without consideration of the variable of follow-up intervals) was 7.5% among all persons aged 55–

Table 6–9 Relationship Between Baseline (NHANES I) Measures and Risk of Hemorrhagic Stroke Over a 10-year Interval for Men and Women

Factor	Relative risk for hemorrhagic stroke
Age (10-year increment)	1.5*
Systolic BP, mmHg	
<127	(1.0)
127–139	0.8
140–148	1.7
149–166	2.0
>166	2.9†
Hemoglobin, g/dl	
<13.4	1.3
13.4–14.1	2.1
14.2–14.9	(1.0)
15.0–15.7	2.0
>15.8	3.5*
Diabetes	
No	(1.0)
Yes	2.9*
Cholesterol, mg/dl	
<201	1.2
201–223	(1.0)
224–246	0.9
247–275	0.8
>275	0.7

Note: (1.0) indicates the reference category for each variable, relative to which the other categories are compared.
*Statistically significant at $p < 0.01$.
†Statistically significant at $p < 0.05$, > 0.01.

64 years, and was 4.7% among those persons who were risk factor negative. For this group the population-attributable proportion estimated at 37% ([7.5–4.7]/7.5). Among participants aged 65–74 years, the comparable estimate was 30%.

STRENGTHS AND LIMITATIONS OF FINDINGS

The findings reported here emphasize the great importance of cerebrovascular disease as a common cause of morbidity, disability, and premature mortality. A dramatic increase in both the prevalence and incidence of cerebrovascular disease with advancing age further reinforces our appreciation of the underlying processes as major pathologic forces in later life.

Neither NHANES I nor NHEFS was specifically designed for investigation of cerebrovascular disease. Our information on the occurrence of these conditions was limited to answers to a few questions and to diagnoses abstracted from death

Table 6–10 Estimates of the Interval Incidence (Approximately a Decade) of Cerebrovascular Disease (CbVD) Comparing Persons from the General Study Population with "Risk Factor-free" Subset (with Systolic Blood Pressure < 149, Hemoglobin < 15.8, and No Evidence of Heart Disease or Diabetes at the Baseline Contact)

Group	Percentage with indicated diagnosis					
	Hemorrhagic stroke	Thromboembolic stroke	Ill-defined CbVD	TIA only	Stroke by history only	All CbVD
Total population aged 55–64	0.6	1.4	2.1	0.7	2.6	7.5
Risk factor-free aged 55–64	0.5	0.8	1.3	0.4	1.6	4.7
Total population aged 65–74	1.1	4.6	6.8	2.7	5.4	20.7
Risk factor-free aged 65–74	0.7	2.0	5.3	2.9	3.5	14.4

certificates and/or hospital or nursing home records. It is well known that clinical records and death certificates are generally a rather poor source of information on cerebrovascular disease events; accuracy and concordance of diagnoses (as death certificate vs. hospital record) are often poor for both the type and the fact of the event (Corwin et al. 1982; Gittelsohn and Senning 1979). Other weaknesses of this study are that only a single set of premorbid observations was available from which to access exposure to risk factors, and the interval between baseline (risk factor ascertainment) and the disease event was variable. The certainty, dose, and duration of risk factor exposures are undefined with relation to the occurrence of the disease events.

The negative effects of these problems must certainly include (1) incomplete ascertainment of cases (missed cases being misclassified as noncases); (2) errors in diagnosis related to type of cerebrovascular disease (especially reciprocal mis-classification between hemorrhagic and thromboembolic stroke); and (3) bias relat-ed to the fact that identified cases are incompletely representative of all true cases in that category. The most usual result to be expected from incomplete ascertainment of cases in research on risk factors for disease is a reduction of power to detect true associations, that is, an increased chance for a true association to be missed. This expectation assumes that the misclassified cases have no other reason for being associated with the factor being tested. Such reduced power reflects both a smaller number of cases than would have been found with complete ascertainment (some true cases being misclassified as unaffected), and dilution of the case group with unaffected persons or persons having a clinically similar condition. Although this problem diminishes the credibility of a negative result somewhat, one generally assumes that statistically significant associations would have been even stronger had case ascertainment been complete.

With incomplete ascertainment and misclassification, the cases identified may not be representative of all true cases in the population (i.e., cases may be systemat-ically missed or misgrouped), and inferences may not be fully generalizable. For example, the risk factor profile identified may be applicable only to the subset of cases identifiable with the methods used. This common epidemiologic problem afflicts nearly all case-control studies and is no greater or lesser a problem in the present investigation.

The meaning of our results related to the ill-defined cerebrovascular disease group is itself ill defined. Persons were included in this category only if they had, in addition to a code indicating acute (ICD9 436–436.9) or chronic (ICD9 437–437.1) ill-defined cerebrovascular disease, no diagnostic codes in the ICD9 series 430–435.9. Thus, excluded from this category were persons who also had a diagnosis of hemorrhagic stroke, thromboembolic stroke, or transient ischemic attacks. None-theless, this category included approximately the same number of persons as identi-fied in the hemorrhagic and thromboembolic stroke categories combined. The prog-nosis associated with this category of cerebrovascular disease was nearly as dismal as that for hemorrhagic stroke; approximately 85 were dead or disabled at follow-up. For reasons mentioned earlier it seems likely that many individuals in this category (especially those with ICD9 code 436) might well have been classified as having thromboembolic or hemorrhagic stroke had the diagnosis been described more precisely.

Despite these several problems, the study remains an extraordinary resource for research on cerebrovascular disease. We know of no other source of data on the predictors of stroke in which unbiased risk factor information has been collected prospectively from a large and nationally representative sample of adults (including a sizable number aged 55–74 years) who were thereafter followed longitudinally for ascertainment of onset of cerebrovascular disease. A close correspondence between these findings and those of earlier studies (Wolf et al. 1986) encourages the interpretation that these data can indeed provide valid epidemiologic information on the risk factors associated with clinically apparent cerebrovascular disease. This in turn encourages us to give credence to the absence of other risk factor associations.

One important, previously identified risk factor association that the present analysis failed to substantiate was that between dietary potassium and stroke. Our observation of no significant association conflicts with a finding reported for the Rancho Bernardo community study implicating lower levels of dietary potassium as a risk factor for increased incidence of disease and mortality due to stroke (Shaw and Barrett-Conner 1987). Both the durations and methods of surveillance for cerebrovascular disease events and the method for ascertaining dietary potassium intake for the Rancho Bernardo study appear to have been similar to those used in the present study. However, unlike the nationally representative sample of persons within whom we sought the association, Rancho Bernardo participants tend to be somewhat self-selected in later life, being predominantly white persons of middle to upper socioeconomic class who reside in a retirement community. In addition, the size of the Rancho Bernardo study population was only about one fifth of the base population for the present report. While it is possible that some as yet undefined common characteristic of the Rancho Bernardo cohort allowed a true protective effect of high levels of dietary potassium to become apparent, our results suggest that the finding is not generalizable to the population of the United States.

As was mentioned earlier, total and age-specific rates of mortality due to stroke have declined precipitously in the United States in recent years. Perhaps the only clue to the causes of these declines has to do with recognition of the importance of hypertension as a risk factor, and the known improvements in detection and treatment of hypertension that have occurred in the past 20–30 years.

In summary, the total incidence of cerebrovascular disease (all categories combined) over the approximately 10-year interval of follow-up was about 21% among participants who were aged 65–74 years at initial contact, and approximately 7.5% among those who were aged 55–64 years. The prognosis associated with incident cerebrovascular disease in this study was poor, risks for death and/or disability being markedly increased after the development of cerebrovascular disease. Proportional hazards multivariate analyses confirmed the association of the two major; types of stroke with previously established risk factors namely, advanced age, elevated blood pressure, diabetes, elevated hemoglobin, a history of heart disease (thromboembolic stroke only), male gender (thromboembolic stroke), and black race (only among males with thromboembolic stroke). No support was found for the previously reported association of high dietary potassium with a lower risk for stroke. We estimate that if it were possible to reduce the risk of cerebrovascular disease for the entire population aged 55–74 years to that now experienced by the segment of the population with none of the major identified risk factors for cerebrovascular disease, the reduction in clinically evident cerebrovascular disease events in a 10-year period of observation would be between 37 and 30%.

REFERENCES

Corwin, L. I., P. A. Wolf, W. B. Kannel, and P. M. McNamara. 1982. "Accuracy of death certification of stroke: The Framingham study." *Stroke* 13:818–821.

Cox, D. R. 1972. "Regression model and life tables." *J R Stat Soc Ser*(B) 34:187–202.

Gittelsohn, A., and H. Senning. 1979. "Studies on the reliability of vital and health records: I. Comparison of cause of death and hospital record diagnoses." *Am J Public Health* 69:680–689.

Kaplan, E. L., and P. Meier. 1958. "Nonparametric estimation from incomplete observations." *J Am Stat Assoc* 53:457–481.

Khaw, K. T., and E. Barrett-Connor. 1987. "Dietary potassium and stroke-associated mortality. A 12-year prospective population study." *N Engl J Med* 316(5):235–240.

Kurtze, J. F. 1985. "Epidemiology of Cerebrovascular disease." In *Cerebrovascular Survey Report 1985*. F. H. McDowell and L. R. Caplan, eds. Available from the National Institute for Neurological and Communicative Disorders and Stroke, National Institute of Helath, Bethesda, MD., pp.1–36.

Pfeiffer, E. 1975. "A short portable mental status questionaire for the assessment of organic brain deficit in elderly patients." *J Am Geriatr Soc* 23:443–441.

Rose, G. A., H. Blackburn, R. F. Gillum, and R. J. Prineas. 1982. "Cardiovascular Survey Methods." Geneva: World Health Organization, pp. 162–165.

Takeya, Y., J. S. Popper, Y. Shimizu, H. Kato, G. Rhoads, and A. Kagan. 1984. "Epidemiologic studies of coronary heart disease and stroke in Japanese men living in Japan, Hawaii and California: Incidence of stroke in Japan and Hawaii." *Stroke* 15:15–33.

Toole, J. F. 1983. In *Cerebrovascular Disease*. M. Revich and H. I. Hurtig, eds. New York: Raven Press, p. 129.

Wolf, P. A. 1985. "Risk factors for stroke." *Stroke* 16:359–360.

Wolf, P. A., W. B. Kannel, and D. L. McGee. 1986. "Prevention of ischemic stroke: Risk factors." In *Stroke: Pathophysiology, Diagnosis and Management*. H. J. M. Barnett, J. P. Mohr, B. Stein, and F. M. Yatsu, eds. New York: Churchill-Livingstone, pp. 967–988.

7

Arthritis

REVA C. LAWRENCE, DONALD F. EVERETT,
AND MARC C. HOCHBERG

The availability of national data on arthritis offers great opportunity for epidemiologic research in arthritis and musculoskeletal diseases. A major source of these data is the National Health and Nutrition Examination Survey (NHANES I) conducted between 1971 and 1975 and the NHANES I Epidemiologic Follow-up Study (NHEFS) conducted between 1982 and 1984 (Lawrence 1989).

NHANES I

In NHANES I arthritis-related questions concerning (1) the presence and character of pain or arching in the back, neck, hip(s), knee(s), and/or other joints for at least one month; (2) swelling of a joint with pain present in that joint for at least one month; (3) stiffness of a joint for at least 15 minutes when arising from bed in the morning; and (4) history of treatment for pain or related disorder were included in the General Medical History Supplement (GMHS) and Arthritis Supplement. The latter was given to 2431 participants who responded positively to at least one of the GMHS questions on arthritis. The specific questions contained in the Arthritis Supplement have been published (National Center for Health Statistics 1979).

The general medical examination that was part of NHANES I included anthropometric measures but did not emphasize arthritis. For study of this condition the physical examination of persons completing detailed components was extended and included specific sections emphasizing the back, hips, knees, and other peripheral joints. The hips were examined for pain on motion, local tenderness, and periarticular muscle wasting; the knees, for bony irregularity, pain on motion, swelling, crepitus, effusion, and periarticular muscle wasting; the back, for deformity, tenderness, limitation of motion and pain on motion; and the other peripheral joints, for tenderness, swelling, deformity, limitation of motion, and pain on motion.

X-ray films of the knees were taken on all but 2.6% of the NHANES I examinees receiving the detailed examination. X-rays of the hips were to be taken

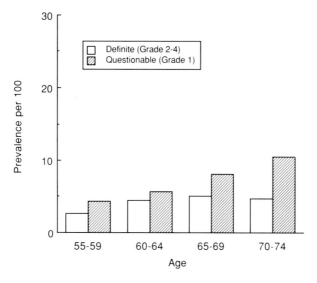

Fig. 7–1. Prevalence rates of questionable and definite osteoarthritis of the knee (radiographic grades 1–4) for men according to age at baseline (NHANES I).

on all male examinees receiving the detailed examination and all females over 50 years of age. However, 6.0% of the hip x-rays were not taken. Radiographs were read independently by two rheumatologists using an ordinal scale (0–4) based on the Atlas of Standard Radiographs, where 0 = normal, 1 = questionable, 2 = minimal abnormality, 3 = moderate abnormality, and 4 = severe abnormality (Atlas of Standard Radiographs 1963).

If an abnormality (score ≥1) was noted by either of the two readers, a final adjudicated reading was made by a third rheumatologist in the presence of the other two readers. These adjudicated readings provided an overall grade of osteoarthritis of the knee and hip, respectively, as well as of other abnormalities, including erosions, osteoporosis, and chondrocalcinosis (National Center for Health Statistics 1979).

The prevalence of questionable (grade 1) and definite (grades 2–4) osteoarthritis may be seen in Fig. 7–1 and 7–2. For both men and women the prevalence of definite and/or questionable osteoarthritis increased with age. However, the frequency of definite and/or questionable osteoarthritis was greater in each age group for women than for men. In addition, the rate of increase by age was greater for women than for men. The proportion of cases with grade 1 findings does not vary with age in the same linear manner as do the cases with grades 2–4 osteoarthritis. It is therefore critical for studies using the NHANES I and NHEFS data sets to specify whether grade 1 cases will be combined with those in grades 2–4 or handled in some other way.

Several previous analyses of the NHANES I data relating to arthritis have been published. The National Center for Health Statistics has released the basic data on prevalence of osteoarthritis of the knees and hips according to overall grade, gender,

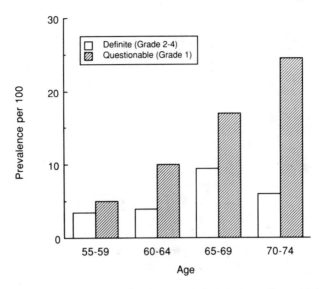

Fig. 7–2. Prevalence rates of questionable and definite osteoarthritis of the knee (radiographic grades 1–4) for women according to age at baseline (NHANES I).

and age in the NHANES I population (National Center for Health Statistics 1979). Cunningham and Kelsey (1984) have reported the epidemiology of disability, as assessed by limitation of physical activity and its relationship to sociodemographic factors, in NHANES I participants who had a clinical diagnosis of osteoarthritis made by the examining physician. Davis (1981) analyzed gender differences in reporting joint symptoms and noted that reporting of symptoms was significantly related to radiographic evidence of osteoarthritis for both genders as well as to two measures of treatment: self-treatment and current treatment by a physician. Acheson (1982) noted an association between body bulk, assessed by ponderal index, and osteoarthritis of the knees in both genders. Hartz and colleagues (1986) made similar observations by using relative weight as a measure of obesity. Hochberg (1984) reported the descriptive epidemiology of chondrocalcinosis of the knee and its relationship to osteoarthritis; these assessments of joint abnormalities were based on the adjudicated x-ray readings. Several additional investigators are in the process of performing secondary analyses of this data set (Anderson and Felson 1986; Davis et al. 1986; Lawrence and Hochberg 1986).

Linkage between NHANES I and the Epidemiologic Follow-up

Questions on symptoms of arthritis from the NHANES I Arthritis Supplement were extensively duplicated in NHEFS. For the most part, identical wording was used in both surveys. However, the structure of NHEFS frequently differed from that of the original survey so as to facilitate rapid administration of the survey instruments. For greater clarity some questions from the original survey were rephrased and subdivided in NHEFS. For example, the original survey question asked, "Have you had pain in either the back or neck on most days for at least one month?" In NHEFS one question asks about back pain and another about neck pain. Questions on medical history, surgical procedures, and hospitalization were the same for both NHANES I and NHEFS. Items dealing with the source and type of treatment that were asked in the original survey were not included in NHEFS. However, NHEFS did include a question regarding hospitalization for joint problems and joint-specific questions on surgical procedures, including joint replacements.

All NHEFS participants were asked the questions on arthritis. In contrast, the original questionnaire was administered to a subsample of the NHANES I participants who were selected for a detailed examination. An understanding of the criteria and conditions for selecting individuals who received the Arthritis Supplement is essential to using the NHANES I data set alone or in tandem with the NHEFS data. According to reports from the National Center for Health Statistics (National Center for Health Statistics 1977, 1979), the Arthritis Supplement was administered to the selected examinees by the physician after completion of the physical examination. The physician was instructed to administer the Arthritis Supplement to those examinees who had answered affirmatively one or more of the screening questions administered at the household interview conducted 1–3 weeks earlier. The screening questions dealt with history of arthritis; pain or aching in joints, neck, back, or hip; and swelling and stiffness of joints.

After an initial period of operation at the beginning of the survey, the examining physicians were instructed not to administer the Arthritis Supplement if repeated questioning of the examinee warranted changing all positive responses to screening questions to negative responses. This procedure was followed for most of the survey. Some of the examining physicians did not recode the original responses to the negative choice to reflect their considered opinion on not giving the Arthritis Supplement. Because of the gate-keeping function of the examining physician and recoding of some medical history questions by the physician after the physical examination, the medical history questions functioned as an imperfect selection tool for the Arthritis Supplement. Not all individuals who responded positively to the arthritis screening questions were given the Arthritis Supplement, and not all participants who gave all negative answers to the arthritis screening questions in the medical history questionnaire were excluded from the group receiving the Arthritis Supplement. In fact, approximately 30% of those who had positive responses recorded for at least one of the medical history questions were not included in the Arthritis Supplement, and 2% of those who had negative responses recorded for all of the gate-keeping questions were given the Arthritis Supplement. Overall, 2431 (35.2%) of the 6913 persons who participated in the detailed component were given the supplement. Table 7–1 provides age-, gender-, and race-specific data for supplement participation for persons aged 55–74 years.

Building on the baseline data collected in NHANES I, NHEFS will greatly enhance the utility of the former's arthritis information by providing a longitudinal view. NHEFS includes not only a detailed arthritis component almost identical to the NHANES I Arthritis Supplement but also data on physical activity, weight,

Table 7-1 Percentage of Individuals Selected to Receive the Arthritis Supplement at NHANES I According to Gender, Race, and Age at Baseline (NHANES I)

Age at baseline	White men		White women		Black men		Black women	
	%	n	%	n	%	n	%	n
55–59	37.0	112	47.2	141	37.8	17	47.6	20
60–64	41.1	99	49.1	135	51.6	16	46.5	20
65–69	39.5	115	52.7	166	45.0	27	53.2	25
70–74	41.7	88	52.1	118	58.1	18	47.7	21

Note: Four individuals between the ages of 55 and 74 were listed as a race other than black or white in the Arthritis Supplement. This was 25% of the "others" in that age group from the component selected for detailed examination.

smoking, alcohol consumption, mental status, use of specific medications, socioeconomic characteristics, hospitalization, and a detailed functional assessment questionnaire containing, in part, the Health Assessment Questionnaire (HAQ). The HAQ is a validated, self-administered questionnaire that measures physical disability in patients with arthritis and related disorders (Brown et al. 1984). The HAQ disability instrument used in NHEFS is divided into eight components: dressing and grooming, arising from an armless straight chair and/or bed, eating, walking, hygiene, reach, grip, and activities. The level of difficulty for the individual and need for aids, devices, or help from another person in carrying out these tasks are also included in NHEFS. Finally, a pain scale from the HAQ is included. Thus, NHEFS provides information on (1) the progression or remission of arthritis symptoms, (2) the relationship of functional impairment and symptoms in persons with radiographic changes of osteoarthritis, and (3) the impact of symptoms and radiographic changes of osteoarthritis on incidences of disability, morbidity (including treatments and hospitalization), and mortality.

Data From NHANES I

Readings of radiographs based on the criteria defined in the Atlas of Standard Radiographs (1963) were used for classification of osteoarthritis of the knee and hip. This system followed the recommendations of Laine concerning diagnostic criteria for population studies of osteoarthritis: "that, for the present time, these be confined to those characteristic x-ray changes described in the Atlas of Standard Radiographs" (Laine 1968). Recently, the American Rheumatism Association (ARA) Subcommittee on Classification Criteria of Osteoarthritis has developed criteria using history, physical examination, laboratory findings, and radiographs for classification of osteoarthritis of the knee (Altman et al. 1986); these criteria have not been utilized herein because of lack of uniform availability of data (physical examination and laboratory findings) and their focus on symptomatic osteoarthritis.

The prevalence rate of osteoarthritis of the knee and hip in surveyed persons aged 55–74 years is shown in Tables 7–2 and 7–3. Overall grade of osteoarthritis is

Table 7–2 Prevalence Rates for Osteoarthritis of the Knee According to Gender and Age at Baseline (NHANES I)

Gender and age at baseline	Percentage with indicated grade of osteoarthritis*				
	0	1	2	3	4
Women					
55–64	89.3	3.5	6.4	0.9	0.0
65–74	75.1	6.9	11.4	6.0	0.6
Men					
55–64	91.7	4.2	3.1	0.7	0.3
65–74	86.3	5.3	6.3	1.8	0.2

Note: This table is adapted from a previous publication (National Center for Health Statistics 1979).

*Definitions of radiographic grades: 0 = normal, 1 = questionable abnormality, 2 = minimal abnormality, 3 = moderate abnormality, 4 = severe abnormality.

based on the adjudicated reading as described earlier. Definite osteoarthritis (grades 2–4) of the knee was present in 83 men and 172 women, whereas that of the hip was present in only 43 men and 35 women in the group aged 55 to 74 years. Because of the small number of cases of osteoarthritis of the hip, we have chosen to focus further analyses, both of the NHANES I and NHEFS data, on osteoarthritis of the knee in this report.

Self-reported pain in or around the knee on most days for at least 1 month was significantly associated with definite osteoarthritis of the knee for both genders (Table 7–4). Thee were no significant age-related differences, in either gender, for the frequency of the presence of pain in persons with osteoarthritis. Among those with normal x-rays, women were almost twice as likely to report pain as men. It is not clear whether this difference reflects physiological or psychosocial differences.

Bony crepitus was found to be the most sensitive physical finding for osteoarthritis of the knee in the ARA subcommittee study of osteoarthritis, occurring in 104 (89%) of 116 patients (Altman et al. 1986). Crepitus was assessed in the

Table 7–3 Prevalence Rates for Osteoarthritis of the Hip According to Gender and Age at Baseline

Gender and age at baseline	Percentage with indicated grade of osteoarthritis*				
	0	1	2	3	4
Women					
55–64	96.3	0.9	1.2	0.8	0.8
65–74	96.1	1.2	1.5	0.6	0.6
Men					
55–64	96.8	0.6	1.9	0.4	0.3
65–74	93.8	1.6	2.3	1.1	1.2

Note: This table is adapted from a previous publication (National Center for Health Statistics 1979).

*Definitions of radiographic grades: 0 = normal, 1 = questionable abnormality, 2 = minimal abnormality, 3 = moderate abnormality, 4 = severe abnormality.

Table 7–4 Percentage of Persons Reporting Knee Pain (on Most Days for at Least 1 Month) According to Definite Osteoarthritis of the Knee (Grades 2–4), Gender, and Age at Baseline (NHANES I)

	Men				Women			
	Normal radiograph		Definite osteoarthritis*		Normal radiograph		Definite osteoarthritis*	
	Grade 0		Grades 2–4		Grade 0		Grades 2–4	
Age at baseline	%	n	%	n	%	n	%	n
55–59	9.6	31	53.3	8	13.6	42	41.2	7
60–64	11.4	28	46.7	7	18.9	53	29.0	9
65–69	9.7	29	42.9	12	23.4	70	53.3	32
70–74	9.0	18	48.0	12	20.9	39	32.8	21
Total	9.9	106	47.0†	39	19.0	204	40.1‡	69

Note: This table is adapted from a previous publication (National Center for Health Statistics 1979).
*Definitions of radiographic grades: 0 = normal, 1 = questionable abnormality, 2 = minimal abnormality, 3 = moderate abnormality, 4 = severe abnormality.
†Mantel-Haenszel test p = <0.001 difference between presence or absence of osteoarthritis for men.
‡Mantel-Haenszel test p = <0.001 difference between presence or absence of osteoarthritis for women.

general physical examination of NHANES I and was significantly associated with the presence of definite osteoarthritis (Table 7–5). Furthermore, crepitus was more common among those with definite osteoarthritis who reported pain than in the remaining persons with definite osteoarthritis who did not report pain (Table 7–6). Nonetheless, among the 255 persons aged 55–74 years who had definite osteoarthritis of the knee, there were still 125 (49%) who lacked both crepitus and

Table 7–5 Percentage of Persons with Definite Osteoarthritis of the Knee (Grades 2–4) According to the Presence of Crepitus on Physical Examination, Gender, and Age at Baseline (NHANES I)

	No. of men (%) with osteoarthritis*				No. of women (%) with osteoarthritis*			
	Crepitus		No crepitus		Crepitus		No crepitus	
Age at baseline	%	n	%	n	%	n	%	n
55–59	13.8	4	3.5	11	14.6	6	3.7	11
60–64	14.3	4	4.5	11	13.8	4	9.6	27
65–69	18.4	7	6.8	21	18.0	9	16.8	51
70–74	15.0	3	10.1	22	44.2	19	20.7	45
Total	15.7	18	6.0†	65	22.0	38	12.2‡	134

Note: This table is adapted from a previous publication (National Center for Health Statistics 1979).
*Definitions of radiographic grades: 0 = normal, 1 = questionable abnormality, 2 = minimal abnormality, 3 = moderate abnormality, 4 = severe abnormality.
†Mantel-Haenszel test p = <0.001 difference between presence or absence of crepitus for men.
‡Mantel-Haenszel test p = <0.01 difference between presence or absence of crepitus for women.

Table 7–6 Percentage of Persons with Definite Osteoarthritis (Grades 2–4)* and Crepitus on Physical Examination According to the Prevalence of Pain, Gender, and Age at Baseline (NHANES I)

	Men				Women			
	Pain		No pain		Pain		No pain	
Age at baseline	%	n	%	n	%	n	%	n
55–59	25.0	2	28.6	2	42.9	3	30.0	3
60–64	28.6	2	25.0	2	33.3	3	4.5	1
65–69	50.0	6	6.3	1	15.6	5	14.3	4
70–74	16.7	2	7.7	1	52.4	11	18.6	8
Total	30.8	12	13.6†	6	31.9	22	15.5‡	16

Note: This table is adapted from a previous publication (National Center for Health Statistics 1979).

*Definitions of radiographic grades: 0 = normal, 1 = questionable abnormality, 2 = minimal abnormality, 3 = moderate abnormality, 4 = severe abnormality.

†Mantel-Haenszel test p = >0.05 difference between presence or absence of pain for men.

‡Mantel-Haenszel test p = <0.01 difference between presence or absence of pain for women.

self-reported pain on most days; this frequency did not differ significantly by gender. Additional studies concerning the association between definite osteoarthritis of the knee with a history of swelling, "locking," or "buckling" of the knee; previous trauma (twisting, sprain, fracture, etc.); or surgery and physical findings (including bony irregularity and/or deformity, pain on motion, and swelling) are feasible via analysis of the NHANES I data tapes.

Data from NHEFS

Analysis of the arthritis component of NHEFS will allow an estimation of the frequency of joint pain at multiple sites (neck, back, hip, knee, other joints) with site-specific descriptors of pain, history of swelling with pain in a peripheral joint, presence of morning stiffness and its duration, history of joint surgery (including replacement arthroplasty), and hospitalization for joint disease (Table 7–7). In addition, the detailed functional status component of NHEFS can be used for comparison of disability and activity status in groups defined in NHEFS (cross-sectional analysis) or in NHANES I (longitudinal analysis). Physical functioning will be reviewed in another chapter of this book and will be described here only in relation to knee pain and radiographic findings at baseline.

Thus, one is able to utilize the NHEFS data to analyze longitudinally outcomes in subgroups of patients defined in NHANES I. These outcomes might include, for example, development or persistence of pain at one or more sites, hospitalization for joint disease and/or joint surgery, and development of functional disability. Because persons were not examined and did not undergo radiographs in NHEFS, a diagnosis of osteoarthritis cannot be made using either the preliminary ARA criteria or radiographic findings.

Table 7–7 Questions Concerning Knee Pain on NHEFS Questionnaire

Question no.	Description
E-04 and 60	Pain in or around the knee on most days for at least 1 month
61	Longest episode of knee pain
62	Age at first episode of recurrent pain
63	Presence of pain at time of interview
64	Last (most recent) episode of pain
65	Pain at rest
66	Swelling, warmth, or redness with pain
67	Locking of the knee
68	Buckling of the knee
69	Twisting of the knee with sprain
79	Surgical procedure on knee
81	Knee joint replacement
82	Morning stiffness
87	Duration of morning stiffness
88	Hospitalization for joint problems

Studies Linking NHANES I and NHEFS

We have chosen to present, as examples, analyses of the relationship of radiological findings of osteoarthritis, pain, and swelling at NHANES I and mortality symptoms and disability at NHEFS.

Mortality

Mortality was assessed in 2384 persons aged 55 and older who had radiographs of the knees during NHANES I and could be traced at NHEFS (Table 7–8). The crude relative risks for cumulative mortality from all causes was 1.72 and 1.23 for women and men, respectively, when persons with questionable (grade 1) or definite (grades 2–4) osteoarthritis were compared with those who had normal knee radiographs. However, these results are not observed consistently when age-specific data from women are analyzed. Furthermore, among men, there is a decrease in relative mortality with increasing age. In addition, the increased mortality among 55–59-year-old women and 55–64-year-old men with osteoarthritis is based on small numbers of cases and is subject to great variability. Despite this, the age-adjusted relative risk for cumulative mortality of 1.45 for women is significantly different from 1.0, a fact suggesting an association of radiographic changes of questionable or definite osteoarthritis with increased mortality among women. Survival analysis (Cox regression) confirmed decreased survival among the 55–59-year-old women. Whether this risk is related to co-morbid conditions associated with osteoarthritis in the population or to effects or complications of treatment is unknown.

In an attempt to address this question, we looked at the association between

Table 7–8 Relationship Between Osteoarthritis (Grades 1–4) at Baseline (NHANES I) and Subsequent Mortality According to Gender and Age

	Men				Women			
	Normal		Osteoarthritis*		Normal		Osteoarthritis*	
Age at baseline	%	n	%	n	%	n	%	n
55–59	16.3†	51	29.2	7	7.0	21	28.6	8
60–64	25.4	61	42.9	12	11.9	31	5.0	2
65–69	36.9	107	41.3	19	25.4	64	28.1	25
70–74	53.6	108	39.4	13	32.6	56	45.6	36
Total	31.6	327	38.9‡	51	17.5	172	30.1§	71

*Definitions of radiographic grades: 0 = normal, 1 = questionable abnormality, 2 = minimal abnormality, 3 = moderate abnormality, 4 = severe abnormality.

†No. (percentage) who died during follow-up interval in age–sex group during NHANES I who were successfully traced in NHEFS.

‡Age-adjusted relative risk = 1.17, $p > 0.05$.

§Age-adjusted relative risk = 1.45, $p > 0.01$, $p < 0.05$.

pain in the knee and mortality, stratifying for presence of radiographic changes of osteoarthritis (Table 7–9). We assumed that individuals who reported pain were more likely to take medication, especially aspirin or other nonsteroidal anti-inflammatory drugs, that might result in adverse effects leading to mortality. Such adverse effects might include peptic ulcer disease or renal insufficiency.

Overall, age-adjusted relative risks of mortality vary from 1.07 for women with normal radiographs to 1.23 for women with questionable or definite osteoarthritis; however, neither are significantly different from 1.0. Similar findings are noted for men. These results do not support an association of self-reported pain at baseline with increased mortality, but they obviously do not exclude an effect of

Table 7–9 Relationship Between Osteoarthritis (Grades 1–4)* with Pain (on Most Days for 1 Month) at Baseline (NHANES I) and Subsequent Mortality According to Gender and Age

	Men				Women			
	No pain		Pain		No pain		Pain	
Age at baseline	%	n	%	n	%	n	%	n
55–59	33.3†	5	22.2	2	33.3	5	23.1	3
60–64	31.2	5	63.6	7	3.3	1	11.1	1
65–69	41.4	12	41.2	7	30.6	15	25.0	10
70–74	38.1	8	41.7	5	37.5	21	65.2	15
Total	37.0	30	42.8‡	21	27.8	42	34.1§	29

*Definitions of radiographic grades: 0 = normal, 1 = questionable abnormality, 2 = minimal abnormality, 3 = moderate abnormality, 4 = severe abnormality.

†No. (percentage) who died during follow-up interval in age–sex group during NHANES I who were successfully traced in NHEFS.

‡Age-adjusted relative risk = 1.27, $p = >.05$.

§Age-adjusted relative risk = 1.23, $p = >.05$.

treatment; data on use of aspirin and other nonsteroidal drugs have not yet been analyzed. These and other analyses can be accomplished by use of the NHEFS data to seek an explanation for the excess mortality among women with radiographic changes characteristic of osteoarthritis of the knee.

Symptoms

NHEFS data permit study of the persistence, progression, and development of knee symptoms relevant to both radiographic changes at NHANES I and to the presence of symptoms such as pain and swelling at baseline.

Using the NHANES I and NHEFS data sets in tandem, we examined how one risk factor, pain at baseline, is associated with symptoms at follow-up. As seen in Table 7–10, about one third of women and one quarter of men who were pain-free at the time of NHANES I had developed knee pain and/or stiffness by the time of NHEFS. Despite this relatively high incidence of symptoms, there exists a strong significant correlation between the presence of knee pain at baseline and knee pain and/or stiffness at time of NHEFS.

Table 7–10 Percentage of Persons Reporting Knee Pain and/or Stiffness* at Follow-up (NHEFS) According to the Presence of Osteoarthritis† (Grades 1–4), Knee Pain, Gender and Age at Baseline (NHANES I)

| | Normal | | | | Grades 1–4† osteoarthritis | | | |
| | No pain | | Pain | | No pain | | Pain | |
Gender, age at baseline	%	n	%	n	%	n	%	n
Women								
25–54	16.1‡	273	53.0	71	60.9	14	82.6	19
55–59	23.8	53	56.3	18	33.3	3	71.4	5
60–64	27.0	48	40.6	13	48.2	13	66.7	6
65–69	24.3	34	33.3	6	38.7	12	76.0	19
70–74	27.6	21	33.3	7	20.0	5	75.0	6
Total	18.6	429	48.5	115	40.9	47	76.4	55
Age-adjusted odds	Reference		3.8		2.4		11.6	
ratios§	group		(3.4,4.4)		(2.0,2.9)		(8.7,15.5)	
Men								
25–54	15.5	207	52.3	68	31.8	7	80.0	8
55–59	20.8	45	45.5	10	33.3	3	100.0	6
60–64	14.4	20	72.2	13	60.0	6	50.0	2
65–69	17.7	26	28.6	4	13.3	2	66.7	6
70–74	14.5	9	20.0	2	44.4	4	50.0	3
Total	16.1	307	51.3	97	33.9	22	71.4	25
Age-adjusted odds	Reference		5.4		2.4		11.7	
ratios§	group		(4.5,6.3)		(1.9,3.2)		(8.0,17.1)	

*Presence or absence of knee pain on most days for 1 month at NHANES I.

†Definitions of radiographic grades: 0 = normal, 1 = questionable abnormality, 2 = minimal abnormality, 3 = moderate abnormality, 4 = severe abnormality.

‡Number (percentage) with knee pain and/or stiffness in age–sex group who completed questionnaire at NHEFS.

§Age-adjusted odds ratios were derived from linear logistic model with reference group being those free of pain and radiographic abnormality at baseline. The 95% confidence intervals are in parentheses.

Table 7–11 Percentage of Persons Reporting Knee Pain at Follow-up (NHEFS) According to the Presence of Osteoarthritis† (Grades 1–4), Knee Pain and Swelling, Gender, and Age at Baseline (NHANES I)

| Gender, age at baseline | Normal radiograph | | | | Grades 1–4* Osteoarthritis | | | |
| | No pain or swelling | | Pain and swelling | | No pain or swelling | | Pain and swelling | |
	%	n	%	n	%	n	%	n
Women								
25–54	12.0	212	47.5	28	51.9	14	83.3	15
55–59	20.8	50	41.2	7	30.8	4	80.0	4
60–64	26.5	53	14.3	2	32.3	10	100.0	4
65–69	19.1	29	33.3	2	41.3	19	70.0	7
70–74	20.4	19	0	0	14.8	4	66.7	4
Total	14.8	363	39.0	39	35.4	51	79.1	34
Age-adjusted odds ratios†	Reference group		3.5 (2.8,4.3)		2.4 (2.0,2.9)		18.0 (12.3,26.3)	
Men								
25–54	13.2	186	50.9	27	36.0	9	85.7	6
55–59	14.2	33	25.0	2	38.5	5	100.0	2
60–64	9.0	13	58.3	7	50.0	6	0	0
65–69	13.3	21	50.0	2	16.7	3	83.3	5
70–74	14.3	9	0	0	50.0	7	0	0
Total	13.0	262	48.1	38	36.7	30	72.2	13
Age-adjusted odds ratios†	Reference group		6.2 (4.9,7.8)		3.7 (2.9,4.8)		16.9 (9.9,28.8)	

*Definitions of radiographic grades: 0 = normal, 1 = questionable abnormality, 2 = minimal abnormality, 3 = moderate abnormality, 4 = severe abnormality.

†Age-adjusted odds ratios were derived from linear logistic model with reference group being those free of pain, swelling, and radiographic abnormality at baseline. The 95% confidence intervals are in parentheses.

It is important to note that among persons not reporting pain during NHANES I, both men and women with radiographic changes of osteoarthritis were more likely to report pain and/or stiffness at NHEFS than were those with normal radiographs. Furthermore, the combination of pain and radiographic change was the best predictor of pain and/or stiffness at follow-up.

The two data sets were also used to examine the predictive value of knee swelling with pain and radiographic findings at baseline and knee pain at follow-up. As seen in Table 7–11, by use of rates unadjusted for age, only 14.8% of women and 13.0% of men who had no pain or swelling and normal radiographs at baseline had pain at follow-up. However, 39.0% of women and 48.1% of men who had normal radiographs with pain and swelling at baseline reported pain at NHEFS. Of the women and men who had questionable or positive radiographs (grades 1–4) but no symptoms of pain or swelling at NHANES I, 35.4% and 36.7%, respectively, had pain at follow-up, whereas 79.1% of women and 72.2% of men who had both positive radiographs and symptoms of pain or swelling at NHANES I reported pain at follow-up.

A linear logistic regression model with adjustment for age showed statistically significant differences in the frequency of knee pain at NHEFS when those who initially had normal radiographs and no symptoms were compared to the three other groups: those with symptoms but no radiographic changes, those with no symptoms but positive radiographs, and those who had both symptoms and radiographic findings. Statistically significant differences were also found in both genders between those who had symptoms and normal radiographs at baseline and those who had both symptoms and abnormal radiographs at baseline.

Functional Limitation

The NHANES I and the NHEFS data can also be used for examination of the relationship between findings at baseline and reported ability to function approximately a decade later. Herein are presented two examples, using the functional domains of walking and arising derived from the Health Assessment Questionnaire (HAQ) at NHEFS, with radiographic data on the knee collected in NHANES I. The walking domain includes questions about difficulty walking from one room to another and walking up and down at least two steps. The arising domain includes

Table 7–12   Percentage of Persons Reporting Difficulty Walking at Follow-up (NHEFS) According to the Presence of Osteoarthritis (Grades 1–4), Knee Pain, Gender, and Age at Baseline (NHANES I)

| | Normal radiograph | | | | Grades 1–4* osteoarthritis | | | |
| | No pain | | Pain | | No pain | | Pain | |
Gender, age at baseline	%	n	%	n	%	n	%	n
Women								
25–54	5.4	94	19.9	27	40.0	10	47.8	11
55–59	11.3	26	18.2	6	33.3	3	57.1	4
60–64	15.4	28	32.4	11	21.4	6	33.3	3
65–69	20.8	32	33.3	6	34.4	11	77.8	21
70–74	42.1	37	54.6	12	33.3	10	75.0	6
Total	9.1	217	25.5	62	32.3	40	60.8	45
Age-adjusted odds	Reference		2.8		2.1		8.6	
ratios†	group		(2.0,3.9)		(1.4,3.2)		(5.1,14.4)	
Men								
25–54	4.1	56	18.9	25	22.7	5	20.0	2
55–59	8.4	19	16.7	4	11.1	1	14.3	1
60–64	14.5	22	31.6	6	30.0	3	50.0	2
65–69	18.7	29	7.1	1	31.3	5	40.0	4
70–74	22.2	16	0.0	0	30.0	3	42.9	3
Total	7.2	142	18.5	36	25.4	17	31.6	12
Age-adjusted odds	Reference		2.8		2.7		3.3	
ratios†	group		(1.9,4.3)		(1.4,4.9)		(1.6,6.9)	

*Definitions of radiographic grades: 0 = normal, 1 = questionable abnormality, 2 = minimal abnormality, 3 = moderate abnormality, 4 = severe abnormality.

†Age-adjusted odds ratios were derived from linear logistic model with reference group being those free of pain and radiographic abnormality at baseline. The 95% confidence intervals are in parentheses.

questions about difficulty standing up from an armless straight chair and getting in and out of bed. A person was classified as having difficulty functioning within a domain if the respondent reported some or much difficulty or was unable to perform a task within the domain.

In Table 7–12 the frequency of reported difficulty walking collected at NHEFS can be examined for subgroups in relation to NHANES I data on radiographic and pain status for the knee. Those individuals who had normal radiographs but reported knee pain at baseline were significantly more likely to experience difficulty walking at follow-up when compared with those who had no reported knee pain and whose radiographs showed freedom from osteoarthritis. Likewise, those who were without knee pain at baseline but had an abnormal radiograph (grades 1–4) also experienced more difficulty walking at the time of NHEFS. The group of individuals who had both abnormal radiographs and reported knee pain at baseline were much more likely to report difficulty walking when compared with those who were free of one or both characteristics.

The frequency of difficulty arising was also examined (Table 7–13). The association between baseline data on radiographic findings and follow-up reports of

Table 7–13 Percentage of Persons Reporting Difficulty Arising at Follow-up (NHEFS) According to the Presence of Osteoarthritis (Grades 1–4), Knee Pain, Gender, and Age at Baseline (NHANES I)

Gender, age at baseline	Normal radiograph				Grades 1–4* osteoarthritis			
	No pain		Pain		No pain		Pain	
	%	n	%	n	%	n	%	n
Women								
25–54	8.8	152	22.1	30	32.0	8	52.2	12
55–59	14.4	33	33.3	11	33.3	3	71.4	5
60–64	19.2	35	35.3	12	32.1	9	22.2	2
65–69	24.7	38	33.3	6	31.3	10	70.4	19
70–74	44.3	39	54.6	12	36.7	11	62.5	5
Total	12.5	297	29.2	71	33.1	41	58.1	43
Age-adjusted odds ratios†	Reference group		2.4 (1.8,3.4)		1.8 (1.2,2.7)		5.9 (3.5,9.8)	
Men								
25–54	6.1	84	22.0	29	22.7	5	30.0	3
55–59	12.9	29	12.5	3	22.2	2	14.3	1
60–64	14.5	22	36.8	7	30.0	3	50.0	2
65–69	20.0	31	21.4	3	18.8	3	60.0	6
70–74	25.0	16	33.3	2	50.0	5	28.6	2
Total	9.3	184	22.6	44	26.9	18	36.8	14
Age-adjusted odds ratios†	Reference group		2.8 (1.9,4.0)		2.3 (1.3,3.5)		3.4 (1.6,6.9)	

*Definitions of radiographic grades: 0 = normal, 1 = questionable abnormality, 2 = minimal abnormality, 3 = moderate abnormality, 4 = severe abnormality.

†Age-adjusted odds ratios were derived from linear logistic model with reference group being those free of pain and radiographic abnormality at baseline. The 95% confidence intervals are in parentheses.

difficulty arising were very similar to those found when the outcome studied was difficulty walking. These findings suggest that pain and radiographic abnormalities of the knee are strongly predictive of disability for weight-bearing tasks a decade later.

Further Research

NHEFS provides a wealth of data related to arthritis, including presence and character of joint symptoms (especially pain), history of hospitalizations (including surgical procedures for joint disease), and functional capacity and activity limitation. In addition, data on co-morbid conditions and treatment, although limited to aspirin, are available for analysis. When NHEFS data are linked with the NHANES I data, longitudinal studies of mortality and morbidity outcomes can be accomplished and used for testing of hypotheses concerning long-term outcome in persons with osteoarthritis and other arthritic conditions.

We have presented brief examples to stimulate the reader to pursue other investigations into this area, utilizing the data available from NHANES I and NHEFS.

Because osteoarthritis and other arthritic/musculoskeletal diseases are a major public health concern, further analyses of these national data will be anticipated with interest and enthusiasm.

REFERENCES

Acheson, R. M. 1982. "Epidemiology and the arthritides." *Ann Rheum Dis* 41:325–334.

Altman, R., E. Asch, D. Bloch et al. 1986. "Development of criteria for the classification and reporting of osteoarthritis: classification of osteoarthritis of the knee." *Arthritis Rheum* 29:1039–1049.

Anderson, J. J., and D. T. Felson. 1986. "Factors associated with knee osteoarthritis (OA) in a national survey." *Amer J Epidemiol* (1988) 128:179–189.

Atlas of Standard Radiographs. 1963. *The Epidemiology of Chronic Rheumatism*, vol. 2. Oxford: Blackwell Scientific Publications.

Brown, J. H., L. E. Kazis, P. W. Spitz et al. 1984. "The dimensions of health outcomes: A cross-validated examination of health status measurement." *A J Pub Health* 74(2):159–161.

Cornoni-Huntley, J., H. E. Barbano, J. A. Brody et al. 1983. "National Health and Nutrition Examination I-Epidemiologic Followup Survey. *Public Health Reports* 98(3):245–251.

Cunningham, L. S., and J. L. Kelsey. 1984. "Epidemiology of musculoskeletal impairments and associated disability." *Am J Public Health* 74(6):574–579.

Davis, M. S. 1981. "Sex differences in reporting osteoarthritic symptoms: A sociomedical approach." *J Health Soc Behavior* 22:298–310.

Davis, M. S., W. H. Ettinger, and J. M. Neuhaus. 1986. "Sex differences in osteoarthritis of the knee (OAK): The role of obesity." *Amer J Epidemiol* 127:1019–1030.

Hartz, A. J., M. E. Fischer, G. Bril, S. Kelber, D. Rupley, Jr., B. Oken, and A. A. Rimm. 1986. "The association of obesity with joint pain and osteoarthritis in the HANES data." *J Chronic Dis* 39:311–319.

Health Resources Administration. 1977. "Plan and operation of the Health and Nutrition Examination Survey—United States, 1971–1973." *Vital and Health Statistics.* Series 1, No. 10B, Washington, DC: U.S. Government Printing Office.

Hochberg, M. C. 1984. "Chondrocalcinosis articularis (CCA) of the knee: Prevalence and association with osteoarthritis (OA) of the knee." *Arthritis Rheum* 27(Suppl):S49.

Laine, V. 1968. "Report from the subcommittee on diagnostic criteria for osteoarthrosis." In *Population Studies of the Rheumatic Diseases.* P. H. Bennett and P. H. N. Wood, eds. Amsterdam: Excerpta Medica Foundation, pp. 417–419.

Lawrence, R. C. 1985. "New research opportunities associated with national data sets." *J Rheumatol* 12:1035–1037.

Lawrence, R. C., and M. C. Hochberg. 1986. "Osteoarthritis of the knee: comparison of signs, symptoms and comorbid conditions in those with and without current knee pain." *Arthritis Rheum* 29(Supple):S16. (Full paper *Seminars Arthritis Rheum:* in press.)

Lawrence, R. C., M. C. Hochberg, J. L. Kelsey et al. 1989. "Estimates of the prevalence of selected arthritic and musculoskeletal diseases in the United States." *J of Rheum* 16:427–441.

National Center for Health Statistics. 1979. "Basic data on arthritis—knee, hip and sacroiliac joints, in adults age 25–74 years: United States, 1971–1975." *Vital and Health Statistics.* Series 11, No. 213. Hyattsville, MD.

III

MORBIDITY AND MORTALITY ASSOCIATED WITH SOCIAL AND PERSONAL CHARACTERISTICS

8

Sociodemographic Differentials in Mortality

DIANE MAKUC, JACOB J. FELDMAN,
JOEL C. KLEINMAN, AND MITCHELL B. PIERRE, JR.

This chapter is a study of the mortality experience of a sample of the U.S. population who were aged 55 years or older when enrolled in the National Health and Nutrition Examination Survey-I (NHANES I). Mortality is analyzed for the period between enrollment in NHANES I during 1971–1975 and interview in the NHANES I Epidemiologic Follow-up Study (NHEFS) during 1982–1984 according to sociodemographic characteristics reported at baseline (i.e, NHANES I). The variables considered are age, race, gender, educational attainment, marital status, and region and metropolitan status of the place of residence at baseline. Educational attainment was selected as a measure of socioeconomic status because it remains relatively constant throughout adulthood. Other measures of socioeconomic status collected at baseline, such as income and occupation, are more likely to be changed by illness at some point prior to death.

NHEFS provides an opportunity to study national differentials in mortality according to socioeconomic and demographic characteristics. This study allows these differentials to be examined for variables that are not usually reported on the death certificate (e.g., educational attainment). The NHEFS also offers advantages for studying mortality by variables that are available on the death certificate (e.g., marital status, age, race, gender), because results are not subject to biases due to reporting differences between death certificates (numerators) and the population estimates derived from the U.S. Census (denominators). In addition, since NHEFS is a prospective study, baseline characteristics were reported before death occurred.

BACKGROUND INFORMATION

A landmark study of differentials in mortality in the United States was carried out nearly three decades ago (Kitagawa and Hauser 1973). In that study, conducted in 1960, a sample of records of deaths that occurred during May through August 1960 was matched with 1960 Census records to obtain socioeconomic data for decedents.

155

The results showed an inverse relationship between years of education and mortality for adults under age 65 in all race and gender groups. Among persons 65 years of age or older, an inverse relationship was found for women but not for men. The 1960 study also found that married persons experienced lower mortality than others among all age, race, and gender groups. However, marital status differentials were much larger for men than for women.

A more recent study of national differentials in mortality was based on linking records from the March 1973 Current Population Survey with deaths on Social Security Administration (SSA) files over a 4-year period (Rosen and Taubman 1979). The study focused on white men 25 years of age or older, because the SSA files can most accurately identify deaths for this group.

The findings of this study differed from those of the 1960 study in that an inverse relationship between education and mortality was found for white men 65 years and older. This study also found that among white men, the widowed, separated, and divorced experienced higher mortality than the married.

Another related study was based on mortality over an 8-year period among adult residents of Washington County, Maryland (Comstock and Tonascia 1977). Information on marital status and education, among other variables, was obtained during a private census of Washington County residents who were at least 25 years of age in 1963. The data showed an inverse relationship between education and mortality that remained significant after adjustment for several other variables. The study also found that married persons had lower mortality rates than unmarried persons.

A major national study of geographic differentials in mortality was based on all deaths in the United States among persons aged 35–74 years during 1968–1972 (National Center for Health Statistics 1980). Among white men the highest death rates were concentrated in the Southeast and the lowest were found west of the Mississippi. Among white women the highest rates were east of the Mississippi, primarily in the Middle Atlantic states. Almost all areas with the lowest death rates were west of the Mississippi. For black persons the lowest death rates were found in the West and the highest in the Southeast. Among white persons death rates were similar for metropolitan and nonmetropolitan residents. Among black persons death rates for cardiovascular diseases were lower in metropolitan areas.

STATISTICAL METHODS

Plots of cumulative survival probabilities (Kaplan and Meier 1958) were used to study survival differentials among sociodemographic subgroups, and proportional hazards regression models (Cox 1972) were used to estimate the relative risk of death among subgroups. Results were calculated by use of the LIFETEST and PHGLM procedures in SAS (SAS Institute, Inc. 1983, 1985). Separate analyses were carried out for age, race, and gender subgroups based on two age categories (55–64 years and 65 years and older), two genders, and two races (white, black). Individual models for all subgroups except white men aged 65–74 years include age in single years as a covariate. Models for white men aged 65–74 years include two age strata based on 5-year intervals because of nonproportional hazards by age for this subgroup.

The sensitivity of the analysis in detecting sociodemographic differences in mortality depends on the sample size and numbers of deaths that occurred during the initial follow-up period. Categories of sociodemographic variables were collapsed, so that results are presented only for categories with at least 20 expected deaths. The power to detect differences in mortality by sociodemographic characteristics varies substantially by age, race, and gender. Results are not presented for black persons aged 55–64 because few deaths have occurred so far in this group (33 among men and 16 among women). The power to detect mortality differentials is greatest among white persons aged 65–74 because of relatively large numbers of deaths (675 for white men and 467 for white women). In contrast, there were only 84 deaths among white women aged 55–64 years. Based on the 84 deaths in this subgroup and an alpha level of ·0.05 (two-tailed test), there is approximately an 80% chance of detecting a relative risk of 2 when comparing mortality among those with less than 12 years of education to those with more than 12 years of education (with two groups of about equal size) (Peto et al. 1976). The chance of detecting a relative risk around 1.5 for this same comparison is less than 50%.

Statistical methods for survival analysis do not directly take into account the complex survey design of the NHANES I. However, the oversampling of the elderly was taken into account by separate analysis of data for this group. The impact of the sample weights within this age group was studied by comparing weighted and unweighted estimates of Cox regression coefficients (Makuc and Kleinman 1986). Weighted and unweighted estimates were similar; therefore, analyses are shown for the unweighted estimates, which have smaller variances. The NHANES I design also incorporates stratification and clustered observations in area-based segments. Design effects calculated using jackknife estimation of variances were approximately 1 for unweighted data; therefore, the analyses presented do not incorporate a design effect (Makuc and Kleinman 1986).

EDUCATIONAL DIFFERENTIALS

Educational attainment was found to vary substantially by age, race, and gender (Table 8–1). Black persons have less education than white persons; persons 65–74 years of age have less education than those 55–64; and men tend to have somewhat less education than women. The percentage with 12 or more years of education is lowest among black men aged 65–74 (9.9%) and highest among white women aged 55–64 (48.6%) The percentage with less than 5 years of education varies from 3.2% among white women aged 55–64 to 49% among black men aged 65–74. The large differences in education distribution by age and race complicate the analysis because of the small numbers of deaths among individuals with certain levels of education. For instance, the number of deaths among black persons 65–74 years of age who are high school graduates is very small (13 men and 10 women). In

Table 8–1 Percentage Distribution of the NHEFS Cohort and Number of Deaths by Educational Attainment According to Race, Gender, and Age at Baseline (NHANES I)

Race and educational attainment	Age 55–64 years		Age 65–74 years	
	Men	Women	Men	Women
No. in sample				
White	741	817	1501	¦680
Black	106	142	313	332
Percentage distribution of the sample				
White				
Total	100.0	100.0	100.0	100.0
0–4 years	6.5	3.2	11.9	8.2
5–8 years	30.6	27.3	43.3	38.6
9–11 years	16.1	20.4	13.2	17.1
12 or more years	46.4	48.6	30.4	35.6
Missing	0.4	0.5	1.1	0.5
Black				
Total	100.0	100.0	100.0	100.0
0–4 years	29.2	19.7	48.6	32.8
5–8 years	35.8	43.0	31.9	40.4
9–11 years	13.2	23.9	7.7	13.3
12 or more years	17.0	12.7	9.9	11.4
Missing	4.7	0.7	1.9	2.1
No. of deaths				
White				
Total	149	84	675	467
0–4 years	12	4	101	56
5–8 years	51	28	305	190
9–11 years	32	17	87	81
12 or more years	54	35	176	138
Missing	0	0	6	2
Black				
Total	33	16	145	110
0–4 years	13	2	74	41
5–8 years	7	6	44	39
9–11 years	8	6	11	17
12 or more years	3	2	13	10
Missing	2	0	3	3

addition, the meaning of a particular educational level as a measure of socioeconomic status may differ substantially across subgroups. For these reasons different education categories are used for different age–race subgroups. For white persons aged 65–74 years the education categories analyzed are 0–4 years, 5–8 years, 9–11 years, and 12 or more years. Preliminary analyses for white persons showed no differences in mortality between those with 12 years of education and those with more than 12 years; therefore, these categories were collapsed. For black persons aged 65–74 years, the highest education category considered is 9 or more years because of the small numbers of deaths at higher levels of education. Among black persons aged 65–74 years, 17.6% of men and 24.7% of women have 9 or more years of education. For white persons aged 55–64 years, two education groups were compared: 0–1'1 years and 12 or more years.

Estimates of survival among groups with different educational attainments are compared graphically in Figs. 8–1 and 8–2 for white men and women 65–74 years of age at baseline. Survival rates are greater for both men and women who have more education. Among white women aged 65–74, those with 0–4 years of education have a particularly low survival rate. For white men aged 65–74 the probabilities of death after 8 years of follow-up are 0.294 for the most educated (12 or more years), 0.345 and 0.366 for the two middle categories, and 0.450 for the least educated (0–4 years) (Table 8–2). Among white women aged 65–74 the corresponding probabilities of death are 0.170 (12 or more years of education), 0.199 (9–11 years), 0.201 (5–8 years), and 0.307 (0–4 years).

Proportional hazards regression models estimate that among white men aged 65–74 the relative risk of death is 1.56 (95% confidence interval = 1.22–2.00) for those with 0–4 years of education as compared with men having 12 or more years of education (Table 8–2). Among white women aged 65–74 the corresponding relative risk is somewhat greater: 1.98 (95% confidence interval = 1.45 - 2.71). Thus, it is

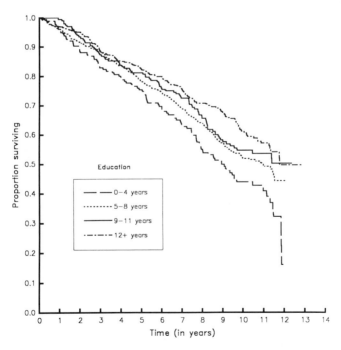

Fig. 8–1. Survival of the NHEFS cohort according to educational attainment for white men 65–74 years of age at baseline (NHANES I).

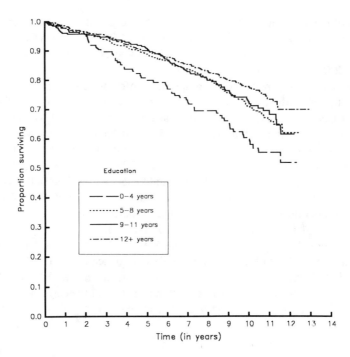

Fig. 8–2. Survival of the NHEFS cohort according to educational attainment for white women 65–74 years of age at baseline (NHANES I).

Table 8–2 Relationships Between Educational Attainment and Subsequent Risk of Death in the NHEFS Cohort According to Race, Gender, and Age at Baseline (NHANES I)

Race, age at baseline, and educational attainment	Kaplan–Meier estimates Probability of death after 8 years (SE)		Cox regression results Relative risk (95% CI)	
	Men	Women	Men	Women
White, age 55–64 years				
0–11 years	0.192 (0.020)	0.080 (0.014)	1.52 (1.09–2.13)	1.35 (0.87–2.08)
12 or more years	0.146 (0.019)	0.077 (0.013)	1.00	1.00
White, age 65–74 years				
0–4 years	0.450 (0.038)	0.307 (0.040)	1.56 (1.22–2.00)	1.98 (1.45–2.71)
5–8 yeras	0.366 (0.019)	0.201 (0.016)	1.26 (1.04–1.51)	1.25 (1.00–1.56)
9–11 years	0.345 (0.034)	0.199 (0.024)	1.13 (0.87–1.46)	1.20 (0.91–1.58)
12 or more years	0.294 (0.022)	0.170 (0.016)	1.00	1.00
Black, age 65–74 years				
0–4 years	0.424 (0.042)	0.317 (0.046)	1.12 (0.72–1.73)	1.51 (0.93–2.47)
5–8 years	0.374 (0.051)	0.197 (0.035)	0.97 (0.60–1.58)	1.05 (0.64–1.73)
9 or more years	0.381 (0.069)	0.264 (0.051)	1.00	1.00

clear that for both men and women the relative risk of death decreases with increasing education.

In contrast to the results for elderly white persons, survival was not clearly associated with educational attainment among black persons 65–74 years of age (Table 8–2). Among elderly black women the risk of death appears to be greatest for those with the least education, but the difference is not statistically significant. The relative risk estimate is 1.51 for black women with 0–4 years of education as compared with those who have 9 or more years of education, but the 95% confidence interval ranges from 0.93 to 2.47. The inability to detect a relationship may be due to the small numbers of deaths (110 deaths among black women and 145 deaths among black men).

The relative risk of death was 52% greater among white men aged 55–64 years who had 0–11 years of education as compared with men of the same age and racial group who had 12 or more years of education (95% confidence interval = 1.09–2.13). Among white women aged 55–64 years the estimated relative risk is 1.35, but the 95% confidence interval includes 1 (0.87–2.08) (Table 8–2).

MARITAL STATUS DIFFERENTIALS

The distribution of marital status at baseline in the NHEFS sample also varies considerably by age, race, and gender (Table 8–3). The proportion married at baseline ranges from 35.8% among black women 65–74 years of age to 85.8% among white men aged 55–64 years. The percentage widowed at baseline is much higher among women than among men; it varies from 20% of white women aged 55–64 to 54.5% of black women 65–74 years of age. Only among white persons 65–74 years are there sufficient numbers of deaths to present mortality results for subgroups of the unmarried (never married, widowed, separated, divorced). For other age and race groups the married have been compared with all of the unmarried.

Survival among married white men aged 65–74 is higher than for the widowed, never married, or separated/divorced. Survival among the three unmarried groups is similar for elderly white men (Fig. 8–3). The probability of death after 8 years is 0.341 for married elderly white men, as compared with 0.406 for the unmarried. The corresponding probabilities for white men 55–64 years of age are 0.160 and 0.233. The results of the proportional hazards regression model (Table 8–4) indicate that the relative risk of death for unmarried white men aged 65–74, as compared with married white men of the same age, is 1.26 (95% confidence interval = 1.05–1.52). The corresponding differential for white men aged 55–64 years is even larger; that is, a relative risk of 1.71 (95% confidence interval = 1.15–2.56). The relative risk of death for unmarried white men in both age groups remains about the same after adjustment for educational attainment.

The relationship between marital status at baseline and mortality for white women differs from the pattern observed for white men. Among white women 65–74 years of age, survival is highest among the never married (Fig. 8–4), especially

Table 8–3 Percentage Distribution of the NHEFS Cohort and Number of Deaths by Marital Status According to Race, Gender and Age at Baseline (NHANES I)

Race and marital status	Age 55–64 years		Age 65–74 years	
	Men	Women	Men	Women
	Percentage distribution of the sample			
White				
Total	100.0	100.0 '	100.0	100.0
Married	85.8	71.4	81.9	49.2
Widowed	3.2	20.0	7.9	41.1
Never married	5.3	3.9	6.3	5.8
Divorced/separated	5.7	4.8	3.8	3.9
Missing	0.1	—	0.1	0.1
Black				
Total	100.0	100.0	100.0	100.0
Married	66.7	49.6	70.3	35.8
Widowed	8.6	27.0	15.7	54.5
Never married	3.8	4.3	5.1	3.3
Divorced/separated	21.0	19.1	8.9	6.4
Missing	1.0	0.7	—	0.6
	No. of deaths			
White				
Total	149	84	675	467
Married	119	55	532	225
Widowed	6	22	62	206
Never married	9	3	50	20
Divorced/separated	15	4	31	16
Missing	0	0	0	0
Black				
Total	33	16	145	110
Married	17	10	104	30
Widowed	3	3	23	70
Never married	2	1	8	2
Divorced/separated	10	2	10	6
Missing	1	0	0	2

after 4 years of follow-up. Survival estimates for separated and divorced elderly white women are not shown because of the small sample size and few expected deaths in this group. The relative risk of death among never-married white women aged 65–74, as compared with ever-married women, is 0.64 (95% confidence interval = 0.41–1.01). Adjustment for education decreases the marital status differential slightly to 0.69 (95% confidence interval = 0.44–1.09).

Among white women aged 55–64 years, differences in mortality by marital status at baseline were not significant. The probability of death after 8 years was 0.069 for the married and 0.103 for the unmarried, most of whom were widowed. The relative risk of death for the unmarried compared to the married was 1.32 (95% confidence interval = 0.84–2.08).

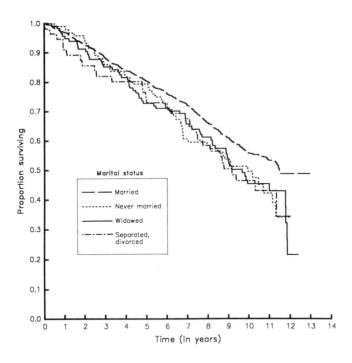

Fig. 8–3. Survival of the NHEFS cohort according to marital status at baseline (NHANES I) for white men 65–74 years of age at baseline (NHANES I).

Table 8–4 Relationship Between Marital Status and Risk of Subsequent Death in NHEFS Cohort According to Race, Gender and Age at Baseline (NHANES I)

Race, age at baseline, and marital status	Kaplan–Meier estimates Probability of death after 8 years (SE)		Cox regression results Relative risk (95% CI)	
	Men	Women	Men	Women
White, age 55–64 years				
Unmarried	0.233 (0.043)	0.103 (0.020)	1.71 (1.15–2.56)	1.32 (0.84–2.08)
Married	0.160 (0.015)	0.069 (0.011)	1.00	1.00
White, age 65–74 years				
Unmarried	0.406 (0.031)	0.214 (0.014)	1.26 (1.05–1.52)	1.00 (0.83–1.20)
Married	0.341 (0.014)	0.181 (0.014)	1.00	1.00
Widowed	0.390 (0.046)	0.228 (0.016)	1.18 (0.91–1.54)	1.06 (0.87–1.28)
Never married	0.418 (0.052)	0.137 (0.035)	1.31 (0.98–1.76)	0.68 (0.43–1.08)
Divorced/separated	0.418 (0.067)	0.190 (0.049)	1.36 (0.94–1.95)	0.89 (0.54–1.48)
Black, age 65–74 years				
Unmarried	0.454 (0.058)	0.291 (0.033)	1.16 (0.81–1.67)	1.46 (0.95–2.24)
Married	0.376 (0.034)	0.198 (0.038)	1.00	1.00

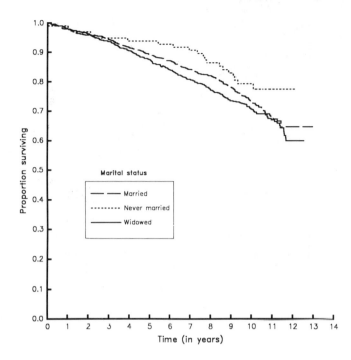

Fig. 8—4. Survival of the NHEFS cohort according to marital status at baseline (NHANES I) for white women 65—74 years of age at baseline (NHANES I).

There were also no significant differences in mortality by marital status at baseline for black persons aged 65–74. However, among elderly black women there was some evidence of an increased risk of death among the unmarried, most of whom were widowed. Unmarried black women have a relative risk of death of 1.46 as compared with the married, but the 95% confidence interval is 0.95 to 2.24. The probability of death after 8 years is 0.291 for the unmarried, as compared with 0.198 for married elderly black women.

GEOGRAPHIC DIFFERENTIALS

The distribution of the sample by selected geographic characteristics of the place of residence at baseline is shown in Table 8–5. Region and metropolitan status distributions vary by age and race, but not by gender. The highest percentage of persons in all age and race groups resided in the South at baseline, but the proportion is highest for black persons aged 65–74 (57.4%). This pattern is similar to the distribution for the U.S. population. There are also large racial differences in the percentage of persons living in the central cities of standard metropolitan statistical areas (SMSA). More than half of the black persons in both age groups live in the central city as compared with 25–28% of white persons. Furthermore, less than

Table 8–5 Percentage Distribution of the NHEFS Cohort by Place of Residence According to Race, Gender, and Age at Baseline (NHANES I)

Region and metropolitan status of place of residence at baseline	Age 55–64 years		Age 65–74 years	
	White	Black	White	Black
	No. in sample			
Total	1558	248	3181	645
Males	741	106	1501	313
Females	817	142	1680	332
	Percentage distribution of the sample			
Region				
Northeast	23.7	21.4	21.9	13.0
Midwest	26.3	21.8	24.9	18.0
South	29.1	45.6	31.3	57.4
West	20.9	11.3	21.8	11.6
Metropolitan status				
SMSA,* central city	25.1	63.7	28.0	53.5
SMSA, not central city	30.0	9.3	24.6	6.7
Non-SMSA	44.9	27.0	47.3	39.8

*Standard Metropolitan Statistical Area.

10% of black persons live outside the central cities of SMSA, as compared with 25–30% of white persons in the two age groups.

Figures 8–5 and 8–6 present cumulative survival distributions by region for white persons aged 65–74. White men 65–74 years of age residing in the South appear to have lower rates of survival than those in the other regions. The Cox regression analysis indicates that for elderly white men the relative risk of death is 0.83 for those residing outside the South (95% confidence interval = 0.71–0.98) (Table 8–6). The relative risks of death are similar for each of the three regions outside the South (Northeast, Midwest, and West). This result remains the same after adjustment for both education and residence in a poverty area.

Among white women aged 65–74 years, cumulative survival in the Midwest region appears higher than that for any of the other regions (Fig. 8–6). The regression model also indicates that residents of this age and gender group in the Midwest region have a lower relative risk of death than those living in other regions, all of which have similar survival rates for this subgroup.

Mortality in the South does not differ from mortality outside the South for white persons aged 55–64 or for black persons 65–74 years old at baseline. However, among elderly black men there is some evidence of lower mortality in the South. The proportion of elderly black men dying after 8 years in the South is 0.364, as compared with 0.440 outside the South. The numbers of deaths in these subgroups are too small to make additional regional comparisons.

There are no significant differences in mortality between populations of metropolitan areas and those of nonmetropolitan areas, except among black women aged

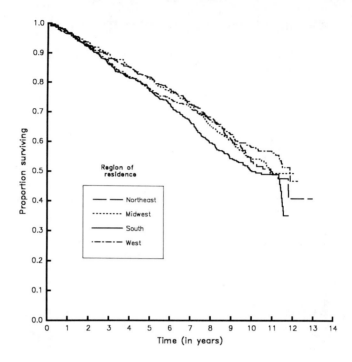

Fig. 8–5. Survival of the NHEFS cohort according to region of residence at baseline (NHANES I) for white men 65–74 years of age at baseline (NHANES I).

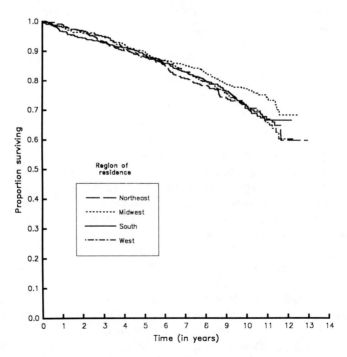

Fig. 8–6. Survival of the NHEFS cohort according to region of residence at baseline (NHANES I) for white women 65–74 years of age at baseline (NHANES I).

Table 8–6 Relationship Between Region of Residence and Risk of Subsequent Death in the NHEFS Cohort According to Race, Gender and Age at Baseline (NHANES I)

Race, age at baseline, and region of residence at baseline	Kaplan–Meier estimates		Cox regression results	
	Probability of death after 8 years (SE)		Relative risk (95% CI)	
	Men	Women	Men	Women
White, age 55–64 years				
Outside South	0.163 (0.016)	0.083 (0.012)	0.92 (0.65–1.30)	1.10 (0.68–1.78)
South	0.187 (0.027)	0.067 (0.017)	1.00	1.00
White, age 65–74 years				
Outside South	0.330 (0.015)	0.197 (0.012)	0.83 (0.71–0.98)	0.92 (0.76–1.11)
South	0.402 (0.023)	0.200 (0.018)	1.00	1.00
Northeast	0.317 (0.026)	0.217 (0.022)	0.86 (0.69–1.06)	1.01 (0.79–1.30)
Midwest	0.347 (0.025)	0.174 (0.019)	0.84 (0.69–1.03)	0.77 (0.60–0.99)
West	0.324 (0.025)	0.203 (0.022)	0.80 (0.65–0.99)	1.02 (0.80–1.30)
Black, age 65–74 years				
Outside South	0.440 (0.045)	0.229 (0.038)	1.28 (0.92–1.77)	0.94 (0.63–1.38)
South	0.364 (0.038)	0.274 (0.033)	1.00	1.00

65–74 (Table 8–7). For this group the relative risk of death is 0.67 in metropolitan areas, as compared with nonmetropolitan areas (95% confidence interval = 0.46–0.98). As indicated earlier, almost all black residents of metropolitan areas live in the central city rather than outside of the city. It is unclear why this mortality differential should be limited to elderly black women, the vast majority (85%) of whom resided at baseline in poverty areas regardless of metropolitan status.

The analysis for white persons 65–74 years of age further divides the populations of metropolitan areas into those within and those outside the central city. Cumulative survival curves for white men and women 65–74 years of age show that survival is greatest among residents outside the central city (Figs. 8–7 and 8–8).

The Cox regression analysis (Table 8–7) indicates that among white men 65–74 years of age the risk of death is 0.83 for metropolitan area residents outside the central city, as compared with nonmetropolitan residents (95% confidence interval = 0.68–1.00). Among white women 65–74 years of age, the relative risk estimate is similar (0.81), but the 95% confidence interval is somewhat larger (0.64–1.04). However, after adjustment for education and residence in poverty areas, these differentials decrease substantially for both men and women. The adjusted risk estimates are 0.89 for elderly white men and 0.88 for elderly white women, and these values are not significantly different from 1.

SUMMARY OF NHEFS MORTALITY FINDINGS

The sociodemographic differentials in mortality found in NHEFS are generally consistent with results from previous studies. A significant inverse relationship between education and mortality was found for white men and women 65–74 years

Table 8-7 Relationship Between Metropolitan Status of Residence and Risk of Subsequent Death in the NHEFS Cohort According to Race, Gender, and Age at Baseline (NHANES I)

Race, age at baseline, and metropolitan status of residence at baseline	Kaplan–Meier estimates		Cox regression results	
	Probability of death after 8 years (SE)		Relative risk (95% CI)	
	Men	Women	Men	Women
White, age 55–64 years				
Metropolitan	0.168 (0.019)	0.089 (0.014)	0.96 (0.70–1.33)	1.17 (0.76–1.81)
Nonmetropolitan	0.173 (0.021)	0.066 (0.013)	1.00	1.00
White, age 65–74 years				
Metropolitan	0.333 (0.017)	0.190 (0.014)	0.89 (0.77–1.04)	0.95 (0.79–1.14)
Nonmetropolitan	0.372 (0.018)	0.205 (0.014)	1.00	1.00
Central city, metropolitan	0.350 (0.024)	0.213 (0.019)	0.96 (0.80–1.15)	1.07 (0.87–1.32)
Other metropolitan	0.316 (0.024)	0.162 (0.019)	0.83 (0.68–1.00)	0.81 (0.64–1.04)
Black, age 65–74 years				
Metropolitan	0.401 (0.038)	0.216 (0.031)	1.09 (0.78–1.52)	0.67 (0.46–0.98)
Nonmetropolitan	0.390 (0.045)	0.313 (0.041)	1.00	1.00

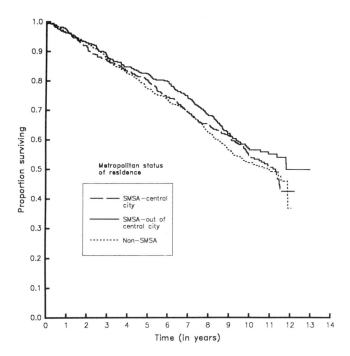

Fig. 8–7. Survival of the NHEFS cohort according to metropolitan (standard metropolitan statistical area; SMSA) status of residence at baseline (NHANES I) for white men 65–74 years of age at baseline (NHANES I).

of age and for white men aged 55–64. Additional years of mortality follow-up are needed to further evaluate educational differentials in mortality among persons in the other age, race, and gender subgroups. The results for white men aged 65–74 years differ from the 1960 matched-records study (Kitagawa and Hauser 1973), in which no educational differential was found for elderly white men. A study of national trends in educational differentials in mortality based on the 1960 matched-records study and the NHEFS shows that among white men death rates have declined more rapidly for the more educated than the less educated (Feldman et al. 1989). In contrast, among white women death rates have declined at about the same rate, regardless of educational attainment. Trends in educational differentials for heart disease mortality are responsible for much of the change for all causes of death (Feldman et al. 1989).

Statistically significant mortality differentials by marital status were found in the same age, race, and gender subgroups as for education. In general, the unmarried had a higher risk of mortality than the married. As in the 1960 study, marital status differentials were stronger for men than for women (Kitagawa and Hauser 1973). Among white men differences between the married and unmarried were greater for the 55–64-year-old age group than for those aged 65–74 years. Among

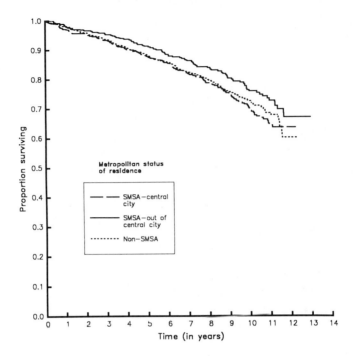

Fig. 8–8. Survival of the NHEFS cohort according to metropolitan (standard metropolitan statistical area; SMSA) status of residence at baseline (NHANES I) for white women 65–74 years of age at baseline (NHANES I).

white women aged 65–74 years, the never married experienced somewhat lower mortality than those who were ever married, although this difference was of marginal significance.

The geographic mortality differentials noted for white persons aged 65–74 years are consistent with the patterns found by Sauer (National Center for Health Statistics 1980). Among elderly white men the South had higher mortality than other regions, and among elderly white women the Midwest region had somewhat lower mortality than other regions. For white persons, there were no differences in mortality between metropolitan and nonmetropolitan areas; this finding confirms the observations of Sauer. Regional variation in disease risk factors, medical care, and socioeconomic factors may explain some of the regional differences in mortality. However, a study of regional variation in ischemic heart disease (IHD) mortality among white men 55 years and over based on the NHEFS found that regional variation in cardiovascular risk factors could not explain regional variation in IHD mortality (Garg et al. 1989). Additional research is needed to understand better the reasons for educational, marital status, and geographic differences in mortality.

REFERENCES

Comstock, G. W., and J. A. Tonascia. 1977. "Education and mortality in Washington County, Maryland." *J Health Soc Behav* 18:54–61.

Cox, D. R. 1972. "Regression models and life tables" (with discussion). *J Roy Statist Soc B* 34:187–220.

Feldman, J. J., D. M. Makuc, J. C. Kleinman, and J. Cornoni-Huntley. 1989. "National trends in educational differentials in mortality." *Amer J Epidemiol* 129:919–933.

Garg, R., J. H. Madans, J. C. Kleinman, and C. Cox. 1989. "Regional variation in mortality associated with IHD." Presented at the 1989 Epidemic Intelligence Service Conference.

Kaplan, E. L., and P. Meier. 1958. "Nonparametric estimation from incomplete observations." *J Am Stat Assoc* 53:457–481.

Kitagawa, E. M., and P. M. Hauser, 1973. *Differential Mortality in the United States: A Study in Socioeconomic Epidemiology.* Cambridge, MA: Harvard University Press.

Makuc, D., and J. C. Kleinman. 1986. "Survival analysis using complex survey data: examples from the NHANES I Epidemiologic Follow-up Study." Presented at the 1986 Annual Meeting of the American Statistical Association.

National Center for Health Statistics. 1980. Sauer, H. I. Geographic Patterns in the Risk of Dying and Associated Factors, Ages 35–74 years, United States 1968–1972. *Vital and Health Statistics.* Series 3., No. 18. DHHS Pub. No. (PHS) 80-1402. Washington, DC: U.S. Government Printing Office.

Peto, R., M. C. Pike, P. Armitage et al. 1976. "Design and analysis of randomized clinical trials requiring prolonged observation of each patient." *Br J Cancer* 34:585–612.

Rosen, S., and P. Taubman. 1979. "Changes in the impact of education and income on mortality in the U.S." In *Statistical Uses of Administrative Records with Emphasis on Mortality and Disability Research.* U.S. DHEW, Washington, DC: U.S. Government Printing Office.

SAS Institute, Inc. 1983. *SAS Supplemental Library User's Guide,* 1983 ed. Cary, NC.

SAS Institute, Inc. 1985. *SAS User's Guide: Statistics,* Version 5 Edition. Cary, NC.

9

Use of Alcohol and Tobacco

MARY DUFOUR, JAMES COLLIVER,
M. BETH GRIGSON, AND FREDERICK STINSON

It is estimated that between 1984 and 2050 the total population of the United States will increase by a third, whereas the number of those 55 and over is expected to more than double (U.S. Administration on Aging 1988). With this increase in the elderly population, alcohol- and tobacco-related morbidity and mortality may increase also. To date, few studies have focused upon the use over time of alcohol and tobacco products or the health-related consequences of such usage among older individuals. Discussion in this chapter encompasses the patterns of alcohol use and smoking of persons aged 55 and older, changes in these patterns over time, the relationship of alcohol consumption to cigarette smoking, and mortality associated with the use of these substances.

ALCOHOL CONSUMPTION

Information gathered on alcohol consumption was limited in the National Health and Nutrition Examination Survey (NHANES I). The items dealing with alcohol consumption were incorporated into the medical history questionnaire. Questions on alcohol consumption were much more detailed in the NHANES I Epidemiologic Follow-up Study (NHEFS) and were prefaced by the explanation that alcoholic beverages include liquor, such as whiskey, rum, gin, or vodka, as well as beer and wine. Additional items included respondents' self-perceived drinking level and their usual drinking pattern at ages 25, 35, 45, 55, 65, and 75, as applicable. The beverage portion of the nutrition questionnaire included additional questions on average consumption of beer, wine, and liquor.

Drinking levels for each respondent were determined on the basis of average daily consumption of absolute alcohol computed from responses to items regarding the quantity and frequency (QF) of drinking. The average daily number of drinks, determined directly from QF data, was converted to ounces of pure ethanol by assuming that each drink contains 0.5 oz of alcohol.

172

To establish levels of drinking for analyses, ranges of average daily consumption were used for classification of respondents into the following four categories: (1) abstainer, (2) light drinker, (3) moderate drinker, 4) heavy drinker. The ranges of ethanol consumption for these categories were an average of less than 0.01 oz of ethanol daily for abstainers (<7.3 drinks a year); 0.01–0.21 oz for light drinkers (one drink every 3–50 days); 0.22–0.99 oz for moderate drinkers (more than one drink every 3 days but less than two drinks per day); and 1.00 oz or more per day for heavy drinkers (at least two drinks per day). This classification scheme has been used in recent surveys by other researchers (Johnson et al. 1977). Despite some limitations, it has been shown that the reliability of QF scores is quite high when this methodology is used (Williams, Malin, and Aitken 1985).

It is important to note that "heavy drinking" does not mean excessive or problem drinking. In addition, it should be noted that the category "abstainer" includes more than "nondrinkers." Although in both surveys the "abstainer" category represented persons who drank <0.01 ounce of ethanol per day, the sequence of questions used to differentiate drinkers from abstainers differed between the NHANES I and the NHEFS. In NHANES I, to be classed as an abstainer, respondents had to have reported less than one drink of beer, wine, or liquor in the previous year. In the NHEFS, respondents were asked if they had consumed at least 12 drinks of any kind of alcoholic beverage in any one year and at least one drink in the past year. Those answering affirmatively were considered to be drinkers. People who did not meet these criteria were designated abstainers.

Questions are often raised about the reliability and validity of survey data on alcohol consumption. The NHEFS provides an opportunity to examine reliability and internal consistency because, in addition to the items in the alcohol section, alcohol consumption questions appear in the nutrition section. A comparison of the responses from these two sections indicates that people are consistent in the categorized levels of alcohol consumption they report. Eighty-eight percent of the respondents fell into the same drinking category in both the alcohol and nutrition sections. Of the remaining respondents, approximately half reported drinking more on the nutrition portion and half reported drinking less. In most cases the differences were not large, varying by only one category (e.g., abstainer vs. light drinker). Large discrepancies between the quantities reported in the two sections were found for only 11 individuals.

Also of interest are the respondents' self-perceived levels of alcohol consumption as compared with the previously described drinking categories. When information provided by proxy respondents is excluded, 27.3% of abstainers, 93.0% of light drinkers, 17.1% of moderate drinkers, and 2.0% of heavy drinkers fell into the same category in both classification schemes. The majority (81.9%) of the moderate drinkers perceived themselves to be light drinkers, whereas, of the heavy drinkers, 49.6% categorized themselves as moderate drinkers and 48.1% considered themselves to be light drinkers. Although the constructed categories are valuable for analyses of trends and to facilitate comparisons with many other studies, the discrepancy between the constructed and the self-reported drinking levels needs further examination. It is quite probable that the public has more liberal definitions of the

Table 9–1 Percentage Distribution of Drinking Patterns at NHEFS, According to Gender and Race

Drinking categories	White men (n = 1271)	Black men (n = 185)	White women (n = 1734)	Black women (n = 295)
Abstainers and light	73.7	86.5	90.5	95.9
Moderate and heavy	26.3	13.5	9.5	4.1

Note: Numbers for NHEFS exclude data from respondents for whom information was obtained only from a proxy.

terms moderate and heavy drinking than those used in constructing the categories in research on alcohol use (Malin, Wilson, and Williams 1985).

Patterns of alcohol consumption were examined for all respondents to NHANES I and all respondents to NHEFS; however, subjects who responded via proxies were excluded. Table 9–1 summarizes the drinking patterns at NHEFS by race and gender. These patterns conform to the results from numerous other studies that have shown marked differences in drinking patterns between men and women and between blacks and whites; there were substantially larger numbers of moderate or heavy drinkers among whites and among men (National Institute on Alcohol Abuse and Alcoholism 1984; Malin et al. 1986; Wilsnack, Wilsnack, and Klassen 1984). At both surveys, black women had the highest proportion of abstainers and the lowest proportion of heavy drinkers. Among men, both blacks and whites had similar proportions of light and moderate drinkers; however, black men had higher rates of abstention and lower rates of heavy drinking.

Since the lower limit of the heavy drinking category, two drinks per day, is conservative, this category was divided into three subcategories for close characterization of the heaviest consumers. The three categories chosen, in ounces of pure ethanol per day were (1) 1.000–1.999, (2) 2.000–2.999, and (3) ≥3.000. Table 9–2 shows the distribution of white persons by gender in these categories. Not surprisingly, most individuals in the heavy-drinking category fell into the lowest level in the subclassification scheme, with proportions of respondents decreasing as the consumption levels increased. Similar trends were seen for black persons, but the numbers were very small.

Since drinking levels are dynamic over time, changes in patterns of alcohol consumption for individuals from NHANES I to NHEFS are of special interest. For this portion of the analysis, individuals for whom proxy respondents provided

Table 9–2 Percentage of White Persons in the Heavy Drinking Category by Daily Alcohol Consumption According to Gender

Pure ethanol (oz/day)	White men (n = 178)	White women (n = 59)
1–1.999	71.3	86.4
2–2.999	16.9	10.2
≥3.000	11.8	3.4

Table 9–3 Changes in Alcohol Consumption Between NHANES I and NHEFS According to Gender and Age at Baseline (NHANES I)

Drinking category at baseline (NHANES I)	Percentage (No.) in indicated drinking category at NHEFS			
	Abstainer/light drinker		Moderate/heavy drinker	
	%	n	%	n
Men				
55–64				
Abstainer/light drinker	55.9	349	10.6	66
Moderate/heavy drinker	12.2	76	21.3	133
65–74				
Abstainer/light drinker	68.8	583	6.2	53
Moderate/heavy drinker	11.9	101	13.1	111
Women				
55–64				
Abstainer/light drinker	82.4	643	5.1	40
Moderate/heavy drinker	6.2	48	6.3	49
65–74				
Abstainer/light drinker	89.3	1120	2.7	34
Moderate/heavy drinker	3.8	48	4.2	52

information were excluded from both the baseline and follow-up analyses. In addition to the aggregate categories shown in Table 9–3, several patterns of change in drinking categories were examined in detail, including (1) baseline drinkers who had become abstainers at follow-up (11.2% of the sample); (2) abstainers and light drinkers who became moderate or heavy drinkers (7.9%); (3) continued heavy drinkers (3.8%); (4) new heavy drinkers (3.5%); (5) continued light/moderate drinkers (27.4%); and (6) lifetime abstainers (51.9%). Most (87.3%) of the baseline abstainers, approximately half of the light and heavy drinkers, and a quarter of the moderate drinkers fell into the same category at follow-up. In addition, a third of those classified as light drinkers at NHANES I fell into the abstainer class at NHEFS. Also becoming abstainers at follow-up were 17.8% of the moderate drinkers at baseline and 13.8% of the heavy drinkers at baseline. Respondents who were abstainers or light drinkers at baseline and became moderate to heavy drinkers at follow-up represented 7.9% of the sample.

Among lifetime abstainers, nearly half (50.2%) gave "don't care to/dislike alcoholic beverages" as their reason for not drinking. The second most common reason for not drinking was equally divided among "not necessary," "religious/moral reasons," and "upbringing," each representing approximately 14% of the responses. Among persons who were former drinkers but had abstained for at least one year prior to the NHEFS (13.4% of the total sample), the most common reason for not drinking was "health reasons" (35.2%), followed by "don't care to/dislike" (28.1%), "not necessary" (17.3%), and "religious/moral reasons" (10.7%). Only 1.3% of these former drinkers specifically mentioned being an alcoholic as the reason for not drinking, although a portion of those listing health reasons might be individuals suffering from medical consequences of alcohol abuse.

Statements can be found in the literature to the effect that people tend to drink less as they age (Gomberg 1982; Straus 1984); however, little research has actually addressed the question of whether individuals decrease alcohol consumption with age or whether the observed differences result from a cohort phenomenon reflecting changes in societal drinking practices and attitudes over time. In the NHEFS the answers to questions on lifetime drinking history at 10-year intervals provide a unique opportunity to address this issue.

Examination of lifetime patterns of drinking is summarized in Figs. 9–1 and 9–2. Data from two groups of respondents were compared: those 65–74 years of age and those 75–84 years of age at follow-up. The percentage of abstainers is shown in Fig. 9–1 for the two cohorts. Although more members of the older cohort reported that they had been abstainers at age 25, there were minimal differences in the percentage of abstainers at the other 10-year age intervals. Many in the older cohort would have been age 25 during Prohibition. Perhaps Prohibition did deter some young people from beginning to drink during those years.

Figure 9–2 shows the percentage of heavy drinkers for the two age groups. The trend of an increasing percentage of heavy drinkers among persons up to 45–55 years of age followed by a decrease at age 65 is seen for both cohorts. However, the percentage of heavy drinkers at each age is consistently less for the older cohort.

Contradictory information provided by a few respondents drew attention to possible validity issues in the historical data. Assuming that respondents desire to make truthful responses, it is logical to expect that one would remember more

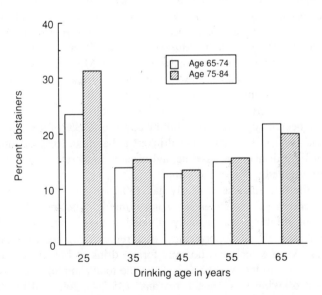

Fig. 9–1. Percentage of abstainers according to cohort and age (proxy respondents included).

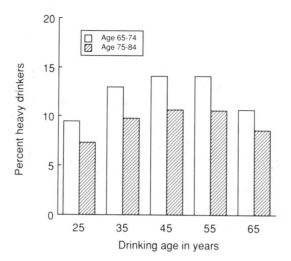

Fig. 9–2. Percentage of heavy drinkers according to cohort and age (proxy respondents included).

accurately how one drank over the year prior to questioning than one could recall drinking 10, 20, or even 50 years prior to an interview. Nevertheless, although one might not recall the exact consumption pattern at precisely age 25, most mentally intact individuals probably have a general idea of approximately when in their lives their highest and lowest levels of drinking actually occurred. However, the people who provided conflicting data were those who were categorized as moderate or light drinkers at the initial examination but who at the follow-up interview gave long histories of continuous, very heavy consumption that overlapped the baseline period of supposedly lower consumption. For example, a white man who was 55 years old at baseline was classed as a moderate drinker on the basis of data provided by the NHANES I interview. At the follow-up interview, however, he reported that he averaged six to eight drinks per day at age 55, and this level of consumption was identical to the one that he reported for ages 25, 35, and 45. This drinking level is well above the two drinks-per-day cutoff necessary to be classified as a heavy drinker. It may be that he, and the few other respondents who reported in a similar manner, might have felt that it is more socially acceptable to admit that one was a heavy drinker in the past than to acknowledge that one is currently a heavy drinker. This data set will provide a valuable opportunity to investigate such issues in more detail.

TOBACCO CONSUMPTION

Questions on tobacco use appeared in the general medical history supplement of NHANES I; this supplement was given only to individuals participating in the detailed component of the examination. This procedure is significant methodologically because only half of the individuals were asked the questions on both alcohol and tobacco. Persons who had smoked at least 100 cigarettes in their lifetimes were designated as smokers. Questions also were asked for cigar and pipe use. Questions on use of other tobacco products were more limited.

Questions on the NHEFS instrument regarding cigarette use were very similar to those asked at NHANES I, but items on the use of other forms of tobacco were more restricted. At follow-up (NHEFS) the questions on smoking were asked of all respondents and included items on the ages at which persons stopped and resumed smoking. Because of the lack of data on smoking for many NHANES I participants, staff of the National Center for Health Statistics developed a methodology for imputing smoking status at baseline from data on smoking history obtained at NHEFS. By use of the ages of cessation and resumption (which covered up to four episodes of smoking and nonsmoking), the total number of years respondents had smoked up to NHEFS was determined, and lifetime nonsmokers were identified. For most respondents this same information was used for determination of baseline smoking status and years smoked up to the age at baseline.

The most meaningful analyses of tobacco consumption as a factor contributing to various health-related conditions have incorporated a cumulative quantity–frequency measure, such as "pack-years." Although detailed data on cigarette consumption per year were not obtained at baseline, estimates of "pack years" can be obtained from information on the smoking history included in the follow-up questionnaire. Even when such a measure is not available at baseline, it is desirable to identify indexes that treat tobacco consumption in several categories, ideally ordinal or interval rather than as a simple dichotomous variable. At the most basic level, a person who is currently a nonsmoker but who smoked previously cannot be classified with lifetime nonsmokers.

For these reasons, a decision was made to categorize persons who had ever smoked as having smoked for (1) the median or more years ("High Smoking") or (2) less than the median number of years ("Low Smoking") for persons of their 5-year age group who had ever smoked. The third descriptive category was assigned to persons who never smoked ("Never Smoked"). All available data for all respondents, including those responding via a proxy, were used in the following analyses.

Distributions of smoking status by age, gender, and race were nearly identical for both studies; therefore, only the data from the NHEFS will be presented (Table 9–4). The percentage of persons who never smoked shows a clear cohort effect, with more persons who never smoked in the older groups. The percentages who had never smoked were as follows: 39.7% of men and 79.0% of women in the oldest group (70–74 years old at baseline); 32.0% of men and 73.7% of women in the group aged 65–69 years; 28.2% of men and 66.3% of women in the group aged 60–64 years; and 23.1% of men and 59.8% of women in the group aged 55–59 years. A higher percentage of lifetime nonsmokers was found among blacks.

Many current smokers at NHANES I had become former smokers at NHEFS. Only 1.4% of former smokers at baseline had resumed the practice at follow-up, and still fewer (0.1%) of those who had never smoked up to the time of baseline were current smokers at NHEFS.

Table 9–4 Distribution by Smoking Status at NHEFS According to Age at Baseline (NHANES I)

Age at NHANES I (years)	Total no. of respondents (n)	Percentage in indicated category			
		Lifetime nonsmokers	Former smokers	Current smokers	Unknown
55–59	880	43.9	36.4	18.4	1.3
60–64	762	52.2	32.4	12.9	2.5
65–69	1911	60.0	30.7	8.0	1.3
70–74	1375	69.4	26.9	3.1	0.6

Note: Data for persons responding through proxies are included.

Marked differences in patterns of alcohol consumption were seen in these different groups of smokers, particularly if the groups were disaggregated by gender (Table 9–5). Many of those who never smoked were also found to be abstainers from alcohol at NHEFS. The two groups of former smokers show patterns of alcohol consumption falling between those of the lifetime nonsmokers and the current smokers. Abstainers had the smallest number of continuing smokers. These findings reconfirm the well-known association between use of tobacco and alcohol (Maletsky and Kotler 1974; Rothman and Keller 1972; Walton 1972).

Information on consumption of tobacco products other than cigarettes is more limited and is primarily descriptive. Approximately a quarter of the people aged 60 years and over and 30% of the 55–59-year-olds (at baseline) reported that they had ever smoked a pipe or cigars. Slightly over half of the men reported ever having used cigars or a pipe, but only 2.2% of the women did. Proportionately, the races were equally represented. Far fewer individuals reported current pipe or cigar usage. There was a slight decrease in usage between NHANES I and NHEFS, with 5.0% of the younger group and only 2.0% of the older group reporting current usage. More men (19.8%) than women (8.2%) who had ever used a pipe or cigars reported current usage. Among blacks who had ever used a pipe or cigars, 36.6% reported current usage, compared with 16.6% of whites.

Approximately 8.8% of the sample reported ever using snuff, with no clear difference over the age groups. Proportionately, almost as many women as men reported using snuff, but nearly three times as many blacks as whites fell into this category (18.7% of blacks vs. 7.2% of whites). About one eighth of the respondents reported ever having used chewing tobacco, regardless of age. The majority of chewing tobacco users were men (85.0%), and proportionately twice as many blacks (23.3%) as whites (11.7%) reported usage.

EFFECT OF ALCOHOL AND TOBACCO USE ON MORTALITY

For assessment of the effects of smoking, drinking, gender, and race on mortality from selected underlying causes of death, survival analysis was used to generate mortality indicators for each 5-year age group. This procedure yielded cumulative probabilities of not dying from specific causes within 5 or 8 years following the

Table 9–5 Percentage Distribution by Change in Smoking Categories Between Baseline (NHANES I) and Follow-up (NHEFS) According to Drinking Categories at Baseline (NHANES I) and Gender

Drinking category at NHANES I	Percentage (no.) of subjects in indicated smoking category									
	Never smoked		Nonsmoker at NHANES I and NHEFS*		Smoker at NHANES, nonsmoker at NHEFS		Smoker at both NHANES I and NHEFS		Total sample	
	%	n	%	n	%	n	%	n	%	n
Men										
Abstainer	37.4	409	26.5	290	17.0	186	7.0	77	100	1073
Light	29.5	179	28.3	172	22.1	134	11.2	68	100	607
Moderate	25.2	85	30.8	104	21.3	72	14.2	48	100	338
Heavy	24.7	72	24.7	72	22.6	66	15.8	46	100	292
Total	32.0	745	27.4	638	19.7	458	10.3	239	100	2330
Women										
Abstainer	78.1	1482	6.5	124	6.7	127	5.0	94	100	1898
Light	61.8	283	9.6	44	12.5	57	12.7	58	100	458
Moderate	41.0	64	15.4	24	12.8	20	20.5	32	100	156
Heavy	35.6	31	16.1	14	19.5	17	18.4	16	100	87
Total	71.6	1860	7.9	206	8.5	221	7.7	200	100	2599

Note: Numbers may not total to 100.0% due to rounding.
* As given, these people reported that although they were nonsmokers at the time of both surveys, they had smoked during some period of their lives (to be distinguished from lifetime nonsmokers, i.e., *Never Smoked*).

baseline examination. Separate rates were generated for each age group and for gender, race, smoking, and drinking categories at baseline. In creating the curves, cases were considered in the at-risk group starting with baseline, and mortality and survival rates for each year were calculated as the ratio of the number surviving through the year relative to the number alive at the beginning of the year. Only deaths from the specific cause were considered in calculating the number surviving; deaths from other causes were handled by right-censoring these deaths (i.e., removing them from both the at-risk and surviving groups for the next year). Individuals from whom follow-up data were collected during the 5- or 8-year period were also right-censored, according to the usual procedure for survival analysis. The cumulative probability of surviving through a specific year after baseline was determined by the Kaplan–Meier product-moment method (i.e., by taking the product of the probabilities of surviving in each year from the first through the target year). Estimates of survival rates were generated for the 5- or 8-year periods following baseline (Maddens et al. 1986). Numerous causes of death were investigated using this methodology. Only highlights of the findings related to alcohol and tobacco consumption will be presented here.

Analysis of the probability of dying from any cause in relation to drinking categories showed little effect for women. Among men of the younger age groups (ages 55–64), drinking status also had little effect. In the 70–74-year age group, however, men who were heavy drinkers were more likely to have died than those in the other groups (probabilities of 5-year survival: 0.749 for male abstainers and 0.689 for male heavy drinkers). All-cause mortality rates for men by drinking category were distributed as follows: abstainers, 32.8/100; light drinkers, 24.4/100; moderate drinkers, 21.3/100; and heavy drinkers, 31.6/100. All-cause mortality rates for men aged 70–74 years at baseline were not only higher overall but markedly higher for heavy drinkers as well: abstainers, 50.2/100, light drinkers, 41.0/100, moderate drinkers, 41.5/100, and heavy drinkers, 55.3/100. Deaths from cirrhosis of the liver were relatively rare, but the 10-year mortality rate for abstainers was 0.1/100 as compared with 0.9/100 for heavy drinkers.

With regard to smoking status, men in the high-smoking group had a much lower probability of survival than did either the never-smokers or the low-smoking group. For males aged 70–74 years at baseline, the probability of survival was 0.579 for high smokers and 0.609 for never-smokers.

Men had a much higher probability of dying from chronic lung disease (emphysema or chronic bronchitis) than did women. The 10-year mortality rate for men was 0.3/100, as compared with 0.1/100 for women. Heavy drinkers of both genders were much more likely to die from chronic lung disease than were persons in the other three drinking categories, which had similar mortality due to this cause. For example, among women, the death rate for abstainers was 0.2/100, while that for heavy drinkers was 1.3/100. A clear gradient was seen with regard to smoking status for men; those in the high-smoking group had a mortality rate (2.9/100), four times that of never smokers (0.7/100).

Men had a 10-year mortality rate from lung cancer four times higher than the rate for women (1.6/100 vs. 0.4/100). A striking relationship to smoking status was seen for men dying of lung cancer, with the high-smoking group (3.2/100) having mortality rates over 10 years that were nearly 11 times those of never-smokers (0.3/100).

With regard to acute myocardial infarction, women (3.7/100) had 10-year mortality rates half those of men (6.7/100). Among men, abstainers had the highest death rates (7.6/100) and light (4.8/100) and heavy drinkers (4.5/100), the lowest. Among women, on the other hand, minimal differences were seen across the drinking categories. Mortality from acute myocardial infarction showed no discernible trend by smoking categories.

An analysis of the NHEFS data on alcohol consumption and mortality from breast cancer is discussed in detail in Chapter 5. The results suggest that moderate alcohol consumption is associated with at least a 50% increase in the risk of breast cancer.

SUMMARY

Discussion in this chapter has encompassed the alcohol and smoking patterns of persons aged 55 years and older, changes in these over time, the relationship of alcohol consumption to cigarette smoking, and their relationship to subsequent mortality. These data confirm other research showing that women and blacks are more likely to be abstainers. The findings also support the hypothesis that alcohol and tobacco consumption are lower among older persons. Smoking and drinking practices were related to one another. Persons who abstained from one tended to abstain from the other.

The probability of dying from any cause was increased in heavy drinkers after age 70. Relationships of drinking and smoking to the chances of survival from various diseases were examined. Deaths from cirrhosis of the liver showed a strongly positive association with alcohol consumption among males. Likelihood of death from chronic lung disease was increased among heavy drinkers and among smokers. Death from breast cancer in women was associated with moderate or heavy use of alcohol.

This chapter has presented analyses based on smoking, alcohol use, and mortality data derived from NHEFS. A number of other analyses can be done, using this data set, especially on the relationship between the use of these substances and the development of morbidity and physical and mental disabilities. See Chapter 12 for a few examples of such analyses.

Another area of interest would be the relationship between use of these substances and self-perceptions of well-being. Additional research is needed to investigate further the factors determining changes in smoking and drinking behavior over time. It is hoped that other investigators will utilize this data set to elucidate further the complex interactions among social characteristics and substance use, on the one hand, and morbidity, disability, and death, on the other.

REFERENCES

Gomberg, E. 1982. Alcohol use and alcohol problems among the elderly. In National Institute on Alcohol Abuse and Alcoholism Alcohol and Health Monograph 4: Department of Health and Human Services Pub. No. (ADM) 82-1193. Rockville, MD: Department of Health and Human Services, pp. 263–290.

Herd, D. 1989. The epidemiology of drinking patterns and alcohol related problems among U.S. blacks. In National Institute on Alcohol Abuse and Alcoholism Research Monograph 18: *Alcohol Use Among U.S. Ethnic Minorities*. Department of Health and Human Services Pub. No. (ADM) 88-1435, Rockville, MD: Department of Health and Human Services, pp. 3–50.

Johnson, P., D. Armor, S. Polich, and H. Stambul. 1977. "U.S. adult drinking practices: time trends, social correlates and sex roles." Working note prepared for NIAAA. Contract No. ADM-281-76-0020. Santa Monica, CA: Rand Corp., pp. 7–8.

Maddens, J., C. Cox, J. Kleinman, D. Makuc, J. Feldman, F. Finucune, H. Barbano, and J. Cornoni-Huntley. 1986. "Ten years after HANES I: mortality experience at initial followup 1982–1984." *Public Health Rep* 101:474–481.

Maletzky, R., and J. Klotter. 1974. "Smoking and alcoholism." *Am J Psychiatry* 131:445–447.

Malin, H., R. Wilson, and G. Williams. 1985. "1983 NHIS Alcohol/Health Practices Supplement: preliminary findings." In *Proceedings of the 1985 Public Health Conference on Records and Statistics*. U.S. Department of Health and Human Services, Hyattsville, MD: Pub. No. (PHS) 86-1214. National Center for Health Statistics, pp. 490–495.

Malin, H., R. Wilson, G. Williams, and S. Aitken. 1986. "1983 alcohol/health practices supplement." *Alcohol Health Res World* 10:48–50.

National Institute on Alcohol Abuse and Alcoholism, 1984. Fifth Special Report to the U.S. Congress on Alcohol and Health from the Secretary of Health and Human Services, Department of Health and Human Services. Pub. No. (ADM) 84-1291. Rockville, MD: Department of Health and Human Services, pp. 2–3.

Rothman, K., and A. Keller. 1972. "The effect of joint exposure to alcohol and tobacco on risk of cancer of the mouth and pharynx." *J Chronic Dis* 25:711–716.

Straus, R. 1984. Alcohol problems among the elderly: the need for a biobehavioral perspective. In National Institute on Alcohol Abuse and Alcoholism Research Monograph No. 14. *Nature and Extent of Alcohol Problems Among the Elderly*. DHHS Pub. No. (ADM) 84-1321. Rockville, MD: Department of Health and Human Services, pp. 263–290.

U.S. Administration on Aging, 1988. *Aging America. Trends and Projections U.S.*, 1987–1988 ed. Washington, DC: Department of Health and Human Services, pp. 8–11.

Walton, R. 1972. "Smoking and alcoholism. A brief report." *Am J. Psychiatry* 1287:1455–1456.

Williams, G., H. Malin, and S. Aitken. 1985. "Reliability of self-reported drinking in a general population survey." *J Stud Alcohol* 46:223–227.

Wilsnack, R., S. Wilsnack, and A. Klassen. 1984. "Women's drinking and drinking problems: patterns from a 1981 national survey." *Am J Public Health* 74:1231–1238.

10

Dietary Patterns

SUZANNE P. MURPHY, DONALD F. EVERETT,
AND CONNIE M. DRESSER

Aging, by definition, involves change. Affecting the aging process are numerous physiologic, psychologic, and economic factors that may also influence the body's nutritional status (Posner 1979). Also important are the individual's genetic make-up, physical activity, education level, use of medications (Lamy 1981), and living arrangements (Davis et al. 1985). However, little is known conclusively about the interaction between aging and nutrition. Although it is generally accepted that aging causes decreased metabolic and organ function and is accompanied by reduced resistance to infection and diminished competence of the immune system, it is not clear how the foods we eat or long-term consumption practices influence the rate of aging and the course of diet-related diseases. It is evident, however, that malnutrition, in the form of either under- or overnutrition, is one of the most pervasive and potentially debilitating problems among the elderly in the United States. Perhaps the changes in energy intake that occur during aging impede the procurement of nutrients needed to retard aging and sustain good health. Prior to the 1982–1984 follow-up of the first National Health and Nutrition Examination Survey (NHANES I), most cross-sectional population studies did not include the longitudinal component necessary to evaluate or assess changes in patterns of food consumption. The NHANES I Epidemiologic Follow-up Study (NHEFS) has provided this opportunity to examine the changes in consumption profiles.

Several specific concerns have been expressed about the nutritional status of the elderly. On the one hand, there is concern about dietary practices that may lead to deficiencies of selected nutrients. However, there is also concern about practices that may lead to health-related excesses (e.g., energy intakes that are associated with obesity, intakes of fats and cholesterol that may be associated with cardiovascular diseases and with various cancers, and intakes of sugars and alcohol that may be associated with various types of morbidity).

Since caloric intakes tend to decrease with age (Kokkonen and Barrows 1986), there is concern that intakes of other nutrients may also decrease. The Nationwide

Food Consumption Survey conducted during 1977–1978 showed marginal intakes of several nutrients by the elderly; these estimates were based on 3-day dietary data: calcium (especially for women), magnesium, and vitamin B_6 (Pao et al. 1985). Another study, based on 7-day food diaries, showed that intakes of zinc, magnesium, and copper were also low (Zabik et al. 1983). Thus, dietary guidance for the elderly has focused on increasing intakes of nutrient-dense food, such as fruits and vegetables, legumes, whole grains, and low-fat dairy products.

To combat the problems associated with high levels of certain serum lipids, the American Heart Association continues to offer dietary guidance aimed at reducing intake of total fat, saturated fat, and cholesterol and at increasing the relative intake of polyunsaturated fats and complex carbohydrates (Grundy et al. 1982). In terms of foods, this advice has been to reduce intakes of foods that are the major source of saturated fats: animal fats, some vegetable oils (palm oil, coconut oil, cocoa butter, and heavily hydrogenated margarines and shortenings), high fat dairy products (whole milk, cream, butter, ice cream, and cheese), and many bakery goods.

Since it appears that cancer of most major sites is influenced by dietary patterns, the Committee on Diet, Nutrition, and Cancer of the National Research Council has suggested its own dietary guidelines (Committee on Diet, Nutrition, and Cancer, National Research Council 1982). The guidelines include reducing intakes of fat; including fruits (especially citrus), vegetables (especially carotene-rich and cruciferous), and whole-grain cereal products in the daily diet; minimizing consumption of salt-cured or smoked foods; and consuming alcoholic beverages in moderation, if at all.

Although many controversies surround the question of what is the optimal amount of fiber in diets, moderate increases over currently common levels are associated with benefits to gastrointestinal function and with possibly lower risk of colon cancer, cardiovascular disease, and diabetes (Slavin 1983). Thus, the elderly have been advised to increase the fiber content of their diets by eating more whole-grain products, particularly those containing bran.

These and other considerations led to publication of two widely circulated documents during the interval between NHANES I and NHEFS. The first was referred to as the Dietary Goals (Select Committee on Nutrition and Human Needs, U.S. Senate 1971). The seven goals set forth in this publication focused on avoiding obesity, increasing consumption of complex carbohydrates, and reducing consumption of simple sugars, total and saturated fat, cholesterol, and sodium. The second document, *Dietary Guidelines for Americans,* was published jointly by two government agencies (U.S. Department of Agriculture and U.S. Department of Health and Human Services 1980). These guidelines offered the same general advice as did the *Dietary Goals,* but without specifying levels of intake. In addition, the *Dietary Guidelines* recommended eating a variety of foods and consuming alcohol in moderation. It might be expected that the wide circulation of these two publications affected the food selections of the elderly. Thus, a comparison of data on intake of items from the different food groups as reported in the baseline survey (NHANES I) and in NHEFS, 10 years later, might be useful in determining whether the guidance offered did indeed change the dietary patterns of the elderly.

DESCRIPTION OF THE DATA

The NHANES I, conducted during 1971–1974, was the first program to collect measures of nutritional status from a sample scientifically designed to be representative of the noninstitutionalized civilian population aged 1–74 years (National Center for Health Statistics 1973, 1977). For assessment of dietary patterns, both a single 24-hour recall and a 3-month food frequency determination were used. The 3 months covered were those prior to the interview and reflected "usual" consumption habits that excluded periods of illness or self-imposed dieting. Daily and weekly frequencies and nonuse of foods were specified. The food groups were adapted from the Ten-State Survey and consisted of 13 major categories with six subdivisions (C. M. Dresser, unpublished data). Foods were assigned to categories on the basis of descriptive and nutrient content similarities. Enough food groups were included to enable the investigation of association between consumption patterns, health status, and socioeconomic variables.

The 10-minute food frequency questionnaire was administered by trained personnel, usually registered dietitians, who were members of a field staff employed by the National Center for Health Statistics. The interviews were conducted in specially equipped mobile units that traveled to 65 sites in the United States between 1971 and 1974. The dietary data were recorded according to an instruction manual and verified by comparison of the answers on the food frequency questionnaire with the foods reported on the individual's 24-hour recall (National Center for Health Statistics 1972). Personnel in the headquarters of the Division of Data Services and Health Examination Statistics trained and supervised the interviewers. Quality control of the data was accomplished by on-site evaluations and review of questionnaires and taped interviews (Dresser 1983).

An extended food frequency questionnaire was used in the NHANES I Epidemiologic Follow-up Study. The design of this questionnaire facilitated comparison with the food frequency data from NHANES I and addressed hypotheses focusing on the relationship of fats, fiber, salt, nitrate, cruciferous vegetables, and vitamins A and C to occurrence of disease and cultural correlates (C. M. Dresser, unpublished data). A merged tape containing 24-hour recall data from the NHANES I and NHANES II surveys was used to assess the foods consumed most often. The selection of the NHEFS food list was based on frequency of report, contribution by weight in grams to total intake, and major contributions of macro- and micronutrients.

In NHEFS an attempt was made to interview all respondents who participated in NHANES I (Cornoni-Huntley et al. 1983; Madans et al. 1986). Proxy interviews were obtained for deceased or incapacitated individuals, but the dietary questionnaire was not administered. Contracted professional interviewers, not trained in nutrition, recorded the dietary data according to detailed guidelines for food group assignments (National Center for Health Statistics 1987). The interview took 30 minutes to administer, the same time required for recording the NHANES I 24-hour recall and food frequency. Unlike NHANES I, in NHEFS subjects were interviewed wherever they were living (e.g., home, hospitals, or related health care facilities).

Telephone interviews were completed for some respondents. Interviewers were trained and supervised by regional field staff, and quality control was conducted by the interviewer and the field office. Respondents were contacted again if there were discrepancies or missing information.

Uses and Limitations of the Dietary Data

The goal of NHANES I was to measure the health and nutritional status of the U.S. population at a particular time. Its design did not permit characterization of dietary profiles of individuals with the precision required for analyses of risk factors. Day-to-day variations make a "single day's" intake inadequate to characterize long-term eating patterns. Thus, for NHEFS, modifications were made in the nutrition questions, and an extended food frequency battery was employed. The major objective of determining dietary intake in NHEFS was to assess the relationship between diet and disease. However, the data collected on food frequencies in NHANES I and NHEFS surveys can assist in identifying segments of the population who may be at nutritional risk by virtue of the types and frequencies of food consumed.

The food frequency method is a way of seeking evidence for possible associations between diseases and diet in general, rather than of detecting the association of disease with the intake of specific nutrients. Food consumption characteristics among groups or individuals can be tested for associations with disease. However, studies have indicated that the validity of the data may vary by sex, age, ethnic group, and level of education (Block 1982). The method's major limitations have been its inability to produce estimates of intakes of specific nutrients and of quantities of food consumed.

Time constraints in NHANES I limited the contents of the food frequency questions; consequently, subjects with a limited knowledge of foods or a short-lived memory of their "usual" consumption pattern were unable to translate their personal definition of foods into groups designated by the interviewer.

Misclassification may have resulted from an insufficient number of food categories. When the data from NHANES I are compared with those of NHEFS, any discrepancies may be attributed, in part, to the differences in specificity of questionnaire content and in the time period addressed.

The frequency data from NHANES I may be used for addressing the types of food categories that were consumed daily or weekly, their major contributing nutrients, and foods that were never eaten during the 3-month period before the respondent's interview. General consumption patterns for groups can be developed and related to health measures, that is, diseases and health habits. The expanded food frequency questionnaire in NHEFS made it possible to estimate consumption of a wider variety of foods and to examine foods that are never eaten; those that are consumed daily, weekly, and monthly over a year's time; foods that are consumed in season; and long-term food preparation habits (Dresser et al. 1982). The detail of the questionnaire makes it possible to devise schemes for scoring the nutrient values of the foods and food groups and to assess the relationship of food consumption patterns of groups or individuals to disease and health habits.

Information Available

The study population was defined as all persons aged 55 or older at the time of NHANES I who had satisfactory dietary records on both NHANES I and NHEFS data sets. Satisfactory dietary records were those with completion codes scored as satisfactory by the interviewer. Of the 4627 elderly individuals with satisfactory food frequency records in NHANES I, 2653 also had NHEFS interviews that were scored as satisfactory and that contained food frequency data. Proxy interviews did not contain food intake information. For these 2653 elderly people, the following parameters were used in the analyses. Unless otherwise noted, the parameters are from the NHEFS questionnaire.

Dietary Parameters

Daily number of servings for NHANES I and NHEFS food groups were calculated by quantifying the responses (daily, weekly, monthly, etc.) and adjusting for seasonal intake. For example, a food item consumed once a week would be considered one seventh of a daily serving. Servings of fruits and vegetables reported as consumed seasonally would be divided by 4 (assuming the item is consumed three out of the 12 months in a year). Because information on portion sizes was not collected, actual amounts could not be quantified. Thus, the size of a daily serving will vary among individuals.

Daily consumption and nonconsumption of food groups at the time of both surveys was investigated.

Users and nonusers of supplements were identified. Users were defined as individuals who reported that they were currently taking any one of the following: a multivitamin, vitamin C, vitamin A, vitamin E, fish liver oil, other vitamins or minerals, or other nutritional supplements.

Demographic Parameters

The study population included 1103 men and 1550 women. There were 2264 whites and 373 blacks (and 16 of other races).

Of these elderly, 922 were 55–64 years of age and 1731 were 65 or older at the baseline (NHANES I) examination. Individuals would be approximately 10 years older at the time of NHEFS.

City dwellers and rural dwellers were identified from the response to the question, "Where have you lived most of your life?" Those responding "city suburbs" were not included in either category.

There were 1317 married elderly and 1336 nonmarried elderly in the study population.

Those who lived alone versus those who lived with others (number in household was greater than 1) were also identified.

Health Parameters

Elderly with self-reported hypertension were identified from the response to the question, "Have you ever been told by a doctor that you have hypertension or high blood pressure?" A similar question was asked during both surveys.

In a similar manner, elderly with hip fracture; colitis or enteritis; peptic, stomach, or duodenal ulcer; or diabetes at the time of either survey were identified. A question about diverticulitis was asked only during NHEFS; therefore, the reported date of onset was used to determine whether the condition had been present at the time of NHANES I.

Dental status was categorized in both surveys by reported presence or absence of teeth in either the upper or lower jaw.

Participants reported their general opinion of their health status during the NHEFS interview: those responding "excellent" or "very good" were compared to those responding "fair" or "poor" (those responding "good" were not included in this comparison).

Those who exercised little or not at all were compared to those who exercised moderately (based on the response to a question about recreational exercise).

Anthropometric Parameters

Body weight and height were measured at baseline, and body weight was measured during the NHEFS interview.

Body mass index was calculated as the ratio of weight (kg) to height (m) squared (height at baseline was used for both surveys). Those in the top 25% were classified as overweight, and those in the bottom 25% were considered underweight. Persons in the middle 50% were classified as normal weight.

Economic Parameters

A poverty index ratio was not calculated on the NHEFS data tapes. Family income over the past 12 months was used for identification of those with incomes of $15,000 and over ($n = 578$) and under $15,000 ($n = 1777$).

DESCRIPTIONS OF FOOD GROUP INTAKES BY THE ELDERLY

Use of Statistical Weights

For estimation of the number of nonsampled individuals represented by the person actually sampled, statistical weights were assigned to each respondent in HNANES I. The weight is a composite of the individual's selection probability, adjustments for nonresponse, and poststratification adjustments (National Center for Health Statistics 1982). If all descriptions and analyses include age, sex, and income as variables, the weights are not critical. However, several of the tables in this chapter present data on food groups for the entire population of elderly. Thus, although the statistical weights are not theoretically correct when a subpopulation of the original NHANES I population is examined, it was felt that descriptions of the food group intakes without the weights might be misleading. Thus, all calculations of means in this and the following sections of this chapter were performed with the weights.

Table 10–1 shows the average servings per day for the 86 NHEFS food groups that could be combined into the Basic Four food groups (U.S. Department of

Table 10–1 Mean Daily Servings of Food Groups Reported at Follow-up (NHEFS)

NHEFS food group	Daily servings	NHEFS food group	Daily servings
Milk (whole)	0.50	Oranges	0.22
Sauces	0.10	Orange juice	0.53
Milk (skim)	0.62	Orange juice (substitute)	0.03
Yogurt	0.04	Grapefruit	0.14
		Grapefruit juice	0.09
Poultry	0.26	Cantaloupe	0.09
Beef	0.43	Watermelon	0.05
Liver	0.04	Strawberries	0.08
Liverwurst	0.02	Vitamin C drinks	0.05
Lunchmeat	0.18	Broccoli	0.08
Pork	0.10	Cauliflower	0.06
Bacon/sausage	0.21	Brussel sprouts	0.02
		Red peppers	0.04
Shellfish	0.04	Green peppers	0.12
Fresh/frozen fish	0.10	Tomatoes, fresh	0.35
Canned fish	0.08	Tomatoes, cooked	0.16
Eggs	0.53	Rice	0.14
Cheese	0.30	Pasta	0.11
Cottage cheese	0.16	Whole wheat bread	0.63
		White bread	0.78
Legumes	0.07	Quick bread	0.12
Peanuts	0.26	Cornbread	0.09
Nuts	0.07	Tortillas	0.01
		Toaster tarts	0.01
Apples	0.31		
Pears	0.08	Cold cereal	0.39
Bananas	0.45	Hot cereal	0.21
Plums	0.06		
Prunes	0.12	Butter/margarine	1.35
Canned fruit	0.25	Salad dressing	0.44
Peas	0.14		
Green beans	0.19	Sweets, candy	0.59
Okra	0.03	Colas (sweetened, unsweetened)	0.23
Corn	0.13	Artificially sweetened beverages	0.10
Squash (summer)	0.07		
Cucumbers	0.15	Coffee, instant decaffeinated	0.56
Lettuce, head	0.43	Coffee, instant	0.40
Lettuce, leaf	0.12	Coffee, ground decaffeinated	0.21
Cabbage	0.12	Coffee, ground	0.96
Potatoes, instant	0.04	Tea, herb	0.04
Potatoes, cooked	0.37	Tea	0.60
Potatoes, fried	0.08		
Vegetable soup	0.10	Salty snacks	0.15
Peaches	0.14	Beer	0.17
Apricots	0.04	Wine	0.08
Squash (winter)	0.03	Liquor	0.19
Carrots	0.24		
Spinach	0.09		
Sweet potatoes	0.06		

Agriculture 1979), which are discussed in a later section. These averages include both consumers and nonconsumers (those who reported they never eat a food item) of the food groups but exclude individuals who did not know their usual intake, or for whom a usual intake was not ascertained. Seasonal adjustments are applied for those foods that were reported as consumed only during certain seasons. Groups with averages of more than 0.5 (consumed on the average at least every other day) were: butter/margarine (1.35), ground coffee (0.96), white bread (0.78), whole wheat bread (0.63), skim milk (0.62), tea (0.60), candy/sweets (0.59), instant decaffeinated coffee (0.56), eggs (0.53), orange juice (0.53), and whole milk (0.50).

For the general descriptive purposes of this chapter, the data on consumption have been presented as mean daily servings. Presentation of the distribution was not feasible here, but it is important to note that a mean value does not provide any details on how consumption is distributed about the mean, and thus has potential limitations. For example, mean daily servings of liver of 0.04 (Table 10–1) is correctly interpreted to mean that if this elderly population was randomly surveyed, 4 out of 100 one-day diets would contain liver. It is not the case that each individual consumed liver an average of 4 times every 100 days. The distribution is skewed by a large number of individuals who never consume liver, and a few who consume liver regularly. Furthermore, consumption patterns of various subpopulations (delineated by sex, race, income, etc.) may not cluster around the mean for the entire group, but may cluster at the extremes. Thus, when conducting detailed analyses, one should consider these distributions and possibly exploit them.

Comparison of NHANES I and NHEFS Food Group Servings

The average number of servings per day of 18 food groups, as reported by this same population during the NHANES I survey, is shown in Table 10–2. Food groups with the highest number of daily servings were coffee/tea (2.39), fruits/vegetables (2.11), and bread (1.79).

For comparison of data on food intakes in NHANES I and NHEFS, a subset of the NHEFS food groups was used to form 14 groups that were similar to those used in NHANES I; for the remaining four NHANES I groups (eggs, vitamin A–rich and vitamin C–rich fruits and vegetables, and sweetened beverages), there were no directly comparable sets of questions on the NHEFS questionnaire. In two cases, the NHANES I groups were collapsed to provide comparability with the NHEFS questions: whole milk and skim milk were combined (since lowfat milk was included with whole milk for NHANES I and with skim milk for NHEFS), and candy and desserts were combined. The differences in number of servings per day between the 14 NHANES I food groups and the NHEFS combined food groups are compared in the last column of Table 10–2. A negative sign indicates that the number of servings decreased in NHEFS; a positive sign indicates an increase. For many food groups, the average number of daily servings increased between NHANES I and NHEFS. Exceptions were a 36% decrease in candy/sweets, a 23% decrease in artificially sweetened beverages, a 12% decrease in alcoholic beverages, and an 8% decrease in breads. It is important to note that differences in actual amounts con-

Table 10–2 Mean Daily Servings at Baseline (NHANES I) and at Follow-up (NHEFS) for 18 Baseline Food Groups

NHANES I food group	NHANES I servings	NHEFS servings	Percentage difference
Milk (whole and skim)	0.99	1.12	13
Meat/poultry	1.22	1.26	3
Fish/shellfish	0.14	0.21	50
Eggs	0.42	N/A	
Cheese	0.38	0.45	19
Legumes/nuts	0.21	0.40	90
Fruits/vegetables	2.11	2.57	22
Vitamin A–rich fruits/vegetables	0.31	N/A	
Vitamin C–rich fruits/vegetables	0.83	N/A	
Bread	1.79	1.64	−8
Cereal	0.38	0.61	61
Butter/margarine	1.30	1.35	4
Candy/sweets	0.92	0.59	−36
Sweetened beverages	0.31	N/A	
Artificially sweetened beverages	0.13	0.10	−23
Coffee/tea	2.39	2.82	18
Salty snacks	0.12	0.15	25
Alcoholic beverages	0.49	0.43	−12

Note: N/A = no comparable NHEFS food group. Percentage difference = ((NHEFS − NHANES I)/NHANES I) times 100.

sumed cannot be determined from these data, because information on portion size was not collected. However, if portion sizes do not vary substantially, then number of servings will be a good predictor of total intake.

Figures 10–1 through 10–5 summarize the differences in daily servings between surveys and among different subgroups of the elderly (based on gender, race, age, and marital status) for 5 baseline food groups. (1) Servings of meat increased slightly for the population as a whole, as well as for men, for both races, for the older elderly, and for both married and unmarried individuals. Number of servings decreased for women and the younger elderly. (2) Number of servings of cheese were similar across all populations, except for the relatively small number of servings consumed by blacks. (3) Number of servings of sweets and candy declined for all populations and were lowest for blacks. (4) Number of servings of cereal increased for all populations, with the greatest increase occurring in blacks. (5) Number of servings of alcoholic beverages declined slightly between surveys and were highest for men, whites, the younger elderly, and the married.

These data may be used for evaluation of the impact of dietary guidance publicized by several national health organizations and federal agencies concerned with public health. The changes summarized in Table 10–2 indicate the following conclusions. (1) There was an increase in milk and cheese servings, possibly in response to guidance suggesting increases in calcium intakes. (2) There was little change in total number of servings of meat, although there may have been changes

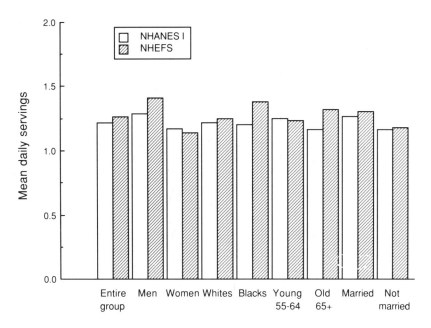

Fig. 10–1. Mean daily servings of meat and poultry reported at baseline (NHANES I) and at follow-up (NHEFS).

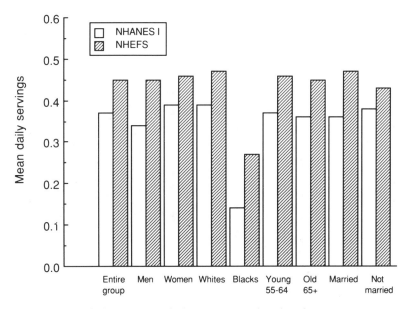

Fig. 10–2. Mean daily servings of cheese reported at baseline (NHANES I) and at follow-up (NHEFS).

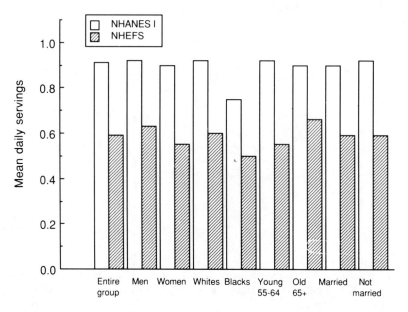

Fig. 10–3. Mean daily servings of sweets reported at baseline (NHANES I) and at follow-up (NHEFS).

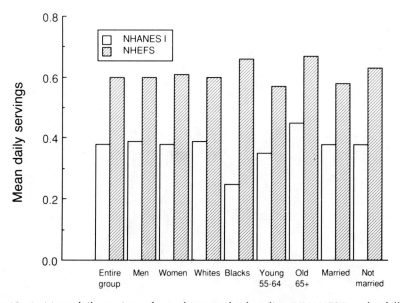

Fig. 10–4. Mean daily servings of cereal reported at baseline (NHANES I) and at follow-up (NHEFS).

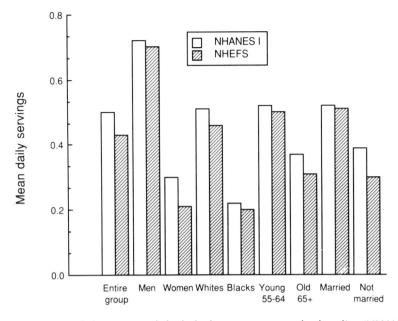

Fig. 10–5. Mean daily servings of alcoholic beverages reported at baseline (NHANES I) and at follow-up (NHEFS).

in the choices within this group. Thus, the appropriate response to advice to lower intakes of fatty meats cannot be evaluated. (3) The increase in number of servings of fish/shellfish servings may indicate response to advice to increase consumption of low-fat sources of protein. (4) The increases in number of servings of fruits and vegetables, cereals, and legumes/nuts may be a response to advice to increase intake of complex carbohydrates and dietary fiber. (5) The decrease in number of servings of sweets and candy may indicate an increased willingness to reduce intakes of simple sugars. (6) The decrease in number of servings of alcohol beverages may be a response to guidance to moderate consumption of alcohol. (7) Because servings of butter/margarine and of salty snacks increased slightly between the surveys, the elderly appear not to be responding to advice to decrease their intakes of fats and salty foods.

Daily Servings of 32 NHEFS Food Groups

It was determined that the NHANES I groups contained some food items that were nutritionally dissimilar and that more detail was required to address nutritional questions of importance to the elderly. However, the full set of over 100 NHEFS food groups was thought to be too detailed for analysis of dietary patterns. Therefore, 32 new food groups were defined on the basis of nutrient composition of component foods and their relevance to current nutritional issues. Table 10–3 lists these 32 NHEFS combined groups. The combined groups with the largest daily

Table 10–3 Mean Daily Servings by Food Groups (Combined) Reported at Follow-up (NHEFS)

Combined food group	Servings per day	Combined food group	Servings per day
1. Milk (whole)	0.50	17. Vitamin A–rich vegetables	0.64
2. Milk (skim)	0.66	18. Cruciferous vegetables	0.20
3. Beef/pork	0.54	19. Citrus fruits	1.07
4. Lunchmeat	0.18	20. Tomatoes	0.51
5. Bacon/sausage	0.21	21. Potatoes	0.50
6. Poultry	0.26	22. Refined grains	1.15
7. Liver	0.06	23. Whole grains	0.74
8. Fish/shellfish	0.21	24. Cereals	0.61
9. Eggs	0.53	25. Animal fats	0.42
10. Cheese	0.45	26. Vegetable fats	1.78
11. Mixed dishes	0.20	27. Sugar products	0.85
12. Legumes	0.07	28. Cola beverages	0.23
13. Nuts	0.33	29. Alcoholic beverages	0.43
14. Other vegetables	0.82	30. Artifically sweetened beverages	0.10
15. Green salads	0.55	31. Coffee/tea	2.82
16. Noncitrus fruits	1.66	32. Salty snacks	0.15

number of servings were coffee/tea (2.82), vegetable fats (1.78), and noncitrus fruits (1.66). Note that the 32 groups cannot be further collapsed into the 18 NHANES I equivalent groups, since the procedures used in developing the 32 groups are, in several cases, incompatible with the methods used during the NHANES I interview. For example, several food items that did not appear on the NHANES I questionnaire are included in the 32 groups. In addition, some of the 32 groups contain food items from multiple NHANES I groups.

Assignment of foods to these 32 groups was based on similar nutrient content, but in some cases food items could have been assigned to more than one group. This was particularly true for vegetables that were high in both vitamins A and C and in some cases were also cruciferous vegetables. Thus, further research might investigate reassignment of some of these food items to see whether the analyses presented here would change.

Differences in mean daily servings exceeding 30% between selected subpopulations included the following. (1) Racial differences were prominent. As compared with whites, blacks reported fewer servings of alcoholic beverages, skim milk, coffee/tea, cheese, green salads, and salty snacks. Whites reported fewer servings of cola beverages, poultry, bacon/sausage, legumes, liver, and eggs than did blacks. (2) Overall, women reported 6% fewer daily servings than men. Items consumed less often by women included alcoholic beverages, eggs, luncheon meat, and bacon/sausage. (3) The older age group of the elderly (i.e., approximately 75 years and older at NHEFS) reported fewer servings of alcoholic beverages and more servings of whole milk than did the younger age group (65–74 years old at NHEFS). (4) Unmarried elderly persons had more frequent intakes of whole milk and less frequent intakes of artificially sweetened beverages, alcohol, and salty snacks than their married counterparts.

There is overlap among individuals in the preceding subpopulations, and it is possible to see that the numbers in each group influence the differences seen. For example, most of the unmarried elderly are women, who consume fewer servings of alcoholic beverages than men. Thus, it is to be expected that the unmarried group would report fewer servings of alcohol than the married one. Likewise, there are more women in the older age group, and thus it is not surprising that a difference in alcoholic beverage servings is seen between the younger and older age groups.

Extension of these initial comparisons among subpopulations of the elderly revealed a number of facts. (1) As compared with those who lived with others, the elderly who lived alone reported more frequent consumption of whole milk and less frequent consumption of alcoholic beverages. These differences resemble those seen for the older age group of the elderly, a finding consistent with the observation that more of the' older elderly live alone. (2) City dwellers consumed green salads and alcoholic beverages more often than did rural dwellers, whereas bacon/sausage and legumes were eaten more frequently by residents of rural areas. (3) None of the food groups servings consumed by elderly with self-reported hypertension differed by more than 30% from those consumed by person without self-reported hypertension. (4) Those who considered themselves to be in excellent or very good health reported consumption of a slightly larger total number of servings of food, as well as less frequent consumption of legumes, cola beverages, and refined grains than those who considered themselves in fair or poor health. (5) As compared with nonusers of supplements, users consumed whole grains more often and cola beverages less often. (6) The elderly who exercised moderately reported more servings of alcohol and green salads than their nonexercising counterparts. (7) Those living in households with family incomes of more than $15,000 (over the past 12 months) reported more than twice as many servings of alcoholic beverages, as well as more servings of artificially sweetened beverages and green salads than did those who belonged to lower-income families.

Thus, there are many dietary differences among the subpopulations of the elderly. However, in some cases, the relative difference may exceed 30%, whereas the absolute difference may be a small number of servings. This situation holds for food groups such as legumes and artificially sweetened beverages, for which the average daily number of servings is small. In these cases, a 30% difference may be less than 0.05 servings per day.

Intake of Basic Four Food Groups: Compliance with Guidelines

Intakes of the NHEFS food groups may be further collapsed into four groups that correspond to the Basic Four food groups (U.S. Department of Agriculture 1979). The average intake of milk group foods (whole and skim milk, cheese) was 1.61 servings per day, or 81% of the recommended two daily servings. Average reported intake of meat group items (meat/fish/poultry, eggs, legumes, nuts) exceeded the recommended two servings per day. The summed responses to 41 individual queries about fruits and vegetables indicated average total fruit and vegetable group intake of 5.9 servings per day; this intake exceeds the recommended four servings per day. However, there was a general NHEFS question about fruit and vegetable intake, with responses averaging 2.6 servings per day. Apparently, the number of servings reported increased with the number of questions asked. Therefore, it is difficult to evaluate how actual intake compared with the recommended four servings per day. Average reported intake of bread group foods (refined and whole grains, cereals) was 2.5 servings per day, or well below the recommended four daily servings.

If we assume that the typical serving sizes of NHEFS subjects do not substantially exceed those recommended as part of the Basic Four, we must conclude that these elderly are not consuming enough of the milk and bread groups. Dietary guidance might focus on increasing intakes of these two groups. The USDA's Daily Food Guide (U.S. Department of Agriculture 1979) also describes a fifth group, the fats/sweets/alcohol group, and it recommends that individuals concentrate on the Basic Four first, and use this fifth group only as a calorie supplement. The elderly participants in NHEFS reported an average of 3.71 servings per day from the fats/sweets/alcohol group; this figure is higher than that for any of the Basic Four groups (except for the sum of the individual fruits and vegetables). Dietary guidance suggesting lowered consumption of these energy-rich foods would be appropriate for many individuals.

RELATION OF CHANGES IN INTAKE TO CHANGE IN HEALTH STATUS AND LIVING ARRANGEMENTS

This section examines changes in food group intakes during the interval between the two surveys and the associations between changes in intake and other changes in the life-style or health of this elderly population. Tables 10–4, 10–4a, and 10–5 are examples of how the longitudinal nature of these data can be exploited. A full examination of these associations would require a multivariate approach to each analysis, in which all variables that might influence the selected dependent variable are included. Thus, the bivariate tables shown here are the exploratory first steps that would precede more in-depth procedures.

Changes Examined

Change in Intake of 18 NHANES I Food Groups

For these analyses, the comparable 18 NHEFS food groups were redefined slightly from those used in Table 10–2, so as to include more of the details from NHEFS. Although the NHANES I and NHEFS food groups were not exactly comparable in several cases, it was still of interest to look at comparative changes among different subpopulations of the elderly. Thus, when examining differences in changes, the exact comparability of the groups is of less concern; the relative differences in the changes are of more interest than the absolute value of the changes.

The categorical variables examined represent change from "never consume" to

Table 10–4 Changes in Mean Daily Servings of Food Groups by Change in Household Composition

Food group	Alone to with others (n = 126)	With others to alone (n = 479)	No change (n = 2048)
Milk	0.17	0.24	0.19
Meat/poultry	0.36	0.05	0.12
Fish/shellfish	0.11	0.06	0.08
Eggs	0.13	0.10	0.12
Cheese	0.07	0.13	0.09
Legumes/nuts	0.23	0.18	0.18
Fruits/vegetables	1.18	1.06	1.24
Vitamin A–rich fruits/vegetables	0.30	0.30	0.31
Vitamin C–rich fruits/vegetables	1.27	1.29	1.32
Bread	0.39	0.17	0.19
Cereal	0.22	0.31	0.25
Butter/margarine	0.53	0.47	0.51
Candy/sweets	−0.22	−0.27	−0.25
Sweetened beverages	0.03	−0.05	−0.05
Artificially sweetened beverages	0.03	0.00	0.01
Coffee/tea	0.23	0.31	0.47
Salty snacks	0.07	0.03	0.03
Alcoholic beverages	−0.25	0.01	−0.04

Table 10–4a Changes in Mean Daily Servings of Food Groups by Change in Marital Status

Food group	Married to not married (n = 522)	Not married to married (n = 43)	No change (n = 2088)
Milk	0.27	0.05	0.18
Meat/poultry	0.07	0.39	0.13
Fish/shellfish	0.07	0.11	0.08
Eggs	0.11	0.06	0.12
Cheese	0.10	0.24	0.09
Legumes/nuts	0.17	0.11	0.18
Fruits/vegetables	1.12	1.87	1.21
Vitamin A–rich fruits/vegetables	0.25	0.26	0.32
Vitamin C–rich fruits/vegetables	1.26	1.57	1.32
Bread	0.19	0.14	0.20
Cereal	0.31	0.26	0.24
Butter/margarine	0.50	0.34	0.51
Candy/sweets	−0.26	−0.16	−0.26
Sweetened beverages	−0.05	0.15	−0.05
Artificially sweetened beverages	0.01	0.05	0.01
Coffee/tea	0.28	0.15	0.47
Salty snacks	0.03	0.05	0.04
Alcoholic beverages	0.03	−0.11	−0.06

Table 10–5 Changes in Mean Daily Servings of Food Groups by Change in Health Status (Diabetes and Diverticulitis)*

Food group	Diabetes (n = 175)	No diabetes (n = 2478)	Diverticulitis (n = 128)	No diverticulitis (n = 2425)
Milk	0.50	0.17	−0.09	0.21
Meat/poultry			−0.09	0.13
Fruits/vegetables	1.47	1.19		
Artificially sweetened beverages	0.15	−0.00		
Sweetened beverages			0.05	−0.05
Coffee/tea	0.04	0.45		
Candy/sweets	−0.47	−0.24	−0.42	−0.25
Alcoholic beverages	−0.28	−0.03		

*Includes only changes which were different between health status categories (*p*-value of <0.05).

"consume daily," from "consume daily" to "never consume," and all other change categories combined. The continuous variables represent change in daily number of servings.

Change in Living Arrangements

The categorical variable for change in the number of persons in the household was living alone to living with others, living with others to living alone, and no change. For change in marital status the categorical variable was married to not married, not married to married, and no change.

Change in Health Status

Although it is possible to explore the development of a variety of health conditions between the two surveys (i.e., hip fracture, hypertension, colitis, ulcers), only two conditions are presented here: diabetes and diverticulitis. The diabetes variable is based on answers to the question, "Has a doctor ever told you that you have the following condition?" Those who answered no at NHANES I and yes at NHEFS were compared to all others. No question on diverticulitis was asked at NHANES I. However, if at the time of the follow-up survey the subject reported diverticulitis and reported being first told about this condition at a date later than the baseline examination date, then a change was assumed.

Change in Dental Status

Two categorical variables were defined, one for teeth in the upper jaw, and the other for teeth in the lower jaw. Subjects with some teeth at NHANES I and no teeth at NHEFS were compared to all others.

Patterns of Change

In general, very few of these elderly NHEFS participants changed their intake patterns drastically, either from daily consumption to no consumption or vice versa. Among the 18 NHANES I food groups, the greatest numeric change was that for the cereal group: 149 individuals (0.6% of the population) changed from no consumption to daily intake. Thus, there were too few individuals in these categories to allow analyses of this type of change.

Tables 10–4 and 10–4a show differences in changes in mean number of daily servings for subpopulations that changed either the number in their households or their marital status. Almost one fifth (479) of these participants changed from living with others to living alone. Fewer than 5% (126) changed from living alone to living with others. When changes in eating patterns were examined, several differences of more than 0.2 servings per day were seen. As compared with persons who had lived with others and changed to living alone, those who changed to living with others had larger increases of daily servings of meat/poultry (0.36 vs. 0.05) and bread (0.39 vs. 0.17) and a decrease in servings of alcoholic beverage servings (-0.25 vs. $+0.01$). In addition, those who changed to living with others increased their total number of food servings more than did the other two subpopulations. These differences would generally be viewed as associated with improvements in the nutritional quality of the diet, since the increases were in number of servings of foods that are important sources of nutrients that may be deficient in the diets of elderly persons.

When those elderly who changed their marital status from not married to married were compared with those changing from married to not married (Table 10–4a), the former group had a smaller increase in daily servings of milk (0.05 vs. 0.27) as well as larger increases in daily servings of fruits and vegetables (1.87 vs. 1.12), of vitamin C–rich fruits and vegetables (1.57 vs. 1.26), and of sweetened beverages ($+0.15$ vs. -0.05). The group changing from unmarried to married also increased total servings of foods more than did the other two groups of elderly. Although the increases in fruit and vegetable servings as well as in total servings would be viewed as nutritional improvements, the apparent substitution of sweetened beverages for milk servings does not correspond to current dietary guidance.

Changes in food group servings were examined for elderly who reported a change in certain health parameters. The significance of the changes was determined by use of an unweighted Student's t-test. The true statistical significance of these changes must be interpreted with caution. The effect of the clustered design of NHANES I should be considered in performing statistical tests, since the size of the sampling variance is likely to be underestimated, and thereby lead to false rejection of the null hypothesis. In this discussion we are using a p-value of 0.05 as a convenient cutoff point for presentation of data rather than as an indictor of statistically significant differences.

Elderly people who had been told that they were diabetic showed changes different from those of the remaining population for six food groups (Table 10–5). Diabetics reported larger increases in servings of milk, fruits and vegetables, and artificially sweetened beverages. They reported larger decreases in servings of candy and sweets and alcoholic beverages and much smaller increases in coffee and tea servings. Most of these changes are clearly associated with the dietary guidance given to diabetic patients: decrease intakes of simple sugars, increase intake of complex carbohydrates, and moderate intake of alcohol. These changes may also be associated with advice to reduce energy intakes as part of a weight loss regime. However, the change in total number of servings was almost identical in those with and without diabetes; both groups reported an increase of 4.7 servings per day.

Those elderly who had been told that they had diverticulitis decreased the number of daily servings of milk and meat/poultry, whereas the rest of the population increased the number of servings of these foods (Table 10–5). The former group also showed a larger decrease in servings of candy and sweets, but they increased rather than decreased the number of servings of sweetened beverages. Perhaps the most important difference was a much smaller increase in total number of servings per day: 3.5 for those with diverticulitis vs. 4.7 for the rest of the elderly. It appears that diverticulitis is associated with a general decrease in food group servings and a substitution of foods that are perceived as easily digestible (such as sweetened beverages). It is interesting to note that these individuals do not appear to be increasing their servings of foods high in dietary fiber, as is often recommended (Slavin 1983).

Loss of all teeth in the upper jaw was reported by 243 elderly, and in the lower jaw by 225. Tooth loss did not result in significantly different changes in food group servings except for consumption of the legumes/nuts group by those who lost teeth from the lower jaw. However, changes in intake of legumes/nuts closely approached significance for those who had lost teeth from the upper jaw ($P = 0.051$). There were smaller increases in legumes/nuts servings in both cases: 0.13 per day for those with upper tooth loss versus 0.18 for the rest of the elderly, and 0.11 for those with lower tooth loss versus 0.19 for the rest of the elderly. There appears to be an association between difficulty in chewing and the change in intake of the legumes/nuts group.

OBESITY AND EATING PATTERNS

Measurement of Overweight and Underweight

It is generally agreed that obesity is widespread in the United States, that it is difficult to treat, and that it is associated with increases in morbidity and mortality (Jeffay 1982). An increase in body weight and body fat is common among the elderly. These changes may be due to decreases in metabolic rate and physical activity that are not accompanied by decreases in food intake. Although a standard definition of obesity is "an excess of body fat," the methods of measuring this excess are not commonly agreed upon. In population studies percentage of ideal body weight is often used, but unless the reference tables are age-specific, the prevalence of obesity among the elderly may be overestimated (Andres 1984). For this chapter, body mass index or BMI (weight in kilograms divided by height in meters, squared) has been used as a relative measure of obesity. Individuals in the top quartile for BMI were defined as overweight (compared to the remainder of the elderly population), those in the middle two quartiles were defined as normal weight, and those in the bottom quartile were considered underweight. If a BMI of

27 is used as the cutoff for obesity (Jeffay 1982), both men and women in the top quartile would be classified as obese. Servings of foods were then compared across these three categories of BMI.

The median BMI was similar for men (25.8 and 25.4) and women (25.9 and 25.2) in both surveys, but the range for the 75th and 25th percentiles was greater for women. When all ages were combined, the data showed slight downward trends in BMI over time for both men and women. However, the younger elderly (55–64 years at NHANES I) tended to have very little change in BMI during the 10-year interval, whereas the BMI of participants in the older group (65–74 years) tended to decrease.

Eating Patterns of Overweight, Underweight, and Normal-Weight Persons

Tables 10–6 and 10–7 compare consumption of 32 combined NHEFS groups for the overweight (top quartile), normal-weight (middle two quartiles), and underweight (bottom quartile) elderly. Although total number of servings per day was similar for both men and women in all three categories, there were several large differences in number of servings of individual food groups. Overweight women consumed fewer servings of alcoholic beverages than did normal weight and underweight women, while overweight men consumed more servings of alcoholic beverages than did men in the other two groups. Men and women in the overweight group consumed more servings of cola beverages and artificially sweetened beverages than their normal or underweight counterparts.

It is interesting to note that overweight elderly tended to report slightly fewer total servings per day than did normal-weight elderly and that the underweight elderly reported eating the most servings. Furthermore, the types of food consumed by the overweight individuals generally represent the less caloric food groups. These findings correspond with results frequently reported by others (Braitman et al. 1985). Thus, there is no evidence to support the concept that the overweight elderly have a higher caloric intake than others in this age group. It is possible that overweight individuals are more likely than normal-weight persons to underreport intakes of food items of high caloric content; however, other researchers have not found evidence to support this idea (Braitman et al. 1985). If portion sizes do not differ between overweight and normal-weight individuals, factors other than over-eating probably play a key role in the development of obesity in the elderly.

Eating Patterns of Weight Losers vs. Weight Gainers

It is also of interest to compare eating patterns of elderly who gained weight during the 10 years between surveys to patterns of those who lost weight. We chose a 10% change in weight to define subpopulations who either gained or lost weight. Men changed an average of −0.49 lb over the 10 years, with 9% losing more than 10% of their baseline weight and 9% gaining more than 10%. The average change for women was −1.72 lb, with 18% losing and 13% gaining. Differences in food intake at baseline between those who gained and those who lost weight were relatively

Table 10–6 Mean Daily Servings by Food Groups (Combined) Reported at Follow-up (NHEFS) According to Body Mass Index for Men

Food groups	Top 25%	Middle 50%	Bottom 25%	Percentage differences bottom vs. top
1. Milk (whole)	0.34	0.52	0.76	123
2. Milk (skim)	0.69	0.77	0.36	−49
3. Beef/pork	0.59	0.57	0.65	9
4. Lunchmeat	0.22	0.24	0.21	−6
5. Bacon/sausage	0.31	0.22	0.33	7
6. Poultry	0.26	0.26	0.27	3
7. Liver	0.08	0.07	0.06	−24
8. Fish/shellfish	0.20	0.23	0.22	10
9. Eggs	0.69	0.60	0.76	11
10. Cheese	0.46	0.46	0.41	−12
11. Mixed dishes	0.23	0.23	0.23	−0
12. Legumes	0.08	0.08	0.10	23
13. Nuts	0.36	0.32	0.40	9
14. Other vegetables	0.78	0.74	0.79	1
15. Green salads	0.50	0.54	0.50	1
16. Noncitrus fruits	1.64	1 63	1.56	−5
17. Vitamin A–rich vegetables	0.51	0.62	0.68	33
18. Cruciferous vegetables	0.19	0.19	0.16	−14
19. Citrus fruits	1.00	1.04	0.77	−24
20. Tomatoes	0.50	0.50	0.48	−4
21. Potatoes	0.54	0.51	0.58	7
22. Refined grains	1.35	1.20	1.32	−2
23. Whole grains	0.72	0.76	0.82	14
24. Cereals	0.50	0.64	0.65	29
25. Animal fats	0.43	0.33	0.73	71
26. Vegetable fats	1.74	1.85	1.55	−11
27. Sugar products	0.76	0.87	1.13	50
28. Cola beverages	0.40	0.23	0.24	−41
29. Alcoholic beverages	0.80	0.60	0.94	18
30. Artificially sweetened beverages	0.15	0.08	0.05	−66
31. Coffee/tea	2.52	2.87	3.41	35
32. Salty snacks	0.18	0.16	0.18	−3

small for both men and women, averaging about 0.5 servings per day more for the subpopulations that gained. For men the greatest differences were for skim milk and artificially sweetened beverages, both of which were consumed twice as often by those who gained weight. For women, those who gained had more frequent intakes of coffee/tea and legumes/nuts and less frequent intakes of salty snacks. It appears that those who gained weight tended to consume foods that were less calorically dense than did those who lost weight. As was noted previously, these data do not support overconsumption as a cause of weight gain in the elderly.

Table 10–7 Mean Daily Servings by Food Groups (Combined) Reported at Follow-up (NHEFS) According to Body Mass Index for Women

Food groups	Top 25%	Middle 50%	Bottom 25%	Percentage differences bottom vs. top
1. Milk (whole)	0.44	0.41	0.55	25
2. Milk (skim)	0.66	0.66	0.63	−4
3. Beef/pork	0.46	0.48	0.53	16
4. Lunchmeat	0.17	0.14	0.14	−17
5. Bacon/sausage	0.15	0.17	0.22	48
6. Poultry	0.24	0.28	0.24	−0
7. Liver	0.05	0.06	0.07	27
8. Fish/shellfish	0.20	0.21	0.19	−5
9. Eggs	0.45	0.41	0.40	−10
10. Cheese	0.43	0.48	0.44	1
11. Mixed dishes	0.17	0.18	0.19	13
12. Legumes	0.05	0.06	0.07	22
13. Nuts	0.29	0.31	0.41	44
14. Other vegetables	0.82	0.92	0.86	5
15. Green salads	0.52	0.60	0.66	28
16. Noncitrus fruits	1.62	1.63	1.83	13
17. Vitamin A–rich vegetables	0.62	0.68	0.70	13
18. Cruciferous vegetables	0.22	0.21	0.21	−8
19. Citrus fruits	1.17	1.08	1.12	−4
20. Tomatoes	0.52	0.52	0.55	5
21. Potatoes	0.43	0.46	0.50	17
22. Refined grains	1.11	0.99	1.04	−6
23. Whole grains	0.60	0.76	0.79	33
24. Cereals	0.61	0.59	0.60	−2
25. Animal fats	0.31	0.37	0.48	57
26. Vegetable fats	1.66	1.82	1.87	13
27. Sugar products	0.78	0.76	0.93	18
28. Cola beverages	0.24	0.17	0.21	−13
29. Alcoholic beverages	0.15	0.26	0.27	84
30. Artificially sweetened beverages	0.14	0.09	0.06	−60
31. Coffee/tea	2.89	2.84	2.79	−3
32. Salty snacks	0.14	0.14	0.17	21

DIET AND MORTALITY

An obvious use of the dietary data collected as part of NHANES I is the study of associations between diet and various health outcomes. A major potential of the data sets from the two surveys is the ability to study longitudinal changes in morbidity and mortality and relate them to individual intakes at baseline. Although this is a potentially rewarding line of investigation, the scientific and statistical concepts are complex, and the possibility of finding both false positives and false negatives is high. In any analyses involving diet, the lack of a reliable measure of usual intake will be a problem: Because of intraindividual variation, the NHANES I 24-hour recall is not likely to describe usual intake, whereas the food frequency groups from NHANES I are too broad for accurate quantification of nutrients and the serving sizes are unknown. Furthermore, relating intakes to incidence of disease requires sophisticated multivariate techniques, and nondietary factors that may influence the development of disease must be incorporated into the analytic models. For example, a researcher investigating potential risk factors associated with cardiovascular disease may be interested in examining specific food groups. However, the analysis might also include other variables, such as family history, smoking history, blood cholesterol level, and body weight.

Examining mean daily servings may be less productive than examining the characteristics of individuals at the extremes of the distribution. Further exploration of these data might include efforts to categorize individuals with high or low consumption of particular food items. For example, it might be of interest to examine subsequent health outcomes for individuals who regularly consume certain food items, versus those who rarely or never consume them. These analyses might focus on current diet-health relationships such as the following:

> Consumption of fruits and vegetables at the extremes above and below recommended levels (such as four daily servings) and cancer incidence.
> High and low consumption of food high in fat and cholesterol and heart disease incidence.
> High and low consumption of dairy products and osteoporosis.
> Survival of persons with exceptionally high consumption of particular foods, such as coffee and colas.

These types of analyses could either validate reported research or identify new relationships between food consumption and health.

SUMMARY

One purpose of this chapter has been to present dietary variables that may be used by researchers investigating changes in intake over the 10 years between the NHANES I and NHEFS surveys. Thus, 14 food groups were suggested that were approximately comparable between the two surveys. Changes in number of daily servings of these groups may be used to estimate dietary trends, although caution must be used because portion sizes were not obtained.

A second purpose has been to present the number of servings of the various food groups, using several food group definitions. The numbers of servings of 86 food groups from the NHEFS questionnaire were presented, as was a combination of these groups into 32 nutritionally similar groups. Servings of the Basic Four food groups were derived from these 32 groups and were compared to dietary guidance offered to the public. The analysis shows that the mean number of servings of the meat group exceeded the recommended two daily servings, that the number of servings of milk and bread was lower than recommended, and that the number of servings of fruits and vegetables was also low if the composite question was used (a query on intakes of all fruits and vegetables) but exceeded the recommendation if servings of 41 individual items were added together. These results indicate that dietary guidance for the elderly might focus more on increasing intakes of milk and grain products.

A third purpose of this chapter has been to demonstrate the type of analyses that might lead to useful insights about causes of dietary changes in the elderly. Change may be defined as a continuous variable based on number of daily servings, or as a discrete variable based on frequency (such as "never consume" changing to "consume daily"). Thus, changes in health status and changes in food group servings were examined, and several relevant differences were noted among those who were diagnosed as diabetic or as having diverticulitis, as compared with the rest of the elderly.

Finally, the associations between diet and obesity were examined. These data support the conclusions reached by other authors (Braitman et al. 1985); there is no clear evidence that overeating is associated with obesity and that, in fact, the obese elderly tend to report fewer total servings and tend to choose less calorically dense foods than their normal-weight or underweight counterparts.

Can these data be used to determine whether the elderly are responding to dietary guidance offered by federal agencies and national health organizations? Changes in food group selections between the surveys indicate that there are indeed some associated trends. Increased daily servings of fruits and vegetables, cereals, and legumes/nuts may have resulted from advice to increase complex carbohydrates and fiber. Increased servings of fish may imply interest in lower-fat protein sources. The larger number of servings of dairy products may be due to concern about calcium intake. Decreased servings of sweets may be a response to advice about avoiding refined carbohydrates and obesity. However, these data do not show adherence to advice about reducing fat or sodium intakes: servings of butter/margarine and of salty snacks did not decrease and, in fact, slightly increased. Future dietary guidance should emphasize further the health risks associated with high intakes of fat.

In conclusion, the data on food group intakes collected as part of NHANES I and NHEFS may be used in a variety of ways to investigate types of food group choices, changes in these choices, and associations of food group servings with various nondietary factors. The longitudinal nature of these data allow a wide range of analyses not possible with the dietary component of any of the previous national surveys. This chapter has presented some examples of the types of analyses that may be relevant. It is hoped that future researchers will find these examples useful as they investigate the full potential of the data set.

REFERENCES

Andres, R. 1984. "Mortality and obesity: The rationale for age-specific height-weight tables." In *Principles of Geriatric Medicine*. R. Andres, E. L. Bierman, W. R. Hazzard, eds. New York: McGraw-Hill, pp. 311–318.

Block, G. 1982. "A review of validations of dietary assessment methods." *Am J Epidemiol* 115:492–505.

Braitman, L. E., E. V. Adlin, and J. L. Stanton. 1985. "Obesity and caloric intake: The National Health and Nutrition Examination Survey of 1971–1975 (NHANES I)." *J Chronic Dis* 38:727–732.

Committee on Diet, Nutrition, and Cancer. National Research Council. 1982. *Diet, nutrition, and cancer.* Washington, DC: National Academy Press.

Cornoni-Huntley, J., H. E. Barbano, J. A. Brody et al. 1983. National Health and Nutrition Examination I—Epidemiologic Follow-up Survey. *Public Health Rep* 98(3):245–251.

Davis M. A., E. Randall, R. N. Forthofer, E. S. Lee, and S. Margen, 1985. "Living arrangements and dietary patterns of older adults in the United States." *J Gerontol* 40:434–442.

Dresser, C. M., R. Zeigler, J. Madans, and S. Gardner, 1982. Part N: Nutrition. In *NHANES I Epidemiologic Followup Survey Subject Questionnaire*. DHHS. Pub. No. (PHS) 82-T-524. Hyattsville, MD: Public Health Service, pp. 50–60.

Dresser, C. M. 1983. From nutrient data to a data base for a health and nutrition examination survey: Organization, coding, and values—real or imputed. In *Proceedings of the Eighth National Nutrient Data Bank Conference,* R. Tobelmann, ed. Springfield, VA: National Technical Information Service, pp. 92–104.

Grundy, S. M., D. Bilheimer, H. Blackburn et al. 1982. "Rationale of the diet-heart statement of the American Heart Association." *Circulation* 65:839A–854A.

Jeffay, H. 1982. "Obesity and aging." *Am J Clin Nutr* 36:809–811.

Kokkonen, G. C., and C. H. Barrows. 1986. "Aging and nutrition." *Nutr Intl* 2:205–212.

Lamy, P. 1981. "Nutrition, drugs and the elderly." Report of the Institute of Nutrition, the University of North Carolina. 40:434–442.

Madans, J. H., J. C. Kleinman, C. S. Cox et al. 1986. "10 years after NHANES I: Report of initial followup, 1982–84." *Public Health Rep* 101:465–473.

National Center for Health Statistics. 1972. *Examination Staff Procedures Manual for the Health and Nutrition Examination Survey,* 1971–73. Part 15a. Rockville, MD.

National Center for Health Statistics. 1973. Plan and operation of the Health and Nutrition Examination Survey, United States, 1971–1973. *Vital and Health Statistics.* Series 1, No. 10a. DHEW Publication No. (HSM) 79-1310. Washington, DC: U.S. Government Printing Office.

National Center for Health Statistics. 1977. Plan and operation of the Health and Nutrition Examination Survey, United States, 1971–1973. *Vital and Health Statistics.* Series 1, No. 10b. DHEW Publication No. (HSM) 79-1310. Washington, DC: U.S. Government Printing Office.

National Center for Health Statistics. 1982. Landis, R. J., J. M. Lepkowski, S. A. Eklund, and S. A. Stehouwer. A statistical methodology for analyzing data from a complex survey: The first National Health and Nutrition Examination Survey. *Vital and Health Statistics.* Series 2, No. 92. DHHS Publication No. (PHS) 82-1366. Washington DC: U.S. Government Printing Office.

National Center for Health Statistics. 1987. Cohen, B. B., H. E. Barbano, C. S. Cox et al. Plan and operation of the NHANES I Epidemiologic Follow-up Study 1982–84. *Vital and Health Statistics.* Series 1, No. 22. DHHS Publication No. (PHS) 87-1324. Public Health Service. Washington DC: U.S. Government Printing Office.

Pao, E. M., S. J. Mickle, and M. C. Burke. 1985. "One-day and 3-day nutrient intakes by individuals—Nationwide Food Consumption Survey spring 1977." *J Am Diet Assoc* 85:313–324.

Posner, B. M. 1979. *Nutrition and the Elderly: Policy Development, Program Planning, and Evaluation*. Lexington, MA: Lexington Books.

Select Committee on Nutrition and Human Needs, United States Senate. 1977. *Dietary Goals for the United States*. Washington, DC: U.S. Government Printing Office.

Slavin, J. L. 1983. "Dietary fiber." *Dietetic Currents* 10:27–32.

U.S. Department of Agriculture. 1979. *Daily Food Guide*. Home and Garden Bulletin No. 228. Washington, DC: U.S. Government Printing Office.

U.S. Department of Agriculture and U.S. Department of Health and Human Services. 1980. *Dietary Guidelines for Americans*. Home and Garden Bulletin No. 232. Washington, DC: U.S. Government Printing Office.

Zabik, M. E., K. J. Morgan, and K. L. Bundy. 1983. Nutrient intake patterns for individuals 62 years and older based on seven-day food diaries. Research Report 447. East Lansing, MI: Michigan State University, Agricultural Experiment Station.

11

Personality Factors

PAUL T. COSTA, JR., ROBERT R. McCRAE,
AND BEN Z. LOCKE

Although both the National Health and Nutrition Examination Survey-I (NHANES I) and the NHANES I Epidemiologic Follow-up Study (NHEFS) focused on physical health and nutrition, some attention was also paid to psychosocial variables. These variables are of intrinsic interest to students of aging, personality, and mental health; in addition, they may be of use in understanding other aspects of health and health-related behavior.

In the Augmentation Survey portion of the NHANES I (National Center for Health Statistics 1978), 6913 adults completed the General Well-being Schedule (GWB) (Dupuy 1978), an 18-item measure of psychological adjustment and well-being; 2814 of them also completed the Center for Epidemiologic Studies Depression scale (CES-D) (Radloff 1977). In NHEFS, 10 items from the GWB and the full CES-D were administered again. In addition, scales measuring the two personality dimensions of extraversion and openness to experience were also included. This chapter gives a brief description of these scales and descriptive statistics for men and women who were aged 55–84 years at the time of NHEFS.

Not discussed here, but included in NHEFS and of potential interest to users of the NHANES I and NHEFS data bases, are several other variables relevant to psychosocial issues, including a short version of the Framingham type A scale (Haynes et al. 1978), a question on social supports, self-ratings of health, a mental status screening instrument, and a scale measuring ability to perform activities of daily living.

INSTRUMENTS FOR MEASUREMENT AND THEIR DERIVATIONS

General Well-being Schedule

The GWB schedule is an 18-item scale that includes questions concerning freedom from worry about health, energy level, interest in life, cheerful mood, relaxation, and emotional and behavioral control. The scale has been validated against both self-reports on other instruments and clinician ratings (Fazio 1977) and has been used in several studies outside the context of the NHANES surveys (Himmelfarb and Murrell 1983).

Because of time limitations, only 10 of the 18 GWB items were administered in NHEFS; these 10 items can be combined into a scale measuring general well-being (see Appendix D for items and scoring direction). When examined in the original NHANES I sample, the 10-item version of the scale correlates well ($r = 0.98$, $n = 6913$) with the full 18-item scale. Internal consistency reliability for the 10-item scale is 0.86, and the 9-year stability coefficient is 0.48 (Costa et al. 1987).

The ten GWB items can also be rationally grouped into subscales measuring positive affect (three items), negative affect (five items), and health concern (two items). These three subscales have internal consistencies ranging from 0.71 to 0.76, and 9-year stability coefficients ranging from 0.37 to 0.44. They also show some evidence of convergent and discriminant validity (Costa et al. 1987).

Although questions in the GWB ask respondents how they have felt "within the past month," the substantial longitudinal stability of the subscales makes it possible to consider them also as indicators of personality traits. In particular, the negative affect subscale has been validated as a measure of the personality disposition of neuroticism against self-reports and spouse and peer ratings (Costa and McCrae 1986) and will be designated here as Neuroticism/Negative Affect.

The Center for Epidemiologic Studies Depression Scale

The CES-D is a 20-item measure of symptoms of depression that has been widely used in survey research. Responses are scored on a four-point scale from "never" to "most or all of the time (5–7 days in the past week)." The CES-D may be used as a continuous scale, with scores ranging from 0 to 60; data on the reliability and validity of this scale are given by Radloff (1977). Alternatively, cutting points of 16 or more or of 20 or more points can be used to screen those "that would likely have a disorder severe enough to require professional intervention" (Himmelfarb and Murrell 1983). Nine-year retest stability for the CES-D in the full sample is 0.39 ($n = 2076$), and in the initial NHANES I sample, the CES-D had a correlation coefficient of -0.72 ($n = 2814$) with the full GWB.

Table 11–1 gives a cross-tabulation of depression status at NHANES I and at NHEFS for the 960 individuals aged 55 years or older at NHEFS, with complete data from both administrations. With use of a cutoff point of 20 to define probable depression, 7.9% of the men and 10.2% of the women were classified as probably depressed at NHEFS. These values are somewhat lower than the estimates (13.7% and 18.2%, respectively) from a survey of Kentucky residents aged 55 and older (Murrell, Himmelfarb, and Wright 1983). When a score of 16 was used as the cutoff point, 11.9% of the men and 18.5% of the women were classified as probably depressed. Another way of looking at these data would be to note that 17.6% of the women and 11.9% of the men are apparently depressed sometime during the 10 year interval.

Table 11–1 Depression Status at Initial Survey (NHANES I) and at Follow-up (NHEFS)

| | No. (%) with stated follow-up status | | | |
| | Women | | Men | |
Initial status	Depressed	Nondepressed	Depressed	Nondepressed
CES-D cutting point of 20				
Depressed	19	39	10	17
	(3.6%)	(7.4%)	(2.3%)	(4.0%)
Nondepressed	35	437	24	379
	(6.6%)	(82.5%)	(5.6%)	(88.1%)
CES-D cutting point of 16				
Depressed	41	41	13	29
	(7.7%)	(7.7%)	(3.0%)	(6.7%)
Nondepressed	57	391	38	350
	(10.8%)	(73.8%)	(8.8%)	(81.4%)

Note: Percentages are given within gender. All corrected χ^2 are significant at $p < 0.001$.
*CES-D = Center for Epidemiologic Studies Depression Scale (Radloff 1977).

Analyses by the χ^2 test of the data in Table 11–1 for each gender and each cutoff point are significant, indicating an association between depression at the initial survey and at the follow-up. Of the 85 individuals initially scoring 20 or higher, 29 (34.1%) were depressed at follow-up; by contrast, only 6.7% of those not depressed initially were classified as depressed at follow-up. Thus, individuals who were initially depressed were about five times more likely to be classified as depressed a decade later than those who initially were not depressed.

Note that this finding does not mean that these individuals have been continuously depressed during the 10-year interval. Depression often occurs in discrete episodes with intermittent periods of remission. These data suggest, rather, that some individuals are particularly susceptible and are more likely than others to be depressed at any given time. Note also that the great majority of individuals were free of depressive symptoms on both occasions. Although depression is a serious problem for a minority of older men and women, it is clearly not characteristic of older people in general.

These retest results apply, of course, only to respondents who were alive and located for follow-up, and it is of interest to consider whether these observations are affected by differential mortality. This question is of particular importance because it has occasionally been reported that depression is a predictor of some kinds of mortality (Shekelle et al. 1981). Respondents aged 45 years and older at the initial survey were therefore classified by status at follow-up (1230 alive vs. 163 dead), and logistic regression analyses were used to determine whether initial depression was associated with subsequent mortality (Table 11–2). Depression, as measured by the CES-D scale with a score of 16 as the cutoff point, was not significantly related to mortality in a univariate analysis. However, any effects of depression may have been masked by other variables; women, for example, are more likely to be depressed, but also to live longer. The logistic regression was therefore repeated, with

Table 11–2 Relative Risks of Mortality at Follow-up (NHEFS) According to Depression at Baseline (NHANES I) and Other Variables

Predictor	Relative risk	P
Univariate analysis		
CES depression (>15)	1.1	0.754
Multivariate analysis with demographics		
Age (>60)	3.4	0.001
Sex (male)	2.7	0.001
Race (nonwhite)	1.1	0.861
Education (<12 years)	1.7	0.004
CES depression (>15)	1.3	0.311
Multivariate analysis with demographics and self-reported health		
Age (>60)	3.1	0.001
Sex (male)	2.7	0.001
Race (nonwhite)	1.0	0.944
Education (<12 years)	1.5	0.043
Self-reported health	2.4	0.001
CES depression (>15)	1.1	0.614

addition of the following variables: age (>60), gender (female = 0, male = 1), race (white = 0, nonwhite = 1), and education (<12 years); again depression was not significantly associated with mortality. Because psychological characteristics like depressive symptoms may result from problems with physical health, a final logistic regression analysis included self-reported health (excellent or very good = 0; good, fair, or poor = 1) along with demographic variables and CES-D score. Here age, gender, education, and self-reported health were significant predictors of mortality, but again, depression was not.

Extraversion

For NHEFS, 14 new items were added for measurement of the personality traits of extraversion and openness to experience. Along with neuroticism, agreeableness, and conscientiousness, these have been repeatedly shown to form the basic dimensions of normal personality (Digman and Inouye 1986; McCrae and Costa 1985, 1987; Norman 1963). As a measure of extraversion, eight items were selected from the 48 extraversion items of the NEO (Neuroticism, Extraversion, Openness) Personality Inventory (Costa and McCrae 1985) by multiple regression techniques using data from the Augmented Baltimore Longitudinal Study of Aging (Shock et al. 1984). The eight items selected include representatives from the six facets of warmth, gregariousness, assertiveness, activity, excitement-seeking, and positive emotions; both positively and negatively keyed items were included to control for acquiescence. Because multiple regression selects maximally independent predictors of the criterion, internal consistency was predictably low (0.51), but there is considerable evidence of validity when responses are correlated with self-reports from other instruments and with spouse and peer ratings of extraversion (Costa and McCrae 1986; Costa et al. 1986).

Openness to Experience

A six-item scale measuring openness to experience was also derived from the NEO Personality Inventory. It included content from facets measuring openness to fantasy, aesthetics, actions, and ideas. Again, internal consistency was necessarily low (0.42), but the scale showed both convergent and discriminant validity (Costa and McCrae 1986).

It should be noted that these brief scales measuring extraversion and openness, although useful as global indicators for survey research, cannot be considered as substitutes for the longer and more reliable full scales of the NEO Personality Inventory.

Procedures for Administration of Instruments

Both the GWB items and the CES-D items were included in a questionnaire that could be self-administered. About one third of the subjects required some assistance in completing the form, and the interviewer provided that assistance. These differences in method of administration did not seem to affect the scores obtained (Costa et al. 1986).

The scales for extraversion and openness were included as part of the basic NHEFS interview. Respondents were given the following instructions by the interviewer: "Now I'm going to read some statements. Don't worry about the exact meaning of these statements, just give me your first impression. Using the categories on this card, I'd like you to tell me if you strongly disagree, disagree, feel neutral, agree, or strongly agree with each statement." Subjects who failed to answer one or more items from any scale were considered to have missing data for the entire scale; again, these individuals did not seem to differ systematically in personality from those with complete data.

AGE-DIFFERENCES IN WELL-BEING, DEPRESSION, AND PERSONALITY

Cross-sectional analyses of responses to the neuroticism, extraversion, and openness scales for the full age range studied in NHEFS have been reported elsewhere (Costa et al. 1986), as have longitudinal analyses of the GWB scales using data from both NHANES I and NHEFS (Costa et al. 1987). All the analyses demonstrate that age has a very limited impact on these aspects of personality and well-being. There are significant negative correlations with age for all three personality variables, but the correlations are quite modest in magnitude ($r = -0.12$ to -0.19). Age accounts for less than 4% of the variance in neuroticism, extraversion, and openness. In the case of neuroticism–negative affect, longitudinal analyses suggest that even this small effect may be due to generational differences rather than to maturation.

Table 11–3 Mean Levels of Well-being (GWB) and Depression Scale (CES-D) Scores at Follow-up

Age, gender*	Negative affect	Positive affect	Health concern	Total well-being	CES depression
Men					
55–59 (407, 393)	9.34	13.27	3.47	50.56	7.53
60–64 (388, 371)	8.05	13.38	3.53	51.80	6.49
65–69 (326, 313)	7.64	13.37	3.79	51.94	7.48
70–74 (261, 252)	7.36	13.13	3.57	52.20	7.23
75–79 (449, 427)	7.90	12.45	3.75	50.80	9.08
80–84 (252, 235)	8.18	11.84	3.58	50.08	9.16
Total (2083, 1991)	8.14	12.94	3.62	51.19	7.82
SD	6.18	3.91	3.86	11.81	7.73
Women					
55–59 (536, 517)	10.34	12.48	3.62	48.51	9.38
60–64 (497, 477)	9.82	12.63	3.47	49.34	8.86
65–69 (384, 361)	9.88	12.35	4.22	48.25	9.20
70–74 (352, 319)	9.72	11.98	4.07	48.19	9.25
75–79 (628, 591)	10.06	11.56	4.43	47.06	10.38
80–84 (392, 363)	10.03	11.13	4.59	46.51	10.94
Total (2789, 2628)	10.00	12.03	4.05	47.98	9.69
SD	6.90	3.89	4.09	12.68	8.76

Note: Total well-being = positive affect − negative affect − health concern + 50.

*Numbers in parentheses are numbers of participants to whom GWB and CES-D instruments were administered at follow-up.

When analyses are confined to individuals aged 55 and older at the time of NHEFS, a similar pattern is seen. (Because of the very large sample size, only effects with a p-value of <0.001 are considered significant in the discussion that follows). Age is negatively correlated with both extraversion ($r = -0.08$, $n = 4891$) and openness ($r = -0.14$, $n = 4961$), but the correlation between age and neuroticism ($r = -0.02$) is not significant.

Table 11–3 gives mean values at NHEFS for the neuroticism–negative affect, positive affect, health concern, and ten-item total-well-being scales, as well as for the CES-D scale for men and women grouped in 5-year age intervals. There are significant differences by gender in all these scales, with women scoring in the direction of lower well-being, but no age–gender interactions are observed. Age differences are significant for positive affect, with older groups scoring lower, and for health concern and CES-D score, with older groups scoring higher. The magnitude of the effects is small, however, and age accounts for no more than about 2% of the variance in these three variables. There are no significant age differences for the neuroticism–negative affect scale or for total GWB scores.

It is somewhat puzzling that depression increases with age, whereas neuroticism does not, because the two variables are highly correlated. Part of the explanation may lie in the fact that the physical and cognitive changes accompanying aging resemble some symptoms of depression (Zemore and Eames 1979). Three of the four CES-D items that individually showed the strongest correlations with age could be interpreted in this light: "I did not feel like eating; my appetite was poor" ($r =$ 0.11); "I had trouble keeping my mind on what I was doing" ($r = 0.10$); and "I felt that everything that I did was an effort" ($r = 0.09$). (The fourth, "I felt lonely" ($r =$ 0.11), may represent loss of social supports.) Age was not significantly correlated with such items as "I thought my life had been a failure," "I had crying spells," and "I felt that I could not shake off the blues," and age was significantly positively correlated with the item, "I felt that I was just as good as other people." Thus, it seems clear that the full syndrome of depressive symptomatology does not increase with age.

In general, these findings are consistent with results from a growing body of longitudinal studies that show little systematic growth or deterioration in personality after age 30 (McCrae and Costa 1984). However, it is possible that maturational effects are not linear, but instead show curves reflecting different phases of the life cycle. In an earlier publication (Costa et al. 1986), neuroticism, extraversion, and openness to experience were examined year by year for individuals under the age of 55. The literature on the midlife crisis or transition (Levinson et al. 1978; Gould 1978) had suggested that changes in personality, particularly neuroticism, might be seen around age 40. But as in other survey research (Farrell and Rosenberg 1981; Lacy and Hendricks 1980), we found no evidence of age-specific changes in the mean levels of personality variables.

Similar analyses were conducted for men and women aged 55 years and older; results are depicted in Fig. 11–1. Mean values are plotted for each year for men and women separately; cell sizes range from 32 to 104 for men and from 59 to 169 for women. The plots show that there are no clear curvilinear trends. It is particularly noteworthy that there is no systematic alteration of personality variables around age 65, despite both retirement and the relabeling of self as "old" that might be expected to occur then.

SOME DIRECTIONS FOR FUTURE RESEARCH

The psychological variables described in this chapter should be of interest to both epidemiologists and psychologists as predictors of health and health behaviors and as outcomes in their own right. Together with the medical, nutritional, and demographic variables examined in NHANES I and its follow-up (NHEFS), they form a data set in which a number of important questions can be addressed.

One clear direction for research concerns the epidemiology of depression. Although age itself is not a strong predictor of depression within the age range of 55–84 years, age-related events may prove to be significant risk factors. Retirement, bereavement, diminishing social supports, physical illness, and impaired cognitive and physical functioning can all be examined in the NHEFS cohort. Further, because the CES-D scale was administered to a subset of individuals in the original NHANES I survey, baseline data are available; thus, in some cases it is possible to test causal hypotheses.

Similar analyses have been reported for the GWB scales (Costa et al. 1987).

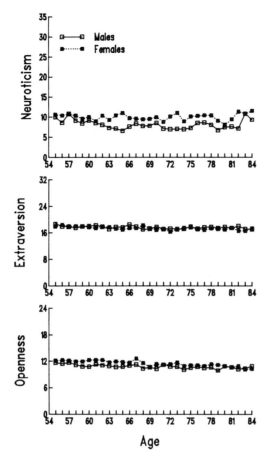

Fig. 11–1. Mean levels of neuroticism, extraversion, and openness to experience according to gender and age at follow-up (NHEFS). Scales for vertical axes are determined by the theoretical range of scores, which is also the observed range for neuroticism. Extraversion scores ranged from 5 to 32, and openness scores ranged from 0 to 22.

The stability of individual differences on the GWB scales was examined for individuals who had or had not experienced changes in marital status, employment status, or state of residence. There were no differences in the retest correlations between the original survey and the follow-up for these groups; this finding suggests that major environmental changes do not have a long-term effect on psychological well-being. The data were interpreted as evidence of the importance of enduring personality dispositions and processes of adaptation in determining levels of well-being.

A large literature has examined the relations between traits in the domain of neuroticism (including anxiety, anger, and depression) and physical disease. However, problems of self-selection and diagnosis based on patient reports have created artifacts that account for some of the reported relations (Costa and McCrae 1987). Most studies designed to overcome these difficulties have focused on coronary artery disease and suggest that while neuroticism is related to somatic complaints, it is not causally related to mortality or cardiovascular disease (Costa et al. 1982; Costa and McCrae 1987). The sampling design, hospitalization histories, and large sample provided by NHEFS make it feasible to examine the associations between neuroticism and a wide range of objectively determined medical conditions. It would also be possible to explore possible links between health and the two personality dispositions of extraversion and openness to experience.

Included among hospitalization data are psychiatric diagnoses. Although scores for neuroticism, extraversion, and openness to experience were obtained only at the conclusion of the NHEFS period and thus cannot unambiguously be seen as predictors of mental illness, their associations with psychiatric diagnostic categories could be of value in understanding the development and differential diagnosis of psychiatric disorders.

Data from NHEFS can be used to test the hypotheses that smoking is associated with extraversion (Eysenck 1963), that heavy drinking is related to neuroticism (Conley 1985), that depression contributes to cancer mortality (Shekelle et al. 1981), or that openness to experience leads to a more varied diet. In these and many more ways, NHEFS can make substantial contributions to an understanding of the relations of personality variables to health and aging.

In summary, the psychosocial variables measured in NHEFS include general well-being, neuroticism, positive affect, health concern, depression, and the personality dispositions of extraversion and openness to experience. Individuals depressed at the initial survey were about five times more likely to be depressed at follow-up as those initially not depressed, but most older respondents were not depressed at either time. Furthermore, depression was not associated with mortality status at follow-up. Cross-sectional analyses of data from individuals aged 55 years and older show a decline in positive affect and increases in health concern and depression with age. Extraversion and openness were negatively correlated with age. However, all these age differences were quite small in magnitude, and plots by 1-year age groups showed no evidence of systematic curvilinear trends. These results are broadly consistent with those of longitudinal studies showing predominant stability of personality in adulthood. The utility of these scales for an understanding of health in older Americans is discussed, and some directions for future research are suggested.

REFERENCES

Conley, J. J. 1985. "A personality theory of adulthood and aging." *Perspectives in Personality,* vol. 1. R. Hogan and W. H. Jones, eds. Greenwich, CT: JAI Press, pp. 81–115.

Costa, P. T., Jr., J. L. Fleg, R. R. McCrae, and E. G. Lakatta. 1982. "Neuroticism, coronary artery disease, and chest pain complaints: Cross-sectional and longitudinal studies." *Exp Aging Res* 8:37–44.

Costa, P. T., Jr., and R. R. McCrae. 1985. *The NEO Personality Inventory Manual.* Odessa, FL: Psychological Assessment Resources.

Costa, P. T., Jr., and R. R. McCrae. 1986. "Cross-sectional studies of personality in a national sample. 1. Development and validation of survey measures." *Psychol Aging* 1:140–143.

Costa, P. T., Jr., and R. R. McCrae. 1987. "Neuroticism, somatic complaints, and disease: Is the bark worse than the bite?" *J Pers* 55:299–316.

Costa, P. T., Jr., R. R. McCrae, and A. B. Zonderman. 1987. "Environmental and dispositional influences on well-being: Longitudinal follow-up of an American national sample." *Br J Psychol* 78:299–306.

Costa, P. T., Jr., R. R. McCrae, A. B. Zonderman, H. E. Barbano, B. Lebowitz, and D. M. Larson. 1986. "Cross-sectional studies of personality in a national sample: 2. Stability in neuroticism, extraversion, and openness." *Psychol Aging* 1:144–149.

Costa, P. T., Jr., A. B. Zonderman, R. R. McCrae, J. Cornoni-Huntley, B. Z. Locke, and H. E. Barbano. 1987. "Longitudinal analyses of psychological well-being in a national sample: Stability of mean levels." *J Gerontol* 42:50–55.

Digman, J. M., and J. Inouye. 1986. "Further specification of the five robust factors of personality." *J Pers Soc Psychol* 50:116–123.

Dupuy, H. J. 1978. "Self-representations of general psychological well-being of American adults." Presented at a meeting of American Public Health Association, Los Angeles, CA.

Eysenck, H. J. 1963. "Smoking, personality, and psychosomatic disorders." *J Psychosom Res* 7:107–130.

Farrell, M. P., and S. D. Rosenberg. 1981. *Men at Midlife*. Boston: Auburn House.

Gould, R. L. 1978. *Transformations*. New York: Simon and Schuster.

Haynes, S. G., S. Levine, N. A. Scotch, M. Feinleib, and W. B. Kannel. 1978. "The relationship of psychosocial factors to coronary disease in the Framingham Study. I. Methods and risk factors." *Am J Epidemiol* 107:362–383.

Himmelfarb, S., and S. A. Murrell. 1983. "Reliability and validity of five mental health scales in older persons." *J Gerontol* 38:333–339.

Lacy, W. B., and J. Hendricks. 1980. "Developmental model of adult life: Myth or reality?" *Aging Hum Dev* 11:89–110.

Levinson, D. J., C. N. Darrow, E. B. Klein, M. L. Levinson, and B. McKee. 1978. *The Seasons of a Man's Life*. New York: Alfred A. Knopf.

McCrae, R. R., and P. T. Costa, Jr. 1984. *Emerging Lives, Enduring Dispositions: Personality in Adulthood*. Boston: Little, Brown.

McCrae, R. R., and P. T. Costa, Jr. 1985. "Updating Norman's "adequate taxonomy": Intelligence and personality dimensions in natural language and in questionnaires." *J Pers Soc Psychol* 49:710–721.

McCrae, R. R., and P. T. Costa, Jr. 1987. "Validation of the five-factor model of personality across instruments and observers." *J Pers Soc Psychol* 52:81–90.

Murrell, S. A., S. Himmelfarb, and K. Wright. 1983. "Prevalence of depression and its correlates in older Americans." *Am J Epidemiol* 117:173–185.

National Center for Health Statistics. 1977. Fazio, A. F. "A concurrent validation study of the NCHS general well-being schedule." *Vital and Health Statistics*. Series 2, No. 73. U.S. DHEW Pub. No. (HRA) 78-1347. Hyattsville, MD: U.S. Government Printing Office.

National Center for Health Statistics. 1978. "Plan and operation of the NHANES I Augmentation Survey of Adults 25–74 years: United States, 1974–1975." U.S. DHEW Pub. No. (PHS) 78-1314. Washington, DC: U.S. Government Printing Office.

Norman, W. T. 1963. "Toward an adequate taxonomy of personality attributes: Replicated factor structure in peer nomination personality ratings." *J Abnorm Soc Psychol* 66:574–583.

Radloff, L. S. 1977. "The CES-D Scale: A self-report depression scale for research in the general population." *Appl Psychol Measurement* 1:385–401.

Shekelle, R. B., W. J. Raynor, A. M. Ostfeld, D. C. Garron, L. A. Bieliauskus, S. C. Liu, C. Maliza, and O. Paul. 1981. "Psychological depression and 17-year risk of death from cancer." *Psychosom Med* 43:117–125.

Shock, N. W., R. C. Greulich, R. Andres, D. Arenberg, P. T. Costa, Jr., E. G. Lakatta, and J. D. Tobin. 1984. *Normal Human Aging: The Baltimore Longitudinal Study of Aging* (NIH) Pub. No. 84-2450. Bethesda, MD: National Institutes of Health.

Zemore, R., and N. Eames. 1979. "Psychic and somatic symptoms of depression among young adults, institutionalized aged and noninstitutionalized aged." *J Gerontol* 34: 716–722.

12

Physical Function

DANIEL J. FOLEY, LAURENCE G. BRANCH,
JENNIFER H. MADANS, DWIGHT B. BROCK,
JACK M. GURALNIK, AND T. FRANKLIN WILLIAMS

Assessment of physical function can provide valuable information about the health status and well-being of the older population (Williams 1983). In evaluating the older patient, the prognosis for physical functioning that is associated with diagnoses of diseases and impairments is critical to sound clinical decision making (Solomon 1988). In general, physical functioning is assessed in terms of the routine self-maintenance activities an individual can do (capacity) or does do (performance) and in terms of the degree of difficulty encountered in performing each activity.

Frequently studied self-maintenance activities include personal care or the activities of daily living (ADL), mobility (i.e., walking or getting around), and home management or the instrumental activities of daily living (IADL) (Katz 1983). The ADL include the self-care functions of bathing, dressing, toileting, transferring from bed to chair, continence, and feeding and were indexed some 25 years ago for assessment of the rehabilitation of disabled patients (Katz et al. 1963). Subsequent conceptual models of functioning incorporated mobility and the IADL (Lawton et al. 1982; Fillenbaum and Smyer 1981). The IADL scale assesses adaptive tasks necessary in an independent living environment such as shopping, cooking, housekeeping, laundry, use of transportation, management of money and medications, and use of the telephone.

Another comprehensive scale of functioning that has received much methodologic investigation and addresses these and other self-maintenance activities is the arthritis-based disability index used in this NHANES I (National Health and Nutrition Examination Survey-I) Epidemiologic Follow-up Study, or NHEFS (Fries et al. 1982; Brown et al. 1984). This index is based on performance in eight domains of self-maintenance: dressing and grooming, hygiene, arising, eating, walking, activities, reach, and grip.

In this chapter the prevalences of two categories of dysfunction, a "disabled" category and a "limited" category, based on the range of values from the disability index scores, are presented for NHANES I survivors participating in NHEFS some 10 years later. The baseline NHANES I survey was conducted between 1971 and

1975, and the NHEFS survey was conducted between 1983 and 1984; therefore, the subjects' ages increased by 7–12 years (average increase, 10 years). In addition, data on symptoms of chronic disease, health perceptions, and health behaviors from the baseline NHANES I survey are used to show associations with mortality during the follow-up and with dysfunction among the survivors.

ANALYTIC METHODOLOGY

For assessment of physical function, NHEFS included 26 self-reported items related to personal care activities and daily routines. Eighteen items were taken from the 20-item disability assessment used in the Health Assessment Questionnaire (HAQ) (Fries et al. 1980). The HAQ is an instrument for outcome assessment developed at Stanford Medical School's Arthritis Research Center and used in clinical studies to evaluate the varied effects of treatment on arthritis. In addition to the disability assessment, the HAQ ascertains outcome in four other areas: death, discomfort, drug toxicity, and dollar costs.

The HAQ disability index represents a summary score for physical functioning based on interim scores in eight domains: dressing and grooming, hygiene, arising, eating, walking, activities, reach, and grip. Each functional domain is assessed by several specific questions related to that domain. Table 12–1 provides an overview of the domains and the component questions. Each item is scored from 0 to 3, representing no difficulty (0), some difficulty (1), much difficulty (2), or unable to do (3), as reported by the subject or his/her proxy. For each domain the item with the individual's poorest score determines the overall score for that domain. The disability index score is the average of the scores for the eight domains. However, unlike the original HAQ disability index, the walking domain in the NHEFS instrument was defined by a different set of questions. For compatibility with the original scoring, some adjustments were made in this domain (see Appendix E). The index values range from 0 to 3, are measured to the first decimal place (i.e., 0.0–3.0), and yield a skewed but continuous measure for physical function.

All subjects ($n = 3517$) who were 55–74 years of age in the NHANES I baseline examination were included in the first part of this analysis. For these subjects the prevalence of dysfunction is described by the degree of difficulty reported in the eight domains of function and the amount of personal help received in these domains. Further, these subjects were grouped and described according to the range of disability index scores. Scores of 1.0–3.0 are used for grouping subjects into a category labeled "disabled," and scores greater than 0 (i.e., no difficulty in all domains) but less than 1.0 are used for grouping subjects into a category labeled "limited." These cutoff points are consistent with the clinical application of the HAQ disability index to describe dysfunction (Fries et al. 1982; Wolfe et al. 1988). A multiple-outcome linear model was used for examination of the associations between age group, gender, and race to the two categories of dysfunction; an approach outlined by Grizzle, Starmer, and Koch was used (Griz-

Table 12–1 The Stanford Health Assessment
Questionnaire Disability Index

Dressing and grooming domain
  Dress yourself, including tying shoes, working zippers
  Shampoo your hair
Hygiene domain
  Wash and dry your whole body
  Get in and out of the bathtub
  Get on and off the toilet
Arising domain
  Stand up from an armless chair
  Get in and out of bed
Eating domain
  Cut your meat
  Lift a full cup or glass to your mouth
  Open a new milk carton
Walking domain*
  Walk a quarter of a mile
  Walk from one room to another on the same level
  Walk up and down at least two steps
Activities domain
  Run errands and shop
  Do light chores such as vacuuming
  Get in and out of a car
Reach domain
  Reach and get down a 5-lb object from above your head
  Bend down and pick up clothing from the floor
Grip domain
  Open push-button car door
  Open jars that have been previously opened
  Turn faucets on and off

---

*Not identical to the HAQ Walking Domain (see Appendix E).

zle, Starmer, and Koch 1969). In the second part of the analyses, a smaller subsample of the NHANES I subjects aged 55–74 years who participated in the Detailed Medical Examination Component (DMEC) was used in evaluating the association of selected chronic diseases present at baseline, health perceptions and health behaviors with subsequent mortality and dysfunction. About 96% of the subjects were successfully traced and used in this outcome analysis ($n = 2415$).

Separate multivariate logistic regression models were used for calculation of the odds ratios among men and women for mortality associated with chronic diseases present at baseline, dysfunction associated with chronic diseases present at baseline (i.e., the ratio of disability index scores greater than zero to scores equal to zero), mortality associated with behaviors and perceptions reported at baseline, and dysfunction associated with behaviors and perceptions reported at baseline (Kleinbaum et al. 1983).

PHYSICAL FUNCTION AT FOLLOW-UP

Table 12–2 presents the rates of difficulty for the eight domains of physical function by age and gender for all NHEFS participants aged 55–74 years at the time of the NHANES I baseline. The categories for "much difficulty" and "unable to do" were collapsed in this table.

In general, for both age groups men reported less difficulty with activities in each domain than did women. However, the prevalence of difficulty increased with age more rapidly for women than for men. For men the lowest prevalence (10%) of difficulty was reported for gripping activities, whereas for women the lowest prevalence (15%) of difficulty was reported for activities in the eating domain. The highest prevalence of difficulty was reported in the activities domain for both men and women–at 23% and 41%, respectively.

Note that the four domains of dressing and grooming, arising, eating, and hygiene are comparable to some of the activities of daily living (ADL). The walking domain addresses the area of mobility, and the activities domain, in a limited way, addresses instrumental activities of daily living (IADL). A fourth area of self-maintenance unique to this arthritis disability index is function of the upper extremities, as described by the reach and grip domains.

Figure 12–1 illustrates the extent to which much difficulty in the eight domains was reported in NHEFS by men and women aged 75 and older. Also illustrated is the proportion of subjects receiving personal help from another person for activities in each domain. The domains for which subjects had most need for personal assistance among those who reported much difficulty or inability to perform included the eating domain (89% and 82% for men and women, respectively); the activities domain (79% for both men and women); and the dressing and grooming domain (68% and 75% respectively, for men and women). These data highlight those areas of disability in which support is most likely to be provided in the form of personal assistance. Except for the walking and the arising domains, most subjects reporting much difficulty received personal assistance in each domain.

Table 12–3 presents the estimated parameters of a multiple-outcome linear model for the two categories of dysfunction: disabled (i.e., disability index score greater than 1.0) and limited (i.e., disability index score greater than 0.0 and less than or equal to 1.0). The parameters for this model are the proportions associated with the age group, gender, race, and interaction between age and gender (i.e., an additional increase among women aged 65–74 at baseline). The model's residual or amount of error not accounted for in the underlying contingency table was not significant ($p = 0.23$); therefore, the model fits the table well.

As indicated in Table 12–3, both the proportion "disabled" and the proportion "limited" increased significantly with age ($p < 0.001$), and both were significantly higher among women ($p < 0.01$ for "disabled" and $p < 0.001$ for "limited"). With respect to race, the proportion "disabled" significantly increased among blacks ($p < 0.01$), but the proportion "limited" did not increase significantly among blacks. In addition, the proportion "disabled" among women aged 65–74 at baseline was significantly larger than the effect of age and gender alone (i.e., a significant

Table 12–2 Percentage of Subjects Reporting Some or Much Difficulty in the Eight Domains of Physical Functioning According to Gender and Age at Baseline (NHANES I)

		Dressing and Grooming		Hygiene		Arising	
		Some difficulty	Much† difficulty	Some difficulty	Much† difficulty	Some difficulty	Much† difficulty
	n*	%	%	%	%	%	%
Men							
55–64	611	7.0	5.1	8.4	4.3	11.5	3.8
65–74	838	11.8	9.4	12.8	11.7	16.5	8.7
Total	1449	9.8	7.6	10.9	8.6	14.4	6.6
Women							
55–64	777	10.0	7.0	11.5	11.1	14.7	6.4
65–74	1247	14.6	18.3	16.5	27.0	22.5	15.6
Total	2024	13.0	13.9	14.6	20.9	19.5	12.1

		Eating		Walking		Activities	
		Some difficulty	Much† difficulty	Some difficulty	Much† difficulty	Some difficulty	Much† difficulty
	n*	%	%	%	%	%	%
Men							
55–64	611	4.4	3.8	8.0	4.8	8.2	7.5
65–74	838	7.3	7.3	10.9	9.9	10.7	17.5
Total	1449	6.1	5.8	9.7	7.7	9.7	13.3
Women							
55–64	777	8.0	3.4	10.8	7.1	14.8	12.9
65–74	1247	11.6	11.5	17.6	20.4	18.3	31.4
Total	2024	10.2	8.4	15.0	15.3	17.0	29.3

		Reach		Grip	
		Some difficulty	Much† difficulty	Some difficulty	Much† difficulty
	n*	%	%	%	%
Men					
55–64	611	13.4	5.4	4.3	2.5
65–74	838	13.4	11.7	7.8	5.5
Total	1449	13.4	9.0	6.3	4.2
Women					
55–64	777	15.6	10.3	8.8	5.8
65–74	1247	18.4	24.6	14.3	13.4
Total	2024	17.3	19.1	12.2	10.5

*Does not include persons with more than five items with missing data ($n = 44$).
†Includes "unable."

interaction between age and gender) ($p < 0.001$), but this association did not hold for the proportion "limited."

Table 12–4 shows the observed percentage distributions for the two categories of dysfunction and the fitted percentage distribution based on the estimated parameters of the model presented in Table 12–3. Most subjects had scores equal to 0

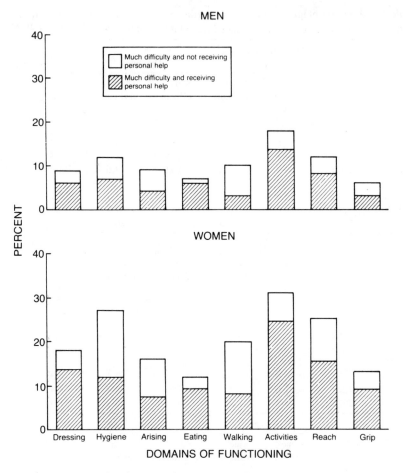

Fig. 12–1. Percentage distribution of persons aged 75 years and older at follow-up (NHEFS) reporting much difficulty and the receipt of personal help for each domain of functioning according to gender.

(i.e., "no difficulty" reported in any domain). These persons were considered to have "good" physical function (58%) and are not reported in the table. Overall, 30% of the subjects were categorized as "limited" in physical function and 12% were categorized as "disabled."

Among men aged 65–74 years at follow-up, the proportion "disabled" among blacks (11%) was nearly double the proportion among whites (6%). Among men aged 75–84 years at follow-up, the differences were less striking; 17% of black men were categorized as "disabled" as compared with 11% of white men. The proportion "disabled" among black women rose from about 11% of those under age 75 to

Table 12–3 Estimated Parameters of a Multiple Outcome Linear Model for Subjects in the Disabled and Limited Categories of Functioning at Follow-up (NHEFS)

| Attributes | Outcomes | | | | | |
| | Disabled* | | | Limited* | | |
Reference group	Parameter estimates	SE	χ^2	Parameter estimates	SE	χ^2
White men aged 55–64 at baseline	0.0568	0.0096	34.88‡	0.2424	0.0174	193.25‡
Persons 65–74 at baseline	0.0578	0.147	15.47‡	0.0872	0.0237	13.5‡
Women	0.0469	0.0146	7.74†	0.0851	0.0241	12.43‡
Black persons	0.0511	0.0183	7.82†	−0.0029	0.0226	0.02
Women aged 65–74 at baseline	0.1032	0.0222	21.63‡	−0.0316	0.0322	0.97

Note: Model goodness of fit: $\chi^2 = 8.14$, $p = 0.23$.

*Disabled = disability index score greater than 1.0; limited = disability index score greater than 0.0 and less than or equal to 1.0.

†$p < 0.01$.

‡$p < .001$.

nearly 32% of those aged 75–84 years at follow-up, as compared with 10% and 26%, respectively, among white women.

The higher rates of disability observed among blacks are consistent with data from other nationally representative studies of physical function (Shanas 1980; Macken 1986). However, some of the racial differences may be attributable to

Table 12–4 Observed Percentage and Model Estimates of Subjects in the Disabled and Limited Categories of Functioning According to Race, Gender, and Age at Baseline (NHANES I)

Race, gender and age*	Number	Disabled		Limited	
White men					
55–64 (65–74)	549	5.6	(5.7)†	23.9	(24.2)†
65–74 (75–84)	717	11.0	(11.5)	34.3	(33.0)
Black men					
55–64 (65–74)	62	11.3	(10.8)	27.4	(24.0)
65–74 (75–84)	121	20.7	(16.6)	25.6	(32.7)
White women					
55–64 (65–74)	667	10.3	(10.4)	31.8	(32.8)
65–74 (75–84)	1062	25.7	(26.5)	38.3	(41.5)
Black women					
55–64 (65–74)	110	10.9	(15.5)	39.1	(32.5)
65–74 (75–84)	185	31.9	(31.6)	37.8	(38.0)

*Ages in parentheses are the approximate ages at the time of the NHEFS.

†Numbers in parentheses are model estimates.

different rates of loss to follow-up for the two races. Among the 893 blacks aged 55 to 74 years at baseline, about 8% were lost to follow-up whereas only 3% of the 4739 white subjects were lost.

Associations of Health Characteristics with Later Mortality and Dysfunction

About 1200 men and 1200 women aged 55–74 years at baseline also participated in the NHANES I Detailed Medical Examination Component (NHANES I DMEC). For this analysis of mortality and dysfunction, chronic disease was defined according to the results of screening subjects in the DMEC. The screening of subjects was based on reported symptoms that led to their subsequent participation in one or more of the cardiovascular, respiratory, and arthritic disease supplements included in the detailed examination. The subjects who were not selected for participation in any of the supplements were used as the control group and were compared with the following groups. Group A included those who participated in the arthritic disease supplement only; Group C/R included those who participated in the cardiovascular and/or the respiratory disease supplement only; and Group A: C/R consisted of subjects who participated in the arthritis supplement and one or both of the cardiovascular and respiratory supplements. This third group is referred to as the co-morbidity group because its members were suspected of having arthritis as well as cardiovascular and/or respiratory disease.

The measures of health perceptions and behaviors at baseline included the subject's self-perceived health status (fair or poor vs. excellent or good); self-perceived level of activity on a usual day aside from recreation (inactive vs. moderately and very active); self-perceived level of exercise in things done for recreation (little or no exercise vs. moderate or much exercise); and smoking status (current vs. never smoked and former vs. never smoked).

Table 12–5 presents the percentage distributions at baseline for the chronic disease supplements, health perceptions, and health behaviors according to age and gender. Screening excluded many persons (38% of men and 35% of women) from participation in any supplement. Sixteen percent of men participated in the arthritis supplement only, and 21% participated in the respiratory and/or the cardiovascular supplement only. The remainder of the men (25%) were in the co-morbidity group (i.e., those subjects participating in the arthritis supplement and either or both of the cardiovascular and respiratory disease supplements). Among women the respective rates were 23%, 15%, and 28%.

As for health perceptions at baseline, about a third of both the men and women perceived their health as fair or poor, and this proportion increased with age, particularly among women. Although both men and women generally reported doing little or no exercise in their recreational activities (40% and 50%, respectively), only 10–15% reported that they were inactive in their usual day.

A large number of the subjects were smokers or former smokers, especially in the younger age group in which 40% of the men and over 25% of the women smoked, and 35% of the men and 11% of the women were former smokers. Rates for current smokers among those aged 65–74 were much lower (28% and 14% for

Table 12–5 Prevalence of Baseline Symptoms, Health Perceptions, and Health Behaviors According to Gender and Age at Baseline (NHANES I)*

Gender and age	Number	Symptoms reported at baseline			
		None %	Arthritis only %	Cardiovascular and/or respiratory only %	Arthritis, cardiovascular and/or respiratory %
Men					
55–64	600	40.8	16.3	18.8	24.0
65–74	569	35.0	15.5	23.9	25.7
Total	1169	38.0	15.9	21.3	24.8
Women					
55–64	636	37.1	20.9	15.2	26.8
65–74	608	33.0	24.3	14.6	28.1
Total	1244	35.1	22.6	14.9	27.5

Gender and age	Number	Health perceptions and behaviors				
		Fair or poor health %	Little exercise in recreation %	Inactive on usual day %	Current smoker %	Former smoker %
Men						
55–64	600	31.2	41.2	10.8	40.4	34.5
65–74	569	35.1	38.6	12.9	28.0	41.8
Total	1169	33.1	39.9	11.8	34.4	38.1
Women						
55–64	636	27.1	48.1	9.9	27.3	11.0
65–74	608	36.8	53.3	14.5	13.8	11.0
Total	1244	31.9	50.6	12.1	20.7	11.0

*Table based on the NHANES I detailed medical examination subsample.

men and women, respectively). Forty-two percent of the men were former smokers as compared with only 11% of the women.

As shown in Table 12–6, an equal majority (55%) of men and women aged 55–64 at baseline retained good function at the time of NHEFS. In this age group, however, twice as many men as women died during the follow-up (22% vs. 10%). Since this interval represents aging from an average age of 60 years to an average of about 70 years, the difference in life expectancy for this age group is directly offset by the difference in the prevalence of dysfunction. Among the cohort 65–74 years of age at baseline, roughly a fourth of the women and a third of the men survived and were categorized as having "good" function; again, more men than women died (44% vs. 31%).

Table 12–7 presents the odds ratios and confidence intervals for mortality and dysfunction from the chronic-disease multiple-logistic regression models. The relative risks of mortality among men and women who participated in the arthritis supplement only (Group A) were lower but not significantly different from the risks of mortality among persons in the control group (odds ratio, 0.8 for men, 0.9 for

Table 12–6 Percentage Distribution by Outcome of Participants in the NHANES I Detailed Medical Examination Subsample According to Gender and Age at Baseline (NHANES I)

	Number	Deceased	Disabled*	Limited*	Good function*
Men					
55–64	600	22.2	4.8	17.7	55.3
65–74	569	44.1	7.2	15.8	32.9
Total	1169	32.9	6.0	16.8	44.4
Women					
55–64	637	9.9	8.8	26.2	55.1
65–74	609	30.9	16.6	25.3	27.3
Total	1246	20.1	12.6	25.8	41.5

*Disabled = disability index score greater than 1.0. Limited = disability index score greater than 0.0 and less than or equal to 1.0. Good function = disability index score of 0.0.

women). However, the odds for dysfunction among these survivors were more than twice the odds for dysfunction among the control group (2.1 and 2.2 for men and women, respectively). The findings among the survivors underscore the debilitating nature of this disease.

For men who participated only in either the cardiovascular or the respiratory supplement or both (Group C/R), the odds ratios for mortality and for dysfunction were roughly two and a half times the odds ratios for the control group (2.4 and 2.6, respectively). Among women in this group, the odds ratio for dysfunction was twice as high as that in the control group (2.0), but there was no difference in the risk of mortality.

With respect to the third group (Group A: C/R), the co-morbidity group, the risk of mortality was higher among men than in the control group (1.6), but again no significant increase was shown for women. Thus, among women the relative risks of mortality associated with any of the chronic disease groups were not significantly

Table 12–7 Odds Ratios and 95% Confidence Intervals for Mortality and Dysfunctioning among Survivors According to Baseline Symptoms and Gender

	Outcome†	
Supplement participation*	Mortality	Dysfunctioning
Men		
Arthritis only	0.8 (0.5–1.2)	2.1 (1.4–3.3)
Cardiovascular and/or respiratory only	2.4 (1.7–3.4)	2.6 (1.7–4.1)
Arthritis, cardiovascular, and/or respiratory	1.6 (1.1–2.2)	3.8 (2.5–5.7)
Women		
Arthritis only	0.9 (0.6–1.4)	2.2 (1.6–3.1)
Cardiovascular and/or respiratory only	1.1 (0.7–1.8)	2.0 (1.4–3.0)
Arthritis, cardiovascular, and/or respiratory	1.4 (1.0–2.0)	3.1 (2.2–4.4)

*Those persons with no symptoms are the reference group for the odds ratios.

†Odds ratios are adjusted for the year of the baseline examination, age, and race.

Table 12–8 Odds Ratios and 95 Percent Confidence Intervals for Mortality and Dysfunctioning among Survivors According to Baseline Health Perceptions and Behaviors and Gender

Health perceptions and behaviors	Outcome*	
	Mortality	Dysfunctioning
Men		
Fair or poor health vs. excellent or good health	1.5 (1.1–2.0)	3.4 (2.4–4.7)
Little or no exercise vs. moderate or much activity	1.5 (1.1–1.9)	1.0 (0.7–1.5)
Inactive on a usual day vs. moderate or much activity	2.2 (1.4–3.3)	1.3 (0.7–2.4)
Current smoker vs. never smoked	1.8 (1.3–2.6)	1.2 (0.8–1.7)
Former smoker vs. never smoked	1.0 (0.7–1.4)	0.9 (0.6–1.3)
Women		
Fair or poor health vs. excellent or good health	1.5 (1.1–2.0)	2.7 (2.0–3.7)
Little or no exercise vs. moderate or much activity	1.2 (0.9–1.7)	1.3 (1.1–1.8)
Inactive on a usual day vs. moderate or much activity	1.2 (0.7–1.8)	1.6 (1.1–2.5)
Current smoker vs. never smoked	1.6 (1.1–2.3)	1.6 (1.1–2.3)
Former smoker vs. never smoked	1.8 (1.1–2.8)	1.1 (0.7–1.7)

*Odds ratios are adjusted for the year of the baseline examination, age, and race.

different from those of the control group after adjustment for the year of the baseline examination, age, and race. However, the odds ratios for dysfunction in this co-morbidity group were over three times greater than those of the control group (3.8 and 3.1 for men and women, respectively).

Table 12–8 presents the odds ratios and 95% confidence intervals for mortality and dysfunction associated with the four health perceptions and behaviors. Except for being a former smoker, all the health perceptions and behaviors among men were associated with higher risks of mortality at the time of the follow-up. The risk of mortality was about 50% higher for men with fair or poor self-perceived health than for those with excellent or good self-perceived health. Likewise, comparison of those reporting little or no exercise in recreational activities with persons reporting moderate or much exercise showed a 50% greater risk of mortality among the former. Men who were inactive in their usual day had a mortality risk that was more than twice the risk for those who were moderately or very active. Men who smoked had an 80% higher risk of mortality than did nonsmokers, but men who were former smokers showed no greater risk of mortality than did nonsmokers. With respect to dysfunction among men, only fair or poor self-perceived health showed a significant increase in the odds ratio (3.4).

Among women, fair or poor self-perceived health was associated with a significant increase in the risk of mortality (odds ratio, about 1.5). For current smokers the odds ratio was 1.6, and for former smokers, 1.8. Aside from former-smoker status, all other health perceptions and behaviors were significantly associated with dysfunction; the odds ratios ranged from 1.3 for little or no exercise to 2.7 for those in fair or poor health.

Discussion

Before the implications of these analyses are considered, it is appropriate to focus on three limitations in the data. First, the HAQ disability index had not been used previously in studies of the health and function of persons in community or nationally representative population, although it is a standard part of the American Rheumatism Association Medical Information System (ARAMIS). These results show that the prevalence of disability, defined by index scores of 1.0 or greater, is substantially higher than prevalences shown in other studies of disability, when it was defined only by the need for assistance in one or more of the activities of daily living (Feller 1986; Macken 1986; Dawson et al. 1987).

At the same time, the disability distributions observed in this study are quite consistent for use of the HAQ instrument in the NHEFS population. Consider that Fries and his colleagues (Fries et al. 1982) reported an average disability index score of 0.6 for 147 patients with osteoarthritis in the community of Stanford, California. The average age of the patients was 69 years. Average disability index scores of similar patients from Phoenix, Wichita, and Saskatoon were reported as 0.4 (Fries et al. 1982). For 294 NHEFS survivors (out of 363 subjects between the ages of 55 and 64 years) who reported having been told by a physician that they had arthritis, the mean age at follow-up was 69 years and the average disability index score was also 0.4.

A second concern lies in the reproducibility and reliability of the information on the chronic diseases reported at baseline. An individual's inclusion in any of the chronic disease supplements is not highly reproducible because examining physicians could (and often did) supersede the screening algorithms for including or excluding a subject from one of the supplements, especially the arthritis supplement. This practice may have contributed a bias associated with the chronic disease groups. Such practices suggest a need for closer scrutiny of the data and caution in generalizing the results. For example, about 27% of the 1036 subjects who reported having been told by a physician that they had arthritis in the NHANES I medical history interview did not participate in the arthritis supplement, whereas 29% of those not reporting such a history did participate.

Third, the absence of comparable baseline data on physical function precludes a clearer temporal understanding of the relationships of health behaviors, health perceptions, and chronic disease to the outcomes of mortality or dysfunction. The severity of one's illness probably influences both subsequent perceptions and behaviors, although some behaviors and perceptions may influence the onset of morbidity, as in the case of smoking and the lack of physical exercise.

Despite such limitations, these findings have substantial implications for the understanding of predictors of both mortality and dysfunction among the young-old (those aged 55–74). The findings do not clarify the conflicting data on whether cessation of smoking among very old smokers is effective in reducing their risks of both mortality and disability in comparison with the risks of those who never smoked. Further study will examine individual pack-years to refine this independent variable and assess cause-specific mortality and the onset of disability to refine the dependent variable. It is interesting to observe, however, that men who were former smokers reduced their risk of mortality to that of never-smokers, but women who were former smokers had a higher risk of mortality than never-smokers. Concerning disability among men, neither current smokers nor former smokers had higher rates of dysfunction than the never-smokers. However, women who were current smokers had risks of dysfunction that were significantly higher than those of women who never smoked, whereas women who were former smokers did not.

Other published studies also have failed to support unequivocally the benefits of smoking cessation among very old smokers, but none can be characterized as definitive. Branch and Jette reported that being a current smoker or a past smoker was not associated with an elevated 5-year mortality rate when compared with never-smokers among men and women who had already survived to age 65 (Branch and Jette 1984). In a study of incident limitations in physical functioning, Branch reported no association with smoking history and incident disability among women who had survived to age 65, but men of the same age who had a positive smoking history (either current or former smokers) were at increased risk of disability after age, health status, income, and other health practices were controlled for (Branch 1985).

In a study of 17-year mortality in Alameda County, California, a model that combined men and women aged 60 and over and adjusted for age, health status, and other practices showed that current smokers had mortality rates that were significantly higher than rates for never-smokers, but the risk for former smokers compared to never-smokers overlapped unity (Kaplan et al. 1987).

The most recently published study (Hermanson et al. 1988) of the outcomes of smoking cessation also presents unified results for those who had already achieved age 65 at the start of their 6-year follow-up (132 men and women who had angiographically documented coronary artery disease). Notwithstanding the authors' report of a lower 6-year survival rate among continuing smokers as compared with former smokers who had coronary artery disease, the reported statistical significance was not definitive for those aged 65–69 ($n = 94$, $p = 0.40$) or for those aged 70 or older ($n = 38$, $p = 0.05$). The beneficial effects of smoking cessation on mortality were more unequivocally supported in the 55–59- and 60–64-year age groups.

Thus, the previous literature on the benefits of smoking cessation among people who have already survived to age 65 years shows mixed results. This study supports the previously observed differences between men and women in the effect of past or present smoking on mortality and disability among older cohorts.

Results from this study of physical function correspond to results obtained by others relating to active life expectancy. In 1983 Katz and his colleagues described the concept of active life expectancy. They observed that although women live longer than men, more of their years of life are compromised by disability (Katz et al. 1983). This study confirms that among the women, chronic disease, morbidity, health perceptions, and behaviors were more predictive of future risks of dysfunction than of risks for mortality.

These data contribute to the growing awareness that co-morbidities among older people require increasing scrutiny (Satariano et al. 1988). There is some suggestion in the literature that the number of co-morbidities might influence dysfunction, independent of the pathways of the specific diseases or conditions. The odds for dysfunction among both men and women participating in one or both of the supplementary cardiovascular and respiratory examinations at NHANES I are 2.0–2.6-fold greater than the odds of dysfunction for those not participating in any supplementary examination, but the odds for those with co-morbidities, as suggested by their participation in multiple supplements, were more than threefold greater than the odds of dysfunction in the control group. The suggestion of an additive influence of co-morbidities is supported by the finding that the group participating in the most supplements had the greatest risk of dysfunction.

The restoration of physical function is one of the fundamental principles in the provision of quality health care for the aged population (Kennie 1983). Although prior research has shown that function can be restored, little is known about factors contributing to restoration (Branch et al. 1984). Most studies of physical function have shown a significant association between dysfunction and adverse and often costly outcomes, including mortality, nursing home care, and informal and formal arrangements for assistance at home (Campbell et al. 1985; Donaldson et al. 1980; Branch and Jette 1982; Branch and Stuart 1984). However, few prospective studies with large representative samples have examined the loss and restoration of these self-maintenance activities in association with morbidity at the older ages.

The 1983–1984 NHEFS is the first of three follow-up contacts on the NHANES I cohort. Two additional follow-ups were conducted in 1985–1986 and in 1987–1988 and will provide data on the course of functional ability through repeated administration of the disability index instrument. These prospective data on function will be related to the prevalence and incidence of self-reported medical conditions and impairments; supplemental information on diagnoses and surgical procedures will be provided through linkage to Medicare utilization files. Moreover, the NHEFS is only one of several national and community-based representative studies whose goal is to provide knowledge on the course of functional ability in self-maintenance activities and its association with morbidity in older persons. Other recent studies include the National Longitudinal Study on Aging (Kovar 1987), the National Long-Term Care Survey (Macken 1986), and the community-based Established Populations for Epidemiologic Studies of the Elderly Study (Cornoni-Huntley et al. 1985).

Results from these studies should help guide developments in health promotion and disease prevention for the older population, particularly those at high risk of losing their independence in self-maintenance activities. Further understanding the disease-to-disability pathway in the rapidly growing older population will assist health care policymakers, planners, and providers in their efforts to emphasize preventive and restorative care and services that will minimize the otherwise predictable increases in the need for acute and long-term care services.

REFERENCES

Branch, L. G., and A. M. Jette. 1982. "A prospective study of long-term care institutionalization among the aged." *Am J Public Health* 72:1373–1379.

Branch, L. G., and N. E. Stuart, 1984. "A five-year history of targeting home care services to prevent institutionalization." *Gerontologist* 24:387–391.

Branch, L. G., S. Katz, K. Kneipman, and J. A. Papsidero. 1984. "A prospective study of functional status among community elders." *Am J Public Health* 74:266–268.

Branch, L. G., and A. M. Jette. 1984. "Personal health practices and mortality among the elderly." *Am J Public Health* 74:1126–1129.

Brown, J. H., L. E. Kazis, P. W. Spitz, P. Gertman, J. F. Fries, and R. F. Meenan. 1984. "The dimensions of health outcomes: A cross-validated examination of health status measurement." *Am J Public Health* 74:159–161.

Campbell, A. J., C. Diep, J. Reinken, and L. McCosh. 1985. "Factors predicting mortality in a total population sample of the elderly." *J Epidemiol Community Health* 39:337–342.

Cornoni-Huntley, J. C., D. J. Foley, L. R. White, R. Suzman, L. F. Berkman, D. A. Evans, and R. B. Wallace, 1985. "Epidemiology of disability in the oldest old: Methodologic issues and preliminary findings." *Milbank Mem Fund Q* 63:350–376.

Donaldson, D., G. Clayton, M. Clarke. 1980. "The elderly in residential care: mortality in relation to functional capacity." *J Epidemiol Community Health* 34:96–101.

Fillenbaum, G. G., and M. A. Smyer. 1981. "The development, validity, and reliability of the OARS multidimensional functional assessment questionnaire." *J Gerontol* 36:428–434.

Fries, J. F., P. Spitz, R. G. Kraines, and H. R. Holman. 1980. "Measurement of patient outcome in arthritis." *Arthritis Rheum* 23:137–145.

Fries, J. F., P. W. Spitz, and D. Y. Young. 1982. "The dimensions of health outcomes: The health assessment questionnaire, disability and pain scales. *J Rheumatol* 9:789–793.

Grizzle, J. E., C. F. Starmer, and G. G. Koch. 1969. Analysis of categorical data by linear models." *Biometrics* 24:489–504.

Hermanson, B., G. S. Omenn, R. A. Kronmal, and B. J. Gersh. 1988. "Beneficial six-year outcome of smoking cessation in older men and women with coronary artery disease: Results from the CASS registry." *N Engl J Med* 319:1365–1369.

Kaplan, G. A., T. E. Seeman, R. D. Cohen, L. P. Knudsen, and J. M. Guralnik. 1987. "Mortality among the elderly in the Alameda County study: Behavioral and demographic risk factors." *Am J Public Health* 77:307–312.

Katz, S., A. B. Ford, R. W. Moskowitz, B. A. Jackson, and M. W. Jaffe. 1963. "Studies of illness in the aged: The Index of ADL, a standardized measure of biological and psychosocial function." *JAMA* 185:914–919.

Katz, S., L. G. Branch, M. H. Branson, J. A. Papsidero, J. C. Beck, and D. S. Greer. 1983. "Active life expectancy." *N Engl J Med* 309:1218–1223.

Katz, S. 1983. "Assessing self-maintenance: Activities of daily living, mobility, and instrumental activities of daily living." *J Am Geriatr Soc* 31:721–727.

Kennie, D. C. 1983. "Good health care for the aged." *JAMA* 249:770–773.

Kleinbaum, D. G., L. L. Kupper, and H. Morgenstern. 1982. "Epidemiologic research: Principles and quantitative methods." New York. Van Nostrand-Reinhold.

Kovar, M. G. 1987. "The Longitudinal study of aging: The 1986 reinterview public-use file." Proceedings of the 1987 Public Health Conference on Records and Statistics.

U.S. Department of Health and Human Services, DHHS, Pub. No. (PHS) 88-1214:45–46.

Lawton, M. P., M. Moss, M. Fulcomer et al. 1982. "A research and service oriented multilevel assessment instrument." *J Gerontol* 37:91–99.

Macken, C. L. 1986. "A profile of functionally impaired elderly persons living in the community." *Health Care Financing Rev* 7:33–49.

National Center for Health Statistics. 1986. Feller, B. A. *Americans Needing Home Care.* Vital and Health Statistics. Series 10, No. 153. U.S. Department of Health and Human Services Pub. No. (PHS) 86-1581. Washington, DC: U.S. Government Printing Office.

National Center for Health Statistics. 1987. Dawson, D., G. Hendershot, and J. Fulton. Aging in the Eighties: Functional Limitations of Individuals Age 65 Years and Over. *Advance Data.* No. 133.

Satariano, W. A., N. E. Ragheb, M. H. Dupuis, 1988. "Co-morbidity in older women with breast cancer: An epidemiologic approach." In R. Yancik and J. Yates, eds. *Cancer in the Elderly: Approach to Early Detection and Treatment.* New York: Springer Verlag.

Shanas, E. 1980. "Self-assessment of physical function: white and black elderly of the United States." In S. G. Haynes and M. Fienleib, eds. *Second Conference on the Epidemiology of Aging.* NIH Publication No. 80-969, pp. 269–281.

Solomon, D. 1988. "Chairman, National Institutes of Health Consensus Development Conference Statement: Geriatric assessment methods for clinical decision-making." *J Am Geriatr Soc* 36:342–347.

Williams, T. F. 1983. "Comprehensive functional assessment: An overview." *J Am Geriatr Soc* 31:637–641.

Wolfe, F., S. M. Kleinheksel, M. A. Cathey et al. 1988. "The clinical value of the Stanford Health Assessment Questionnaire Functional Disability Index in patients with rheumatoid arthritis." *J Rheumatol* 15:1480–1488.

APPENDIX A

NHANES I
Epidemiologic Follow-up Survey

ID NUMBER [ ][ ][ ] - [ ][ ]

OMB No. 0925-0161
Approval Expires 12-31-83

U.S. DEPARTMENT OF HEALTH AND HUMAN SERVICES
PUBLIC HEALTH SERVICE
NATIONAL CENTER FOR HEALTH STATISTICS
NATIONAL INSTITUTE ON AGING
NATIONAL INSTITUTES OF HEALTH

NHANES I EPIDEMIOLOGIC FOLLOWUP SURVEY

SELF-ADMINISTRATION SUBJECT INTERVIEW BOOKLET

ASSURANCE OF CONFIDENTIALITY

All information which would provide identification of the individual will be held in strict confidence, will be used only for purposes of and by persons engaged in the survey, and will not be disclosed or released to others for any purposes in accordance with Section 308(d) of the Public Health Service Act (42 USC 242 m).

PHS T-523
(7-82)

PART A.

TIME BEGAN: _____ AM / PM

Begin A0

[ ] 11-15

BOX A
INTERVIEWER: REVIEW LABEL AND CIRCLE ONE:
S IS UNDER 60 . . . . 1 (Q.A-6)
S IS 60 OR OLDER 2 (Q.A-1)
BOXED QUESTIONNAIRE 3 (Q.A-6)

First I'd like to verify a few facts.

MSQ I

	RESPONSE vs. ACTUAL	SCORE ANSWERS

What is your complete address?

A-1. Number and street _____ (NO.) (R) [ ]   16
_____ (STREET) (R)
(RECORD NUMBER AND STREET NAME FROM LABEL)
_____ (NO.) (A)
_____ (STREET) (A)

A-2. City and State _____ (CITY) (R) [ ]   17
_____ (STATE) (R)
(RECORD CITY AND STATE FROM LABEL)
_____ (CITY) (A)
_____ (STATE) (A)

A-3. How old are you now? _____ (AGE) (R) [ ]   18
(AGE AT LAST BIRTHDAY. RESPONSE SHOULD BE WITHIN ONE YEAR OF ACTUAL AGE.)
(RECORD AGE FROM LABEL.) _____ (A)

When were you born?

A-4. Month? "DAY" (DO NOT SCORE) _____ (R) (A) [ ]   19
_____ (RECORD MONTH)

A-5. Year? _____ (R) (A) l   20

[ ] BOX 1   21

BOX B
INTERVIEWER: REVIEW BOX 1 AND CIRCLE ONE:
BOX 1 IS LESS THAN 3 . . . . . 1 (MSQ II P. 43)
BOX 1 IS 3 OR MORE 2 (Q.A-6)

INTERVIEWER:
INTERVIEWER OBSERVE TYPE OF LIVING QUARTERS AND CIRCLE ONE
PRIVATE RESIDENCE OR APARTMENT BUILDING 1 (Q.A-7)
SHELTERED HOUSING 2 (Q.A-7)
NURSING HOME 3 (Q.A-16)
PERSONAL CARE HOME 4 (Q.A-16)
OTHER INSTITUTION (SPECIFY) 5 (Q.A-16)

...next series of questions is about your household.

ENTER NAME OF S ON LINE a OF QUESTION A-12 BELOW.

A-7. How many people live in your household including yourself?

A-7   ONE.............01
  # PEOPLE:|__|__| (Q.A-9)   22-23

A-8. About how long have you lived alone?

A-8   LESS THAN ONE
  YEAR..........00 (Q.A-25)
  # YEARS: |__|__| (Q.A-25)
  DK............98 (Q.A-25)   24-25

A-9. What is the name of the head of your household? (IF S IS NOT HEAD OF HOUSEHOLD ENTER HH ON LINE 12b AND CIRCLE.)   26

A-10. What (is/are) the name(s) of the other person(s) who live(s) in your household? (RECORD NAMES IN Q.A-12).

A-11. Have I missed anyone who usually lives here but is now away from home?

A-11   YES.............1 (RECORD IN Q.A-12)
  NO..............2

A-12. AFTER LISTING HOUSEHOLD ASK Q.A-13 THROUGH A-15 FOR EACH PERSON, AS APPROPRIATE. NAME (FIRST, MIDDLE INITIAL, LAST).

	A-13. How old was (PERSON) on (his/her) last birthday? YEARS OF AGE	A-14. (ASK SEX IF QUESTIONABLE.) Is (PERSON) male or female? M	F	A-15. How is (PERSON) related to you? RELATIONSHIP	
a.				(SUBJECT)	27-31
b.	YRS: |__|__|	1	2		32-36
c.	YRS: |__|__|	1	2		37-41
d.	YRS: |__|__|	1	2		42-46
e.	YRS: |__|__|	1	2		47-51
f.	YRS: |__|__|	1	2		52-56
g.	YRS: |__|__|	1	2		57-61
h.	YRS: |__|__|	1	2		62-66
i.	YRS: |__|__|	1	2		67-71
j.	YRS: |__|__|	1	2		72-76
k.	YRS: |__|__|	1	2		77-81
l.	YRS: |__|__|	1	2		82-86

INTERVIEWER: GO TO Q.A-25

3

...next series of questions is about the last household in which you lived.

ENTER NAME OF S ON LINE a OF QUESTION A-21 BELOW.

A-16. How many people lived in your household including yourself?

A-16   ONE.............01
  # PEOPLE: |__|__| (Q.A-18)   22-23

A-17. About how long did you live alone?

A-17   LESS THAN ONE
  YEAR..........00 (Q.A-25)
  # YEARS: |__|__| (Q.A-25)
  DK............98 (Q.A-25)   24-25

A-18. What was the name of the head of your household? (IF S IS NOT HEAD OF HOUSEHOLD ENTER HH ON LINE 21b AND CIRCLE.)   26

A-19. What (was/were) the name(s) of the other person(s) who lived in your household? (RECORD NAMES IN Q.A-21).

A-20. Have I missed anyone who usually lived there?

A-20   YES.............1 (RECORD IN Q.A-21)
  NO..............2

A-21. AFTER LISTING HOUSEHOLD ASK Q.A-22 THROUGH A-24 FOR EACH PERSON, AS APPROPRIATE. NAME (FIRST, MIDDLE INITIAL, LAST).

	A-22. How old was (PERSON) just prior to your leaving the household? YEARS OF AGE	A-23. (ASK SEX IF QUESTIONABLE.) Is (PERSON) male or female? M	F	A-24. How is (PERSON) related to you? RELATIONSHIP	
a.				(SUBJECT)	27-31
b.	YRS: |__|__|	1	2		32-36
c.	YRS: |__|__|	1	2		37-41
d.	YRS: |__|__|	1	2		42-46
e.	YRS: |__|__|	1	2		47-51
f.	YRS: |__|__|	1	2		52-56
g.	YRS: |__|__|	1	2		57-61
h.	YRS: |__|__|	1	2		62-66
i.	YRS: |__|__|	1	2		67-71
j.	YRS: |__|__|	1	2		72-76
k.	YRS: |__|__|	1	2		77-81
l.	YRS: |__|__|	1	2		82-86

4

PART B: FAMILY HISTORY

In this part of the questionnaire, I would like to ask you about your relatives. This includes your natural parents, your sisters and brothers and your children. Do not include adopted or step relatives, but do include half relatives.

Begin B0

B-1. How many brothers and sisters living or deceased do you have?

B-1
NONE......... 00 (Q.B-3)
#: |__|__|
DK........... 98 (Q.B-3)

11-12

B-2. How many of these brothers and sisters were born before you?

B-2
S OLDEST...... 00
OLDER:..... |__|__|
DK........... 98

13-14

B-3. How many children living or deceased have you had? Remember not to include adopted or step children.

B-3
NONE......... 00
CHILDREN: |__|__|

15-16

B-4. Is your mother still living?

B-4
YES.......... 1 (Q.B-7)
NO........... 2
DK........... 8 (Q.B-7)

17

B-5. In what year did she die?

B-5
YR: |_1_|_1_|_9_|__|
DK........... 9998

18-21

B-6. Was your mother's death due to an injury or an accident?

B-6
YES.......... 1
NO........... 2
DK........... 8

22

B-7. In what year was your mother born?

B-7
YR: |__|__|__|__|
DK........... 9998

23-26

B-8. Is your father still living?

B-8
YES.......... 1 (Q.B-11)
NO........... 2
DK........... 8 (Q.B-11)

27

B-9. In what year did he die?

B-9
YR: |_1_|_1_|_9_|__|
DK........... 9998

28-31

B-10. Was your father's death due to an injury or an accident?

B-10
YES.......... 1
NO........... 2
DK........... 8

32

B-11. In what year was your father born?

B-11
YR: |__|__|__|__|
DK........... 9998

33-36

B-12. Think about the relatives that you have included in the previous questions, your parents, brothers, sisters, and children. Did a doctor ever say that any of these relatives had cancer?

B-12
YES.......... 1
NO........... 2 (BOX C)
DK........... 8 (BOX C)

37

6

A-25. What is the highest grade or year of school that (HEAD OF HOUSEHOLD) ever completed? Include trade or vocational school.

A-25
NONE............ 10
GRADE 1......... 21
GRADE 2......... 22
GRADE 3......... 23
GRADE 4......... 24
GRADE 5......... 25
GRADE 6......... 26
GRADE 7......... 27
GRADE 8......... 28
GRADE 9......... 31
GRADE 10........ 32
GRADE 11........ 33
GRADE 12........ 34

VOCATIONAL
1 YEAR.......... 01
2 YEARS......... 02
3 YEARS OR MORE. 03

COLLEGE
1 YEAR.......... 41
2 YEARS......... 42
3 YEARS......... 43
4 YEARS......... 44
GRADUATE SCHOOL. 45
DK.............. 98

A-26. (In the last household in which you lived) how many children (did/do) you have who live(d) away from home?

A-26
NONE............ 00 (PART B)
OF CHILDREN: |__|__|

102-103

A-27. (At that time) How many of your children live(d)...

A-27
OF CHILDREN:

a. less than 1/2 hour away?   a |__|__| 104-105

b. about 1/2 hour away?   b |__|__| 106-107

c. about an hour away?   c |__|__| 108-109

d. about two hours away?   d |__|__| 110-111

e. more than two hours away?   e |__|__| 112-113
                                         |__|__| 114-115

OFFICE USE ONLY: |__|__|__|__|__|__| 116-122

PART D: HEALTH/DISEASES AND OPERATIONS

The questions I'm going to ask you now concern your health as well as diseases and operations you might have had.

Begin D1

D-1. Would you say that your health in general is excellent, very good, good, fair, or poor?
EXCELLENT............. 1
VERY GOOD............. 2
GOOD.................. 3
FAIR.................. 4
POOR.................. 5   11

D-2. Have you ever been told by a doctor that you had hypertension or high blood pressure?
YES.................. 1
NO.................. 2 (Q.D-6)
DK.................. 8 (Q.D-6)   12

D-3. In what year were you first told that you had this condition?
YR: |_1_|_9_|__|__| (Q.D-5)
DK.................. 9998   13-16

D-4. Can you remember if it was less than a year ago, between 1 and 5 years ago, between 5 and 10 years ago, or 10 or more years ago?
LESS THAN ONE YEAR....... 1
1 BUT LESS THAN 5 YEARS... 2
5 BUT LESS THAN 10 YEARS. 3
10 OR MORE............... 4
DK....................... 8   17

D-5. Since 1970, have you been hospitalized overnight for problems related to your hypertension or high blood pressure?
YES.................. 1 (CHART)
NO.................. 2   18

D-6. Have you ever had any pain or discomfort in your chest?
YES.................. 1 (Q.D-8)
NO.................. 2   19

D-7. Have you ever had any pressure or heaviness in your chest?
YES.................. 1
NO.................. 2 (Q.D-27)   20

D-8. Do you get this (pain or discomfort/pressure or heaviness) when you walk uphill or hurry?
YES.................. 1
NO.................. 2 (Q.D-19)
NEVER WALKS UPHILL OR HURRIES........ 3   21

D-9. Do you get this (pain or discomfort/pressure or heaviness) when you walk at an ordinary pace on level ground?
YES.................. 1
NO.................. 2   22

D-10. What do you do if you get this pain while you are walking, stop or slow down, take a nitroglycerin, or continue at the same pace? (CIRCLE YES OR NO FOR EACH.)

		YES	NO
a	STOP OR SLOW DOWN.	1	2	23
b	TAKE A NITROGLYCERIN...	1	2	24
c	CONTINUE AT THE SAME PACE.......	1(Q.D-19)	2	25

8

D-11. Could you tell me which relatives have had cancer?
[CIRCLE RELATIONSHIP TO SUBJECT IF S IN COLUMN A.]

COLUMN A — CIRCLE RELATIONSHIP TO SUBJECT
COLUMN B — Could you tell me the site or type of the cancer which your (RELATIVE) had?

a.
MOTHER...... 1
FATHER...... 2
SISTER...... 3
BROTHER..... 4
SON......... 5
DAUGHTER.... 6   38
SITE: _____
OR
TYPE: _____   38-41 / 42-44

b.
MOTHER...... 1
FATHER...... 2
SISTER...... 3
BROTHER..... 4
SON......... 5
DAUGHTER.... 6   45
SITE: _____
OR
TYPE: _____   46-48 / 49-51

c.
MOTHER...... 1
FATHER...... 2
SISTER...... 3
BROTHER..... 4
SON......... 5
DAUGHTER.... 6   52
SITE: _____
OR
TYPE: _____   53-55 / 56-58

d.
MOTHER...... 1
FATHER...... 2
SISTER...... 3
BROTHER..... 4
SON......... 5
DAUGHTER.... 6   59
SITE: _____
OR
TYPE: _____   60-62 / 63-65

e.
MOTHER...... 1
FATHER...... 2
SISTER...... 3
BROTHER..... 4
SON......... 5
DAUGHTER.... 6   66
SITE: _____
OR
TYPE: _____   67-69 / 70-72

PART C

INTERVIEWER: CIRCLE ONE:
S IS FEMALE.......1 (PART C - SELF ADMINISTRATION BOOKLET)
S IS MALE.........2 (PART D)

7

D-11. If you do stop or slow down, is the pain relieved or not?
RELIEVED...........1
NOT RELIEVED.......2 (Q,D-19)   26

D-12. How soon is the pain relieved?
TEN MINUTES OR LESS.. 1
MORE THAN 10 MINUTES. 2 (Q,D-19)   27

D-13. Have you ever had this (pain or discomfort/pressure or heaviness) more than three times?
YES................1
NO.................2   28

D-14. About how old were you when you first had it? (READ AGE CATEGORIES IF NECESSARY.)
LESS THAN 15 YEARS OLD. 01
15 LESS THAN 20 YEARS.. 02
20 LESS THAN 30 YEARS.. 03
30 LESS THAN 40 YEARS.. 04
40 LESS THAN 50 YEARS.. 05
50 LESS THAN 60 YEARS.. 06
60 LESS THAN 70 YEARS.. 07
70 LESS THAN 80 YEARS.. 08
80 YEARS OR OLDER...... 09   29-30

D-15. Have you been bothered by this (pain or discomfort/pressure or heaviness) in the past 12 months?
YES................1 (Q,D-17)
NO.................2   31

D-16. In what year did you last experience the (pain or discomfort/pressure or heaviness)?
YR: |_1_|_9_|_|_|
DK.................9998   32-35

D-17. Please look at this diagram. Do you get this (pain or discomfort/pressure or heaviness) (SHOW DIAGRAM IN SELF-ADMINISTRATION BOOKLET, PAGE 6)

	YES	NO	DK	
a. in region A -- ?	1	2	8	36
b. in region B -- ?	1	2	8	37
c. in region C -- ?	1	2	8	38
d. in region D -- ?	1	2	8	39

D-18. Do you feel it anywhere else?
YES................1 (MARK ON DIAGRAM)
NO.................2   40
]]   41 42

D-19. Have you ever had a severe pain across the front of your chest lasting half an hour or more?
YES................1
NO.................2 (Q,D-27)
DK.................8 (Q,D-27)   43

D-20. Did you see a doctor because of this pain?
YES................1
NO.................2 (Q,D-22)   44

D-21. What did the doctor say it was?
SPECIFY:
_____
_____
DK.................8   ] 45

D-22. How many of these attacks have you had?
ATTACKS: |_|_|
DK.................98   46-47

D-23. In what year was your (first) attack?
YR: |_1_|_9_|_|_|
DK.................9998   48-51

D-24. How long was the episode of pain?
1/2 TO ONE HOUR... 00
HRS: |_|_| 52-53

BOX D
INTERVIEWER: CHECK THE NUMBER OF ATTACKS REPORTED (Q,D-22) AND CIRCLE ONE:
Q,D-22 = 01........1 (Q,D-26b)
OTHERWISE..........2 (Q,D-25)

D-25. In what year was your last attack?
YR: |_1_|_9_|_|_|
DK.................9998   54-57

D-26a. How long was the episode of pain?
1/2 TO ONE HOUR... 00
HRS: |_|_| 58-59

D-26b. Since 1970, have you been hospitalized overnight for (this/these) attack(s)?
YES................1 (CHART)
NO.................2   60

D-27. Do you get pain in either leg when walking?
YES................1
NO.................2 (Q,D-39a)
UNABLE TO WALK.....3 (Q,D-39a)   61

D-28. Does this pain ever begin when you are standing still or sitting?
YES................1 (Q,D-39a)
NO.................2   62

D-29. In what part of your leg do you feel it? (IF CALVES NOT MENTIONED, ASK, "Anywhere else?" IF STILL NOT MENTIONED, CIRCLE 2.)
PAIN INCLUDES CALF/CALVES.....1
PAIN DOES NOT INCLUDE CALF....2 (Q,D-39a)   63

D-30. Do you get this pain when you walk uphill or hurry?
YES................1
NO.................2 (Q,D-39a)
NEVER WALKS UP-HILL OR HURRIES. 3   64

D-31. Do you get this pain when you walk at an ordinary pace on level ground?
YES................1
NO.................2   65

D-32. Does this pain ever disappear while you are still walking?
YES................1 (Q,D-39a)
NO.................2   66

D-33. What do you do if you get this pain while walking, stop or slacken your pace or continue at the same pace?
STOP OR SLACKEN PACE........1
CONTINUE AT SAME PACE.......2 (Q,D-39a)   67

D-34. If you do stop, is the pain relieved or not? [D-34]
RELIEVED.............1
NOT RELIEVED.........2 (Q.D-39a)   68

D-35. How soon after stopping is the pain relieved? [D-35]
TEN MINUTES OR LESS.............1
MORE THAN 10 MINUTES............2   69

D-36. How old were you when you first had it? (READ CATEGORIES IF NECESSARY.) [D-36]
LESS THAN 15 YEARS OLD..01
15 LESS THAN 20 YEARS...02
20 LESS THAN 30 YEARS...03
30 LESS THAN 40 YEARS...04
40 LESS THAN 50 YEARS...05
50 LESS THAN 60 YEARS...06
60 LESS THAN 70 YEARS...07
70 LESS THAN 80 YEARS...08
80 YEARS OR OLDER.......09   70-71

D-37. Have you been bothered by this condition in the past 12 months? [D-37]
YES.............1 (Q.D-39a)
NO..............2   72

D-38. In what year did you last experience this problem? [D-38]
YR: |1|9|_|_|
DK........9998   73-76

READ COLUMN a TO S. IF THE ANSWER TO COLUMN a IS "YES," ASK COLUMN b FOR THE CONDITION. IF "NO," ASK COLUMN a FOR THE NEXT CONDITION.

COLUMN a	COLUMN b
Have you ever had (CONDITION):	Did this condition last longer than 24 hours?

D-39a. A sudden loss of vision?
YES..............1
NO...............2 (Q.D-40a)
D-39b. YES.....1 NO.....2 DK.....8   77-78

D-40a. A sudden loss of speech, difficulty in speaking, or slurred speech?
YES..............1
NO...............2 (Q.D-41a)
D-40b. YES.....1 NO.....2 DK.....8

D-41a. A sudden paralysis or weakness of an arm and/or leg on the same side of the body?
YES..............1
NO...............2 (Q.D-42a)
D-41b. YES.....1 NO.....2 DK.....8   79-80

D-42a. A sudden numbness on one side of the body?
YES..............1
NO...............2 (Q.D-43)
D-42b. YES.....1 NO.....2 DK.....8   81-82 / 83-84

11

D-43. Did a doctor ever tell you that you had gall bladder disease? [D-43]
YES.............1
NO..............2 (BOX E)   85

D-44. In what year were you first told that you had this condition? [D-44]
YR: |1|9|_|_| 86-89

D-45. Did you have surgery or a surgical procedure for this condition? [D-45]
YES.............1
NO..............2 (Q.D-47)   90

D-46. In what year did you first have surgery for this condition? [D-46]
YR: |1|9|_|_| 91-94

D-47. Since 1970, have you been hospitalized overnight for this condition? [D-47]
YES.............1 (CHART)
NO..............2   95

```
                    BOX E

     INTERVIEWER: CIRCLE ONE:

        S IS FEMALE............1 (Q.D-48)
        S IS MALE.............2 (Q.D-55)
```

D-48. Did a doctor ever tell you that you had a lump or cyst in your breast? [D-48]
YES.............1
NO..............2 (Q.D-54)   96

D-49. Did you ever have a biopsy or aspiration for this condition? [D-49]
YES.............1
NO..............2 (Q.D-52)   97

D-50. What is the total number of breast biopsies that you have had? Do not include aspiration where fluid was removed. [D-50]
NO BIOPSIES......00 (Q.D-54)
BIOPSIES: |_|_|
DK...............98   98-99

D-51. In what year did you (first) have a biopsy for a cyst or lump? [D-51]
YR: |1|9|_|_|
DK........9998   100-103

D-52. Did the doctor ever tell you that a lump or cyst in your breast was cancerous or malignant? [D-52]
YES.............1
NO..............2   104

D-53. Have you had one or both of your breasts removed? [D-53]
YES, ONE BREAST.....1
YES, BOTH BREASTS...2
NEITHER.............3   105

D-54. Since 1970 have you been hospitalized overnight for any type of breast condition, female problem or a pregnancy? [D-54]
YES.............1 (CHART)
NO..............2   106

12

These next questions are about skin problems you may have had.

D-55. Have you ever had a skin tumor, growth on your skin, skin ulcer or other skin lesions for which you received medical treatment by a doctor? (Do not include bedsores.)

YES.............. 1
NO............... 2 (Q,D-62)
107

D-56. Since 1970, for how many skin conditions have you received treatment by a doctor?

NONE......... 00 (Q,D-62)
OF CONDITIONS: |__|
DK........... 98
108-109

Now I'd like to ask you about (this/these) (NUMBER) condition(s).

READ D-57 TO D-61 FOR EACH CONDITION.	1st SKIN CONDITION	2nd SKIN CONDITION	3rd SKIN CONDITION Begin D2
D-57. Was the (#SKIN CONDITION) a tumor or growth, a skin ulcer or something else?	TUMOR OR GROWTH..... 01, SKIN ULCER.. 02, MOLE......... 03, CYST......... 04, WART......... 05, OTHER (SPECIFY) 06, DK........ 08 — 11-12	TUMOR OR GROWTH..... 01, SKIN ULCER.. 02, MOLE......... 03, CYST......... 04, WART......... 05, OTHER (SPECIFY) 06, DK........ 08 — 27-28	TUMOR OR GROWTH..... 01, SKIN ULCER.. 02, MOLE......... 03, CYST......... 04, WART......... 05, OTHER (SPECIFY) 06, DK........ 08 — 41-44
D-58. Did the doctor tell you that this condition was cancerous or malignant?	YES.......... 1 NO........... 2 — 13	YES.......... 1 NO........... 2 — 29	YES.......... 1 NO........... 2 — 45
D-59. How many times has this condition recurred which required treatment by a doctor, including surgical removal?	# TIMES: |__| CONTINUOUS.. 96 DK........ 98 — 14-15	# TIMES: |__| CONTINUOUS.. 96 DK........ 98 — 30-31	# TIMES: |__| CONTINUOUS.. 96 DK........ 98 — 46-47
D-60. On what parts of the body was this condition located? (CIRCLE YES OR NO FOR EACH.)	Y N — a. HEAD OR FACE.... 1 2, b. ARMS..... 1 2, c. HANDS... 1 2, d. LEGS.... 1 2, e. FEET.... 1 2, f. OTHER (SPEC.) 1 2 — 16-25	Y N — a. HEAD OR FACE.... 1 2, b. ARMS.... 1 2, c. HANDS.. 1 2, d. LEGS.. 1 2, e. FEET.. 1 2, f. OTHER (SPEC.) 1 2 — 32-41	Y N — a. HEAD OR FACE.... 1 2, b. ARMS.... 1 2, c. HANDS.. 1 2, d. LEGS.. 1 2, e. FEET.. 1 2, f. OTHER (SPEC.) 1 2 — 48-57
D-61. Since 1970, have you ever stayed in a hospital overnight for treatment of this condition?	YES.... 1 (CHART) NO.... 2 (IF ANOTHER CONDITION GO TO D-57) — 26	YES.... 1 (CHART) NO.... 2 (IF ANOTHER CONDITION GO TO D-57) — 42	YES.... 1 (CHART) NO.... 2 (IF ANOTHER CONDITION GO TO D-57) — 58

13

D-62. Did a doctor ever tell you that you had any cancer (other than the cancer we talked about)? (DON'T INCLUDE SKIN CANCER UNLESS MELANOMA.)

YES.............. 1
NO............... 2 (Q,D-66)
75

ASK D-63 AND RECORD EACH SEPARATE DIAGNOSIS OF CANCER, THEN ASK D-64 AND D-65 FOR EACH DIAGNOSIS.

	1st DIAGNOSIS	2nd DIAGNOSIS	3rd DIAGNOSIS
D-63. Where was the cancer or what type of cancer was it? (Have you had any other cancer diagnosed?)	SITE: ___ OR TYPE: ___ — 76-78	SITE: ___ OR TYPE: ___ — 84-86	SITE: ___ OR TYPE: ___ — 92-94
D-64. In what year were you first told that you had (SITE/TYPE)?	YR: |1|9|__|__| DK........ 9998 — 79-82	YR: |1|9|__|__| DK........ 9998 — 87-90	YR: |1|9|__|__| DK........ 9998 — 95-98
D-65. Since 1970, have you been hospitalized overnight for this condition?	YES.... 1 (CHART) NO...... 2 — 83	YES.... 1 (CHART) NO...... 2 — 91	YES.... 1 (CHART) NO...... 2 — 99

These next questions are about respiratory problems.

D-66. Do you usually have a cough? Exclude clearing your throat. (Include a cough when getting up, a cough when going out of doors, a cough with the first smoke, or coughing at all during the rest of the day or night.)

YES.............. 1
NO............... 2 (Q,D-68)
100

D-67. Do you usually cough like this on most days for three consecutive months or more during the year?

YES.............. 1
NO............... 2
101

D-68. Do you usually bring up phlegm from your chest? Exclude bringing up phlegm from your nose. (Include bringing up phlegm at all when getting up in the morning, when first going up out of doors, with the first smoke or bringing up phlegm at all the rest of the day.)

YES.............. 1
NO............... 2 (Q,D-70)
102

D-69. Do you bring up phlegm like this on most days for three consecutive months or more during the year?

YES.............. 1
NO............... 2
103

14

(IF 5 IS UNABLE TO WALK, CODE 3.)

D-70. Are you troubled by shortness of breath when hurrying on level ground or walking up a slight hill?
YES............... 1
NO............... 2 (Q.D-75)
UNABLE TO WALK.... 3 (Q.D-74)
104

D-71. Do you have to walk slower than people of your age on level ground because of breathlessness?
YES............... 1
NO............... 2
105

D-72. Do you ever have to stop for breath when walking at your own pace on level ground?
YES............... 1
NO............... 2
106

D-73. Do you ever have to stop for breath after walking about 100 yards or after a few minutes, on level ground?
YES............... 1
NO............... 2
107

D-74. Are you too breathless to leave the house or breathless on dressing or undressing?
YES............... 1
NO............... 2
108

D-75. Does your chest ever sound wheezy or whistling...

	YES	NO
a. on most days or nights?	1 (Q.D-76)	2	109
b. when you have a cold?	1	2	110
c. occasionally when you don't have a cold?	1	2	111

The next few questions are about ways in which the environment may affect your skin.

D-76. During your adult life, as part of your usual job, were you outdoors in the sun frequently, occasionally, rarely or never?
FREQUENTLY...... 1
OCCASIONALLY.... 2
RARELY.......... 3
NEVER........... 4
DK.............. 8
112

D-77. During your adult life, in your leisure time, including hobbies and sports, were you outdoors in the sun frequently, occasionally, rarely or never?
FREQUENTLY...... 1
OCCASIONALLY.... 2
RARELY.......... 3
NEVER........... 4
DK.............. 8
113

D-78. When you were a child or teenager, were you ever sunburned so badly that your skin blistered?
YES............... 1
NO............... 2
DK.............. 8
114

15

D-79. In the summer, once you have already been in the sun several times, what reaction will your skin have the next time you go out in the sun for two or more hours on a bright day? Would you say you would get no reaction, some redness only, a burn, or a painful burn?
NO REACTION/TAN... 1
SOME REDNESS....... 2
BURN.............. 3
PAINFUL BURN...... 4
DK................ 8
115

D-80. After repeated sun exposures, for example, a two-week vacation outdoors, would your skin become slightly darker, somewhat darker, very dark, or would there be no change?
SLIGHTLY DARKER... 1
SOMEWHAT DARKER... 2
VERY DARK......... 3
NO CHANGE......... 4
DK................ 8
116

D-81. In the past ten years, have you ever been confined to bed for most of the day for at least a two-week period?
YES............... 1
NO............... 2 (PART E)
117

D-82. Have you ever had a bedsore, an open sore caused by being confined to bed for a long time or unable to move about as usual?
YES............... 1
NO............... 2 (PART E)
118

D-83. When this bedsore occurred, were you at home, in a hospital, in a nursing home or somewhere else?
HOME (OWN)........ 1
HOSPITAL.......... 2
NURSING HOME...... 3
OTHER (SPECIFY)... 4
119

TIME ENDED: _____ AM
                       PM

16

TIME BEGAN: _____ AM / PM

PART E: MUSCULOSKELETAL PROBLEMS

These next questions are about some other health problems you might experience from time to time.

Begin E1

E-1. Have you had pain in your neck on most days for at least one month?
YES............. 1 (Q.E-10)
NO.............. 2
11

E-2. Have you had pain in your back on most days for at least one month?
YES............. 1 (Q.E-29)
NO.............. 2
12

E-3. Have you had pain in or around either hip joint, including the buttock, groin and side of upper thigh, on most days for at least one month?
YES............. 1 (Q.E-50)
NO.............. 2
13

E-4a. Have you had pain in or around the knee, including back of knee, on most days for at least one month?
YES............. 1 (Q.E-61)
NO.............. 2 (Q.E-5)
14

E-4b. Which knee?
LEFT............ 1 (Q.E-61)
RIGHT........... 2 (Q.E-61)
BOTH............ 3 (Q.E-61)
15

E-5. Have you had pain or aching in any joint other than the hip, back or knee on most days for at least six weeks?
YES............. 1 (Q.E-72)
NO.............. 2
16

E-6. Have you had any swollen joints which were painful when touched on most days for at least one month?
YES............. 1 (Q.E-74)
NO.............. 2
17

E-7. Have you had stiffness in your joints when first getting out of bed on most mornings for at least one month?
YES............. 1 (Q.E-83)
NO.............. 2
18

E-8. Have you ever been told by a doctor that you fractured a hip?
YES............. 1 (Q.E-91)
NO.............. 2
19

E-9. Have you ever been told by a doctor that you had a dislocated hip?
YES............. 1 (Q.E-96)
NO.............. 2 (PART F)
20

E-10. What was the longest episode of neck pain you ever had? [IF'S INDICATES LESS THAN 1 MONTH, REASK'Q.E-1.]
1 MONTH.......... 1
MORE THAN 1 BUT LESS THAN 6 MONTHS.......... 2
6-12 MONTHS...... 3
MORE THAN 1 YEAR.. 4
21

E-11. How old were you when you first experienced this recurring neck pain? (READ CATEGORIES IF NECESSARY.)
LESS THAN 15 YEARS OLD.......... 01
15 LESS THAN 20 YEARS. 02
20 LESS THAN 30 YEARS. 03
30 LESS THAN 40 YEARS. 04
40 LESS THAN 50 YEARS. 05
50 LESS THAN 60 YEARS. 06
60 LESS THAN 70 YEARS. 07
70 LESS THAN 80 YEARS. 08
80 AND OLDER.......... 09
22-23

E-12. Are you still having this neck pain?
YES............. 1 (Q.E-14)
NO.............. 2
24

E-13. When was the last time you had this pain? (READ CATEGORIES IF NECESSARY.)
LESS THAN 1 YEAR AGO... 1 (Q.E-15)
1 BUT LESS THAN 3...... 2 (Q.E-15)
3 BUT LESS THAN 5...... 3 (Q.E-15)
5 OR MORE YEARS AGO.... 4 (Q.E-15)
DK.................... 5 (Q.E-15)
25

E-14. Does this neck pain occur more frequently than it used to?
YES............. 1
NO.............. 2
26

E-15. (Is/was) the pain present when you (are/were) resting at night?
YES............. 1
NO.............. 2 (Q.E-17)
27

E-16. (Does/did) it awaken you from sleep at night?
YES............. 1
NO.............. 2
28

E-17. (Does/did) the pain seem to spread?
YES............. 1
NO.............. 2 (Q.E-19)
29

E-18. (Does/did) the pain spread to:

	YES	NO	DK
a. the top and back of the head?	a 1	2	8
b. either shoulder?	b 1	2	8
c. the arms or hands?	c 1	2	8

30, 31, 32

E-19. (Is/was) your neck pain made worse...

	YES	NO	DK
a. by coughing, sneezing or deep breathing?	a 1	2	8
b. with bending or twisting motion?	b 1	2	8
c. after prolonged sitting?	c 1	2	8
d. after prolonged standing?	d 1	2	8
e. with other motion?	e 1	2	8

33, 34, 35, 36, 37

E-20. Have you ever had neck pain due to an injury?
YES............. 1
NO.............. 2 (Q.E-23)
38

E-21. Was the neck pain caused by playing a sport, doing your job at work, or some other activity?
PLAYING A SPORT..... 1
DOING YOUR JOB AT WORK.. 2
ANOTHER ACTIVITY.... 3
DK.................. 8
39

E-22.	Have you ever been told by a doctor that you had a "whiplash" injury of the neck?	YES.............. 1 NO.............. 2	(40)
E-23.	Have you ever been told by a doctor that you had a slipped or ruptured disc in your neck?	YES.............. 1 NO.............. 2 (Q.E-25)	(41)
E-24.	Were you in traction to treat this slipped or ruptured disc?	YES.............. 1 NO.............. 2	(42)
E-25.	Have you ever stayed in a hospital overnight for neck pain?	YES.............. 1 NO.............. 2 (Q.E-28)	(43)
E-26.	Was this hospitalization since 1970?	YES.............. 1 (CHART) NO.............. 2	(44)
E-27a.	Did you have any surgery for neck pain?	YES.............. 1 NO.............. 2 (Q.E-28)	(45)
E-27b.	How many times?	# OF TIMES:|___|___|	(46-47)
E-28.	Have you had pain in your back on most days for at least one month?	YES.............. 1 NO.............. 2 (Q.E-49)	(48)
E-29.	What was the longest episode of back pain you have ever had? (IF 5 INDICATES LESS THAN ONE MONTH, REASK Q.E-28)	1 MONTH........... 1 MORE THAN 1 BUT LESS THAN 6 MONTHS....... 2 6-12 MONTHS...... 3 MORE THAN 1 YEAR........ 4	(49)
E-30.	How old were you when you first experienced this recurring back pain? (READ CATEGORIES IF NECESSARY.)	LESS THAN 15 YEARS OLD.......... 01 15 LESS THAN 20 YEARS. 02 20 LESS THAN 30 YEARS. 03 30 LESS THAN 40 YEARS. 04 40 LESS THAN 50 YEARS. 05 50 LESS THAN 60 YEARS. 06 60 LESS THAN 70 YEARS. 07 70 LESS THAN 80 YEARS. 08 80 AND OLDER.......... 09	(50-51)
E-31.	Are you still having this pain?	YES.............. 1 (Q.E-33) NO.............. 2	(52)

19

E-32.	When was the last time you had this pain? (READ CATEGORIES IF NECESSARY.)	LESS THAN 1 YEAR AGO... 1 (Q.E-34) 1 BUT LESS THAN 3...... 2 (Q.E-34) 3 BUT LESS THAN 5...... 3 (Q.E-34) 5 OR MORE YEARS AGO... 4 (Q.E-34) DK................ 8 (Q.E-34)	(53)
E-33.	Does this pain occur more frequently than it used to?	YES.............. 1 NO.............. 2	(54)
E-34.	(Is/was) the pain located in your...	YES NO a. upper back? UPPER BACK 1 2 b. mid-back? MID-BACK 1 2 c. lower back? LOWER BACK 1 2	(55) (56) (57)

BOX F
INTERVIEWER: CHECK E-34a-c AND CIRCLE ONE:

Q.E-34a-c, 2 or more = YES(1)..... 1 (Q.E-35)
OTHERWISE............ 2 (Q.E-36)

E-35.	When you (have/had) this pain, where (is/was) it most intense, in your (upper back/mid/or lower back)?	YES NO a. UPPER BACK.... 1 2 b. MID-BACK...... 1 2 c. LOWER BACK.... 1 2	(58) (59) (60)
E-36.	(Was/is) the pain present when you (are/were) resting at night?	YES.............. 1 NO.............. 2 (Q.E-38)	(61)
E-37.	(Does/did) it awaken you from sleep at night?	YES.............. 1 NO.............. 2	(62)
E-38.	(Does/did) the pain seem to spread?	YES.............. 1 NO.............. 2 (Q.E-40)	(63)
E-39.	(Does/did) the pain spread to:	YES NO DK a. the back of the right leg? 1 2 8 b. the back of the left leg? 1 2 8 c. the top of the head? 1 2 8 d. the sides of the body? 1 2 8	(64) (65) (66) (67)

20

E-51. How old were you when you first experienced this recurring pain in the hip? (READ CATEGORIES IF NECESSARY.)

LESS THAN 15 YEARS......... 01
15 BUT LESS THAN 20 YEARS. 02
20 BUT LESS THAN 30 YEARS. 03
30 BUT LESS THAN 40 YEARS. 04
40 BUT LESS THAN 50 YEARS. 05
50 BUT LESS THAN 60 YEARS. 06
60 BUT LESS THAN 70 YEARS. 07
70 BUT LESS THAN 80 YEARS. 08
80 AND OLDER.............. 09   [84-85]

E-52. Are you still having this hip pain?

YES................. 1 (Q.E-54)
NO.................. 2   [86]

E-53. When was the last time you had the hip pain?

LESS THAN 1 YEAR AGO...... 1
1 BUT LESS THAN 3......... 2
3 BUT LESS THAN 5......... 3
5 OR MORE YEARS AGO....... 4
DK........................ 8   [87]

E-54. In which of these areas of the body (is/was) the hip pain usually most intense:

	YES	NO	DK	
a. right buttock?	1	2	8	[88]
b. left buttock?	1	2	8	[89]
c. right groin?	1	2	8	[90]
d. left groin?	1	2	8	[91]
e. side of right upper thigh?	1	2	8	[92]
f. side of left upper thigh?	1	2	8	[93]
g. somewhere else?	1	2	8	[94]

(SPECIFY)

E-55. From the hip (does/did) the pain tend to spread?

YES................. 1
NO.................. 2 (Q.E-57)   [95-96]

E-56. (Does/did) the pain tend to spread to:

	YES	NO	DK	
a. the inside of your leg?	1	2	8	[98]
b. the front of your leg?	1	2	8	[99]
c. the outside of your leg?	1	2	8	[100]
d. the back of your leg?	1	2	8	[101]
e. somewhere else?	1	2	8	[102]

(SPECIFY)

E-57. (Do/did) you have pain in or around the hip when either coughing or sneezing?

YES................. 1
NO.................. 2   [103-104]

E-58. When this pain (is/was) present, (does/did) it hurt when resting as well as when moving?

YES................. 1
NO.................. 2   [106]

22

E-40. (Is/was) your back pain made worse...

	YES	NO	DK	
a. by coughing, sneezing or deep breathing?	1	2	8	[68]
b. with bending or twisting motion?	1	2	8	[69]
c. after prolonged sitting?	1	2	8	[70]
d. after prolonged standing?	1	2	8	[71]
e. with other motion?	1	2	8	[72]

E-41. Have you ever had back pain due to an injury?

YES................. 1
NO.................. 2 (Q.E-43)   [73]

E-42. Was the back pain caused by playing a sport, doing your job at work or some other activity?

PLAYING A SPORT.......... 1
DOING YOUR JOB
    AT WORK.............. 2
ANOTHER ACTIVITY......... 3
DK....................... 8   [74]

E-43. Have you ever been told by a doctor that you had a slipped or ruptured disc in your back?

YES................. 1
NO.................. 2 (Q.E-45)   [75]

E-44. Were you in traction to treat this slipped or ruptured disc?

YES................. 1
NO.................. 2   [76]

E-45. Have you ever stayed in a hospital overnight for back pain?

YES................. 1
NO.................. 2 (Q.E-49)   [77]

E-46. Was this hospitalization since 1970?

YES................. 1 (CHART)
NO.................. 2   [78]

E-47. Did you have any surgery?

YES................. 1
NO.................. 2 (Q.E-49)   [79]

E-48. How many times?

OF TIMES: |__|__| [80-81]

E-49. Have you had pain in or around either hip joint, including the buttock, groin, and side of the upper thigh on most days for at least one month?

YES................. 1
NO.................. 2 (Q.E-60)   [82]

E-50. What is the longest episode of hip pain you have ever had? [IF S INDICATES LESS THAN ONE MONTH, REASK Q.E-49]

1 MONTH.................. 1
MORE THAN 1 BUT LESS
    THAN 6 MONTHS........ 2
6-12 MONTHS.............. 3
MORE THAN 1 YEAR......... 4   [83]

21

E-59. Since 1970, have you stayed in a hospital overnight for problems related to your hip pain?
YES.............. 1 (CHART)
NO............... 2   107

E-60a. Have you had pain in or around the knee, including the back of the knee, on most days for at least one month?
YES.............. 1
NO............... 2 (Q.E-71)   108

E-60b. Which knee?
LEFT............. 1
RIGHT............ 2
BOTH............. 3   109

E-61. What was the longest episode of knee pain you have ever had? [IF 5 INDICATES LESS THAN ONE MONTH, REASK Q.E-60a]
1 MONTH..................... 1
MORE THAN 4 WEEKS BUT LESS THAN 6 WEEKS..... 2
MORE THAN 6 WEEKS BUT LESS THAN 6 MONTHS.... 3
6-12 MONTHS................. 4
MORE THAN 1 YEAR............ 5   110

E-62. How old were you when you first experienced recurring pain in the knee? (READ CATEGORIES IF NECESSARY.)
LESS THAN 15 YEARS OLD....... 01
15 BUT LESS THAN 20 YEARS.... 02
20 BUT LESS THAN 30 YEARS.... 03
30 BUT LESS THAN 40 YEARS.... 04
40 BUT LESS THAN 50 YEARS.... 05
50 BUT LESS THAN 60 YEARS.... 06
60 BUT LESS THAN 70 YEARS.... 07
70 BUT LESS THAN 80 YEARS.... 08
80 AND OLDER................. 09   111-112

E-63. Are you still having this knee pain?
YES.............. 1 (Q.E-65)
NO............... 2   113

E-64. When was the last time you had this knee pain? (READ CATEGORIES IF NECESSARY.)
LESS THAN 1 YEAR AGO.... 1
1 BUT LESS THAN 3....... 2
3 BUT LESS THAN 5....... 3
5 OR MORE YEARS AGO..... 4
DK..................... 8   114

E-65. When this pain (is/was) present, (does/did) it hurt when resting as well as when moving?
YES.............. 1
NO............... 2   115

E-66. When this knee pain (is/was) present:

	YES	NO	
a. (Is/was) there also swelling of the knee joint?	1	2	116
b. (Is/was) the joint warm to the touch?	1	2	117
c. (Does/did) the joint appear red?	1	2	118

E-67a. Have you ever had "locking" of the knee?
YES.............. 1
NO............... 2 (Q.E-68a)   119

E-67b. Which knee?
LEFT............. 1
RIGHT............ 2
BOTH............. 3   120

E-68a. Has either knee ever "given way" under you?
YES.............. 1
NO............... 2 (Q.E-69)   121

E-68b. Which knee?
LEFT............. 1
RIGHT............ 2
BOTH............. 3   122

E-69. Have you ever had a severe twisting of either knee resulting in a sprain or swelling lasting more than two weeks?
YES.............. 1
NO............... 2 (Q.E-71)   123

E-70. Which knee?
RIGHT............ 1
LEFT............. 2
BOTH............. 3   124

E-71. Have you had pain or aching in any joint other than the hip, back, neck or knee on most days for at least six weeks?
YES.............. 1
NO............... 2 (Q.E-73)   125
Begin E2

E-72. Which joints were painful. . .

			IF "YES"...Was it the right or the left?		
	YES	NO	RIGHT	LEFT	BOTH
a. Finger(s)?	1	2	a 1	2	3	11-12
b. Wrists?	1	2	b 1	2	3	13-14
c. Elbows?	1	2	c 1	2	3	15-16
d. Shoulders?	1	2	d 1	2	3	17-18
e. Ankles?	1	2	e 1	2	3	19-20
f. Toes?	1	2	f 1	2	3	21-22

E-73. Have you ever had any swollen joints which were painful when touched on most days for at least one month?
YES.............. 1
NO............... 2 (Q.E-78)   23

E-74. How old were you when you first experienced swelling of your joints? (READ CATEGORIES IF NECESSARY.)
LESS THAN 15 YEARS OLD....... 01
15 BUT LESS THAN 20 YEARS.... 02
20 BUT LESS THAN 30 YEARS.... 03
30 BUT LESS THAN 40 YEARS.... 04
40 BUT LESS THAN 50 YEARS.... 05
50 BUT LESS THAN 60 YEARS.... 06
60 BUT LESS THAN 70 YEARS.... 07
70 BUT LESS THAN 80 YEARS.... 08
80 AND OLDER................. 09   24-25

E-75. Are you still having this swelling of your joints?
YES.....1 (Q.E-77)
NO.....2

E-76. When was the last time you had this swelling? (READ CATEGORIES IF NECESSARY.)
LESS THAN 1 YEAR AGO.....1
1 BUT LESS THAN 3.....2
3 BUT LESS THAN 5.....3
5 OR MORE YEARS AGO.....4
DK.....8

E-77. Which joints (are/were) usually involved whenever you (have/had) this swelling with tenderness on touching..

IF "YES">...Was it the right or the left?

	YES	NO	RIGHT	LEFT	BOTH
a. Finger(s)?	a 1	2	1	2	3
b. Wrists?	b 1	2	1	2	3
c. Elbows?	c 1	2	1	2	3
d. Shoulders?	d 1	2	1	2	3
e. Hips?	e 1	2	1	2	3
f. Knees?	f 1	2	1	2	3
g. Ankles?	g 1	2	1	2	3
h. Toes?	h 1	2	1	2	3

E-78. Did you ever have a surgical procedure on any of your joints?
YES.....1
NO.....2 (Q.E-82)

E-79. Which joints were operated upon...

IF "YES">...Was it the right or the left?

	YES	NO	RIGHT	LEFT	BOTH
a. Finger(s)?	a 1	2	1	2	3
b. Wrist?	b 1	2	1	2	3
c. Elbow?	c 1	2	1	2	3
d. Shoulder?	d 1	2	1	2	3
e. Hip?	e 1	2	1	2	3
f. Knee?	f 1	2	1	2	3
g. Ankle?	g 1	2	1	2	3
h. Toes?	h 1	2	1	2	3

E-80. Did you have the joints replaced?
YES.....1
NO.....2 (Q.E-82)

E-81. Which joints were replaced...

IF "YES">...How many replacements?

	YES	NO	
a. Finger(s) on right hand?	a 1	2	b
b. Finger(s) on left hand?	b 1	2	b
c. Left hip?	c 1	2	c
d. Right hip?	d 1	2	d
e. Left knee?	e 1	2	e
f. Right knee?	f 1	2	f
g. Any other joints?	g 1	2	g

(SPECIFY)

E-82. Have you had stiffness in your joints when first getting out of bed on most mornings for at least one month?
YES.....1
NO.....2 (Q.E-88)

E-83. How old were you when you first experienced this morning stiffness of your joints? (READ CATEGORIES IF NECESSARY.)
LESS THAN 15 YEARS OLD.....01
15 BUT LESS THAN 20 YEARS.02
20 BUT LESS THAN 30 YEARS.03
30 BUT LESS THAN 40 YEARS.04
40 BUT LESS THAN 50 YEARS.05
50 BUT LESS THAN 60 YEARS.06
60 BUT LESS THAN 70 YEARS.07
70 BUT LESS THAN 80 YEARS.08
80 AND OLDER.....09

E-84. Are you still having this morning stiffness?
YES.....1 (Q.E-86)
NO.....2

E-85. When was the last time you had this morning stiffness? (READ CATEGORIES IF NECESSARY.)
LESS THAN 1 YEAR AGO.....1
1 BUT LESS THAN 4 YEARS AGO.2
4 BUT LESS THAN 10 YEARS AGO.3
10 OR MORE YEARS AGO.....4
DK.....8

E-86. Which joints (are/were) usually involved whenever you (have/had) this morning stiffness...

IF "YES">...Was it the right or the left?

	YES	NO	RIGHT	LEFT	BOTH
a. Finger(s)?	a 1	2	1	2	3
b. Wrists?	b 1	2	1	2	3
c. Elbows?	c 1	2	1	2	3
d. Shoulders?	d 1	2	1	2	3
e. Hips?	e 1	2	1	2	3
f. Knees?	f 1	2	1	2	3
g. Ankles?	g 1	2	1	2	3
h. Toes?	h 1	2	1	2	3
i. Back?	i 1	2			

25

26

			YES		NO	
E-87. After getting up and moving around (did/does) this morning stiffness usually last...	E-87					
a. all day?		a	1 (Q.E-88)		2	109
b. longer than 1/2 hour?		b	1 (Q.E-88)		2	110
c. longer than 15 minutes?		c	1		2	111
E-88. Have you ever stayed overnight in a hospital because of joint problems?	E-88	YES..................	1			
		NO...................	2 (Q.E-90)			112
E-89. Since 1970, have you ever stayed overnight in a hospital because of joint problems?	E-89	YES..................	1 (CHART)			
		NO...................	2			113
E-90. Have you ever been told by a doctor that you had a fractured hip?	E-90	YES..................	1			
		NO...................	2 (Q.E-95)			114
E-91. Which hip was broken?	E-91	RIGHT...............	1			
		LEFT................	2			
		BOTH................	3			115
E-92. How old were you when it happened?	E-92	AGE: |___|___|			
		DK.................	98			116-117
E-93. Did you have surgery?	E-93	YES..................	1			
		NO...................	2			118
E-94. Since 1970, have you stayed in a hospital overnight for a fractured hip?	E-94	YES..................	1 (CHART)			
		NO...................	2			119
E-95. Have you ever been told by a doctor that you had a dislocated hip?	E-95	YES..................	1			
		NO...................	2 (Q.E-100)			120
E-96. Which hip was dislocated?	E-96	RIGHT...............	1			
		LEFT................	2			
		BOTH................	3			121
E-97. How old were you when it happened?	E-97	AGE: |___|___|			
		DK.................	98			122-123
E-98. Did you have surgery?	E-98	YES..................	1			
		NO...................	2			124

133-368 C - 83 - 3

E-99. Since 1970, have you stayed in the hospital overnight for problems related to your dislocation?	E-99	YES.................	1 (CHART)
		NO..................	2
			125

E-100. Now, I'd like you to look at this line in this booklet.

In the past week, how much pain have you had from your joint condition? (GO TO SELF-ADMINISTRATION BOOKLET, PAGE 6.) |___| 126-127

Begin FO

PART F: ACTIVITIES OF DAILY LIVING

NURSING HOME INSTRUCTIONS: CIRCLE ONE:
RESPONDENT CAN ANSWER THIS SECTION. 1
RESPONDENT CANNOT ANSWER THIS SECTION
ASK OF NURSING HOME STAFF. . . . . 2 (PART G)

11

IF S IS BEDRIDDEN, ASK:

F1. Are you usually confined to bed for most of the day?
YES. 1
NO 2 (F-3a)

12

F2. How long have you been confined to bed?
OF MONTHS: |__|__| (ASK * QUESTIONS ONLY)   13-14

OR

OF YEARS: |__|__| (ASK * QUESTIONS ONLY)   15

INTERVIEWER INSTRUCTIONS: ASK F-3a THROUGH F-28a. IF ANY RESPONSE = 3 OR 4, ASK F-3b THROUGH F-28b.
IF b = YES (USES HELP EITHER FROM ANOTHER PERSON OR AN AID) ASK F-3c THROUGH F-24c WHERE INDICATED.

Now I am going to read a list of activities with which some people have difficulty. Using the categories on this card, please tell me if:

HANDS CARD A

	You have no difficulty, some difficulty, much difficulty or are unable to do these activities at all when you are by yourself and without the use of aids.						You said that you (have difficulty/are unable to) (ACTIVITY) by yourself. . . Do you have help from. . .					(ASK ONLY IF HAVE HELP) With help how difficult is it for you to do?			
	No diffi- culty	Some diffi- culty	Much diffi- culty	Unable to do	DK		another person?		a mechanical aid or device i.e., cane?			With no difficulty	Some difficulty	Much difficulty	Unable to do	
							Yes	No	Yes	No						
F-3. Dress yourself, including tying shoes, working zippers and doing buttons?	1	2	3	4	8	F-3	1	2	1	2		1	2	3	4	16-19
F-4. Shampoo your hair?	1	2	3	4	8	F-4	1	2	1	2		1	2	3	4	
F-5. Stand up from an armless straight chair?	1	2	3	4	8	F-5	1	2	1	2		1	2	3	4	
F-6. Get into and out of bed?	1	2	3	4	8	F-6	1	2	1	2		1	2	3	4	
F-7. Prepare your own food?	1	2	3	4	8	F-7	1	2								
*F-8. Cut your meat?	1	2	3	4	8	F-8	1	2								
*F-9. Lift a full cup or glass to your mouth?	1	2	3	4	8	F-9	1	2								
*F-10. Open a new milk carton?	1	2	3	4	8	F-10	1	2								
F-11. Walk a quarter mile (two or three blocks)?	1 (Q,F-13)	2 (Q,F-13)	3	4	8	F-11	1	2				1	2	3	4	
F-12. Walk from one room to another on the same level?	1	2	3	4	8	F-12	1	2	1	2		1	2	3	4	
F-13. Walk up and down at least two steps?	1	2	3	4	8	F-13	1	2	1	2		1	2	3	4	
F-14. Turn faucets on or off?	1	2	3	4	8	F-14	1	2								
F-15. Get in and out of the bathtub?	1	2	3	4	8	F-15	1	2	1	2		1	2	3	4	
F-16. Wash and dry your whole body?	1	2	3	4	8	F-16	1	2	1	2		1	2	3	4	
F-17. Get on and off the toilet?	1	2	3	4	8	F-17	1	2	1	2		1	2	3	4	
*F-18. Comb your hair?	1	2	3	4	8	F-18	1	2								
F-19. Reach and get down a 5 lb. object (bag of sugar) from just above your head?	1	2	3	4	8	F-19	1	2	1	2		1	2	3	4	
F-20. Bend down and pick up clothing from the floor?	1	2	3	4	8	F-20	1	2	1	2		1	2	3	4	
F-21. Open push button car doors?	1	2	3	4	8	F-21	1	2				1	2	3	4	
F-22. Open jars which have been previously opened?	1	2	3	4	8	F-22	1	2								
*F-23. Use a pen or pencil to write with?	1	2	3	4	8	F-23	1	2								
F-24. Get in and out of a car?	1	2	3	4	8	F-24	1	2	1	2		1	2	3	4	
F-25. Run errands and shop?	1	2	3	4	8	F-25	1	2								
F-26. Do light chores such as vacuuming?	1	2	3	4	8	F-26	1	2								
F-27. Lift and carry a full bag of groceries?	1	2	3	4	8	F-27	1	2								
F-28. Do heavy chores around the house or yard, or washing windows, walls or floors?	1	2	3	4	8	F-28	1	2							90-91

BOX G

INTERVIEWER: REVIEW F-3a through F-28a AND CIRCLE ONE:

ALL RESPONSES, F-3a THROUGH F-28a = 1 OR 2. . . . . 1 (PART G)

FOR ANY RESPONSE IN F-3a THROUGH F-28a = 3 OR 4. . . 2 (Q,F-3b)

30

31

PART G: MEDICAL CONDITIONS

INTERVIEWER INSTRUCTIONS: READ G-1a THROUGH G-23a FIRST. IF RESPONSE = YES (1) ASK b AND c.

Begin G1

Did a doctor ever tell you that you had any of the following conditions?	In what year were you first told that you had (CONDITION)?	Since 1970, have you stayed overnight in a hospital for (CONDITION)?	
G-1a. Asthma YES..............1 NO..............2	**G-1b.** YR: |_1_|_9_|__|__| DK...........9998	**G-1c.** YES..............1 (CHART) NO..............2	11-16
G-2a. Chronic bronchitis, emphysema YES..............1 NO..............2	**G-2b.** YR: |_1_|_9_|__|__| DK...........9998	**G-2c.** YES..............1 (CHART) NO..............2	17-22
G-3a. Migraine YES..............1 NO..............2	**G-3b.** YR: |_1_|_9_|__|__| DK...........9998	**G-3c.** YES..............1 (CHART) NO..............2	23-28
G-4a. Psoriasis YES..............1 NO..............2	**G-4b.** YR: |_1_|_9_|__|__| DK...........9998	**G-4c.** YES..............1 (CHART) NO..............2	29-34
G-5a. Ulcers: Peptic, stomach or duodenal YES..............1 NO..............2	**G-5b.** YR: |_1_|_9_|__|__| DK...........9998	**G-5c.** YES..............1 (CHART) NO..............2	35-40
G-6a. Kidney disorder or kidney stones YES..............1 NO..............2	**G-6b.** YR: |_1_|_9_|__|__| DK...........9998	**G-6c.** YES..............1 (CHART) NO..............2	41-46
G-7a. Urinary tract or kidney infection more than 3 times YES..............1 NO..............2	**G-7b.** YR: |_1_|_9_|__|__| DK...........9998	**G-7c.** YES..............1 (CHART) NO..............2	47-52

32

Did a doctor ever tell you that you had any of the following conditions?	In what year were you first told that you had (CONDITION)?	Since 1970, have you stayed overnight in a hospital for (CONDITION)?	
G-8a. Polyps or tumor of the colon YES..............1 NO..............2	**G-8b.** YR: |_1_|_9_|__|__| DK...........9998	**G-8c.** YES..............1 (CHART) NO..............2	53-58
G-9a. Cirrhosis of the liver Yes..............1 No..............2	**G-9b.** YR: |_1_|_9_|__|__| DK...........9998	**G-9c.** YES..............1 (CHART) NO..............2	59-64
G-10a. Parkinson's disease YES..............1 NO..............2	**G-10b.** YR: |_1_|_9_|__|__| DK...........9998	**G-10c.** YES..............1 (CHART) NO..............2	65-70
G-11a. Multiple Sclerosis YES..............1 NO..............2	**G-11b.** YR: |_1_|_9_|__|__| DK...........9998	**G-11c.** YES..............1 (CHART) NO..............2	71-76
G-12a. Nervous breakdown YES..............1 NO..............2	**G-12b.** YR: |_1_|_9_|__|__| DK...........9998	**G-12c.** YES..............1 (CHART) NO..............2	77-82
G-13a. Diverticulitis YES..............1 NO..............2	**G-13b.** YR: |_1_|_9_|__|__| DK...........9998	**G-13c.** YES..............1 (CHART) NO..............2	83-88
G-14a. Colitis, enteritis YES..............1 NO..............2	**G-14b.** YR: |_1_|_9_|__|__| DK...........9998	**G-14c.** YES..............1 (CHART) NO..............2	89-94
G-15a. Heart condition or heart trouble YES..............1 NO..............2	**G-15b.** YR: |_1_|_9_|__|__| DK...........9998	**G-15c.** YES..............1 (CHART) NO..............2	95-100

33

Page 34

Did a doctor ever tell you that you had any of the following conditions?	In what year were you first told that you had (CONDITION)?	Since 1970, have you stayed overnight in a hospital for (CONDITION)?	
G-16a. Angina YES.......... 1 NO............ 2	**G-16b.** YR: |1|9|_|_| DK........ 9998	**G-16c.** YES.......... 1 (CHART) NO............ 2	101–106
G-17a. Heart attack YES.......... 1 NO............ 2	**G-17b.** YR: |1|9|_|_| DK........ 9998	**G-17c.** YES.......... 1 (CHART) NO............ 2	107–112
G-18a. Cataracts YES.......... 1 NO............ 2	**G-18b.** YR: |1|9|_|_| DK........ 9998	**G-18c.** YES.......... 1 (CHART) NO............ 2	113–118
G-19a. Glaucoma YES.......... 1 NO............ 2	**G-19b.** YR: |1|9|_|_| DK........ 9998	**G-19c.** YES.......... 1 (CHART) NO............ 2	119–124
G-20a. Detached retina YES.......... 1 NO............ 2	**G-20b.** YR: |1|9|_|_| DK........ 9998	**G-20c.** YES.......... 1 (CHART) NO............ 2	125–130
G-21a. Small stroke sometimes known as TIA (transient ischemic attack) YES.......... 1 NO............ 2	**G-21b.** YR: |1|9|_|_| DK........ 9998	**G-21c.** YES.......... 1 (CHART) NO............ 2	Begin G2 11–16
G-22a. Stroke (sometimes called a CVA) YES.......... 1 NO............ 2	**G-22b.** YR: |1|9|_|_| DK........ 9998	**G-22c.** YES.......... 1 (CHART) NO............ 2	17–22

BOX H

S IS FEMALE. . . . . 1 (ASK b AND c FOR ANY YES IN Q.G-1a – Q.G-22a, THEN GO TO Q.G-24)

S IS MALE. 2 (Q.G-23a)

34

Page 35

Did a doctor ever tell you that you had any of the following conditions?	In what year were you first told that you had (CONDITION)?	Since 1970, have you stayed overnight in a hospital for (CONDITION)?	
G-23a. Prostate trouble YES.......... 1 NO............ 2	**G-23b.** YR: |1|9|_|_| DK........ 9998	**G-23c.** YES.......... 1 (CHART) NO............ 2	23–28

[FOR Q.G-1a–Q.G-23a, IF YES, ASK b and c.]

These next questions will be about medications that you have taken or are now taking.

READ Q.G-24 TO Q.G-28 FOR ANTACIDS, THEN READ Q.G-24 TO Q.G-27 FOR ASPIRIN

	a. Antacids such as Rolaids, Tums, Digel, Maalox	b. Aspirin, not including aspirin substitutes
G-24. Have you ever taken (MEDICATION) regularly, that is at least once every week?	YES.......... 1 NO.......... 2(Q.G-24b) 29	YES.... 1 NO.... 2(Q.G-29) 37
G-25. For how many years have you regularly taken (MEDICATION)?	# YEARS: |_|_| DK.......... 98 30–31	# YEARS: |_|_| DK......... 98 38–39
G-26. Do you still take (MEDICATION) regularly?	YES.......... 1 NO.......... 2 32	YES.... 1 NO.... 2 40
G-27. (When you took (MEDICATION) regularly) On the average, how many times a day or week (do/did) you take it?	# TIMES/DAY: |_|_| OR # TIMES/WEEK: |_|_| 33–34 |_|35	# TIMES/DAY: |_|_| OR # TIMES/WEEK: |_|_| 41–42 |_|43
G-28. What is the brand name of the antacid you (used/use) most frequently?	MAALOX........ 1 DIGEL......... 2 MYLANTA....... 3 ROLAIDS....... 4 TUMS.......... 5 OTHER (SPECIFY)... 6 36	

35

G-29. Has a doctor ever prescribed digitalis, also called digoxin or lanoxin for you?

G-29	YES................1
	NO...........2 (Q.G-33)
	DK...........8 (Q.G-33)

[44]

G-30. How old were you when this medication was first prescribed?

G-30	AGE: |__|__|

[45-46]

G-31. Is this medication prescribed for you now?

G-31	YES................1
	NO...........2 (Q.G-33)

[47]

G-32. How often do you take this medication?

G-32	#TIMES/DAY: |__|__|
	OR
	#TIMES/WK: |__|__|
	DK.................98

[48-49] [50]

G-33. Has a doctor ever prescribed medication for you for hypertension or high blood pressure?

G-33	YES................1
	NO...........2 (Q.G-36)
	DK...........8 (Q.G-36)

[51]

G-34. Are you now taking medication for this condition?

G-34	YES................1
	NO...........2 (Q.G-36)

[52]

G-35. What is the name of this medication? (CIRCLE ALL THAT APPLY)

G-35		
a	ALDACTAZIDE........1	[53]
b	ALDOMET............1	[54]
c	DIURIL.............1	[55]
d	DYAZIDE............1	[56]
e	HYDROCHLORO-THIAZIDE.......1	[57]
f	HYDRODIURIL........1	[58]
g	HYGROTON...........1	[59]
h	INDERAL............1	[60]
i	LASIX..............1	[61]
j	LOPRESSOR..........1	[62]
k	OTHER (SPECIFY)....1	[63]

[64-65] [66-67] [68-69]

G-36. Did a doctor ever tell you that you had diabetes or sugar diabetes?

G-36	YES................1
	NO...........2 (Q.G-41)
	DK...........8 (Q.G-41)

[70]

G-37. In what year were you first told that you had it?

G-37	YR: |_1_|_9_|__|__|
	DK..............9998

[71-74]

G-38. Are you now taking medication for this condition?

G-38	YES................1
	NO...........2 (Q.G-40)

[75]

36

G-39. What is the name of this medication? (CIRCLE ALL THAT APPLY)

G-39		
a	DIABINESE..........1	[76]
b	INSULIN............1	[77]
c	OTHER (SPECIFY)....1	[78]

[79-80]

G-40. Since 1970, have you been hospitalized overnight for diabetes?

G-40	YES.........1 (CHART)
	NO.................2

[81]

G-41. Did a doctor ever tell you that you had thyroid disease or goiter?

G-41	YES................1
	NO...........2 (Q.G-46)
	DK...........8 (Q.G-46)

[82]

G-42. In what year were you first told that you had it?

G-42	YR: |_1_|_9_|__|__|
	DK..............9998

[83-86]

G-43. Are you now taking medication for this condition?

G-43	YES................1
	NO...........2 (Q.G-45)

[87]

G-44. What is the name of this medication? (CIRCLE ALL THAT APPLY)

G-44		
a	SYNTHROID..........1	[88]
b	THYROID............1	[89]
c	THYROID STRONG.....1	[90]
d	OTHER (SPECIFY)....1	[91]

[92-93]

G-45. Since 1970, have you been hospitalized overnight for this condition?

G-45	YES.........1 (CHART)
	NO.................2

[94]

G-46. Did a doctor ever tell you that you had epilepsy?

G-46	YES................1
	NO...........2 (Q.G-51)
	DK...........8 (Q.G-51)

[95]

G-47. In what year were you first told that you had it?

G-47	YR: |_1_|_9_|__|__|
	DK..............9998

[96-99]

G-48. Are you now taking medication for this condition?

G-48	YES................1
	NO...........2 (Q.G-50)

[100]

G-49. What is the name of this medication? (CIRCLE ALL THAT APPLY)

G-49		
a	DILANTIN...........1	[101]
b	PHENOBARBITAL......1	[102]
c	OTHER (SPECIFY)....1	[103]

[104]

37

G-50. Since 1970, have you been hospitalized overnight for this condition?

G-50 YES.............. 1 (CHART)
　　　 NO.............. 2
105

G-51. Do you currently take any tranquilizers that have been ordered by a doctor such as Valium, Tranxene, Mellaril or Compazine?

G-51 YES.............. 1
　　　 NO.............. 2
106

G-52. Do you currently take any anti-depressants that have been ordered by a doctor such as Elavil, Sinequan, Limbitrol, or Tofranil?

G-52 YES.............. 1
　　　 NO.............. 2
107

We have been talking about specific medications you may have taken. Now I'd like you to think about vitamins you may be taking.

INTERVIEWER INSTRUCTIONS: READ G-53a – G-59a FIRST. FOR EACH "YES" RESPONSE, ASK b–d.

Are you now taking...	What is the exact name of the multi-vitamin you are taking?	How many pills or spoonfuls do you take?	For how many years of the last 10 years have you taken (VITAMIN) on a regular basis?
G-53a Multivitamin pills including thera-peutic and geri-atric multivitamins and Geritol? YES..........1 NO..........2 108	**G-53b** NAME: [ ] NAME: [ ]	**G-53c** (How often?) D W M # [|||] 1 2 3 [|||] 1 2 3	**G-53d** [| |] YEARS: [_|_] 109-115 YEARS: [_|_] 116-122
	How many (UNITS) of (VITAMIN) do you take?	What is the dosage of each (tablet/capsule)?	123-132
G-54a Vitamin C tablets? YES..........1 NO..........2	**G-54b** # OF TABLETS:[|_] A DAY..........1 A WEEK..........2 A MONTH..........3	**G-54c** DOSAGE:[_|_] [|||] mg.	**G-54d** [| |] YEARS: [_|_]
G-55a Vitamin A capsules? YES..........1 NO..........2	**G-55b** # OF CAPSULES:[|_] A DAY..........1 A WEEK..........2 A MONTH..........3	**G-55c** DOSAGE:[_|_] [|||] I.U.	**G-55d** [| |] Begin G3 YEARS: [_|_] 11-21
G-56a Vitamin E capsules? YES..........1 NO..........2	**G-56b** # OF CAPSULES:[|_] A DAY..........1 A WEEK..........2 A MONTH..........3	**G-56c** DOSAGE:[_|_] [|||]I.U.	**G-56d** [| |] YEARS: [_|_] 22-31
G-57a Cod liver oil or other fish liver oils? YES..........1 NO..........2	**G-57b** # OF SPOONFULS OR TABLETS:[|_] A DAY..........1 A WEEK..........2 A MONTH..........3		**G-57d** [| |] YEARS: [_|_] 32-37

40

Page 41

Are you now taking....	G-58b What is the exact name of the other (vitamin or mineral/nutritional supplements) you are taking?	G-58c How many pills or spoonfuls do you take? (How often? D W M)	G-58d For how many years of the last 10 years have you taken (VITAMIN) on a regular basis?
	NAME: |_|_|_|	#|_| |_| 1 2 3	YEARS: |_|_| 39-45
	NAME: |_|_|_|	|_| |_| 1 2 3	YEARS: |_|_| 46-52
	NAME: |_|_|_|	|_| |_| 1 2 3	YEARS: |_|_| 53-59
	NAME: |_|_|_|	|_| |_| 1 2 3	YEARS: |_|_| 60-66

G-58a Any other vitamins or minerals?
YES..........1
NO...........2
38

G-59a Any other nutritional supplements such as lecithin, protein powders, nutritional yeast or selenium?
YES..........1
NO...........2
67

G-59b	G-59d
NAME: |_|_|_|	YEARS: |_|_| 68-71
NAME: |_|_|_|	YEARS: |_|_| 72-75
NAME: |_|_|_|	YEARS: |_|_| 76-79

G-60. For how many years of the last 10 years have you taken any multivitamins on a regular basis?

G-60 # YEARS.............|_|_| 80-81

41

Page 42

82

G-61. I have asked you about various illnesses and whether or not you have been hospitalized for them. Now, I would like you to think back over the time between 1970 and the present, that is the last (NUMBER) years. You would have been about (AGE) in 1970. Have you stayed in a hospital overnight for any other reason (including pregnancies) since you were (AGE)?

G-61   YES.............. 1 (CHART)
NO............... 2 (Q.G-62)

BOX I

HOSPITAL AND HEALTH CARE FACILITY QUESTIONS
(SEE CHART ON BACK COVER OF SELF-ADMINISTRATION BOOKLET).

INTERVIEWER: ASK A-E FOR EACH OVERNIGHT STAY. RECORD ON CHART.

A. What year were you in the (INSTITUTION)? (RECORD YEAR)

B. Why were you in the (INSTITUTION)? (RECORD CONDITION/ILLNESS)

C. What is the name of the (INSTITUTION)? (PROBE FOR FULL NAME AND RECORD TYPE OF INSTITUTION)

D. What is the address of that (INSTITUTION)? (RECORD STREET, CITY AND STATE)

E. Have you stayed in (INSTITUTION) for any other reason? (IF YES, RECORD ON CHART.)

(IF NO, GO TO Q.G-62 IF NOT YET ASKED; OTHERWISE GO TO Q.G-64)

83

G-62. Since 1970 when you were (AGE), have you ever stayed overnight in any other health care facility such as a rest home, a nursing home, a mental health facility or a health care rehabilitation center of any kind?

G-62   YES.............. 1
NO............... 2 (Q.G-64)

G-63. What type of facility was that?
(RECORD TYPE OF FACILITY ON CHART AND ASK A-D IN BOX I FOR EACH STAY)

G-63

84-92

G-64. As part of this survey, I'd like to have your social security number. Provision of this number is voluntary and not providing the number will not have any effect on your receipt of benefits from the Federal Government. This number will be useful in conducting future followup studies. It will be used to match against future mortality records. This information is collected under the authority of Section 306 of the Public Health Service Act. What is your social security number?

SOCIAL SECURITY #: |_|_|_| - |_|_| - |_|_|_|_|

42

PART K: WEIGHT

Begin K0

These questions are about your weight and height.

K-1. When you were about 12-13 years old, compared to other (girls/boys) of the same age, were you considered to be skinny, somewhat slender, average, chubby, or very heavy?

SKINNY	1
SOMEWHAT SLENDER	2
AVERAGE	3
CHUBBY	4
VERY HEAVY	5
DK	8

11

K-2. When you were about 12-13 years old, compared to other (girls/boys) of the same age, were you considered to be very tall, somewhat taller than average, about average, somewhat shorter than average, or very short?

VERY TALL	1
SOMEWHAT TALLER	2
AVERAGE	3
SOMEWHAT SHORTER	4
VERY SHORT	5
DK	8

12

K-3. How does your weight now compare to your weight 6 months ago? Is it at least 10 pounds more, at least 10 pounds less or about the same?

AT LEAST 10 POUNDS MORE	1
AT LEAST 10 POUNDS LESS	2
ABOUT THE SAME	3
DK	8

13

K-4. About how much do you weigh now?

LBS: |__|__|__|

DK 998

14-16

K-5. What was your usual weight at the age of 25?

LBS: |__|__|__|

DK 998

17-19

(IF S IS 41 OR OLDER, ASK:)

K-6. What was your usual weight at the age of 40?

LBS: |__|__|__|

DK 998

20-22

(IF S IS 66 OR OLDER, ASK:)

K-7. What was your usual weight at the age of 65?

LBS: |__|__|__|

DK 998

23-25

44

PART H: MSQ II

MSQ II

BOX J

INTERVIEWER: CHECK S's AGE ON THE LABEL AND CIRCLE ONE:

S IS UNDER 60 YEARS OLD	1 (SELF-ADMINISTRATION BOOKLET, PART I AND PART J)
S IS 60 OR OLDER	2 (Q.H-1)
BOXED QUESTIONNAIRE	3 (PART K)

These next questions ask about particular bits of information that many people seem to forget from time to time. They are routine questions that we ask everyone and may or may not apply to you directly.

Begin H0

MSQ II		Score
H-1. Who is the President of the United States?	(R)	|__| 11
H-2. Who was the President before him?	(R)	|__| 12
H-3. What is today's date?		
a. Month?	(R) _____ MO	|__| 13
b. Day? (within one day)	(R) _____ DAY	|__| 14
c. Year?	(R) _____ YR	|__| 15
	SCORE	|__|
	SCORE FROM PAGE 1	|__|
	TOTAL SCORE	|__| 16

SELF-ADMINISTRATION BOOKLET INSTRUCTIONS

(1) IF S IS YOUNGER THAN 60 OR MSQ SCORE IS 8 OR MORE:

HAND S THE SELF-ADMINISTRATION BOOKLET AND TELL HIM/HER TO START WITH PART I AND TO COMPLETE THE BOOKLET.

WHEN S HAS COMPLETED BOOKLET, CONTINUE WITH INTERVIEW.

(2) IF S MSQ SCORE IS LESS THAN 8:

HAND S THE SELF-ADMINISTRATION BOOKLET AND ASK S TO COMPLETE PART I, J AND THEN ADMINISTER PART P. THEN BRING A CLOSE FRIEND OR RELATIVE TO ASSIST WITH THE INTERVIEW STARTING WITH PART A.

43

PART L: SMOKING HISTORY

This section of the questionnaire deals with your smoking history.

Begin L/0

L-1. Did you ever smoke at least 100 cigarettes or more in your lifetime?
YES..................1
NO...................2 (Q.L-11)
11

L-2a. Do you smoke cigarettes now?
YES..................1 (Q.L-3)
NO...................2
12

L-2b. Did you stop smoking cigarettes in the past year?
YES..................1
NO...................2
13

READ L-3 TO L-6 FOR EACH SMOKING PERIOD	Smoking period #1	Smoking period #2	Smoking period #3
L-3. About how old were you when you (first/next) began to smoke cigarettes regularly?	AGE: |__|__| DK............98 DID NOT SMOKE REGULARLY....00 → (BOX K) 14-15	AGE: |__|__| DK............98 DID NOT SMOKE REGULARLY....00 → (BOX K) 20-21	AGE: |__|__| DK............98 DID NOT SMOKE REGULARLY....00 → (BOX K) 26-27
L-4. Did you ever stop smoking cigarettes (for at least a year (again)?	YES......1 NO.......2 (BOX K) 16	YES......1 NO.......2 (BOX K) 22	YES......1 NO.......2 (BOX K) 28
L-5. How old were you when you (first/next) stopped for at least a year?	AGE: |__|__| DK............98 17-18	AGE: |__|__| DK............98 23-24	AGE: |__|__| DK............98 29-30
L-6. Did you ever start smoking cigarettes again?	YES......1 (Q.L-3) NO.......2 (Q.L-9) 19	YES......1 (Q.L-3) NO.......2 (Q.L-9) 25	YES......1 (Q.L-3) NO.......2 (Q.L-9) 31

BOX K

INTERVIEWER: CHECK IF S SMOKES NOW (L-2a) AND CIRCLE ONE:
L-2a = 1 (YES)...1 (Q.L-7)
L-2a = 2 (NO)....2 (Q.L-9)

L-7. About how many cigarettes a day do you now smoke?
CIGARETTES: \|__\|__\|__\|
LESS THAN ONE A DAY..... 000
32-34

L-8. For how long have you been smoking this amount?
YEARS: \|__\|__\|
OR
MONTHS: \|__\|__\|
35-36
37

L-9. During all the years when you were smoking, about how many cigarettes a day did you usually smoke?
CIGARETTES: \|__\|__\|__\|
LESS THAN ONE A DAY..... 000
DK.....................998
38-40

L-10. (Are/Were) the cigarettes which you have smoked for the longest period of time filtered or nonfiltered?
FILTER..........1
NONFILTER.......2
41

L-11. Did you ever smoke cigars or a pipe?
YES.............1
NO..............2 (Q.L-13)
42

L-12. Do you now smoke cigars or a pipe?
YES.............1
NO..............2
43

L-13. Did you ever use . . .

	YES	NO	
a. snuff?	1	2	44
b. chewing tobacco?	1	2	45

L-14. Have you ever been married to someone who smoked cigarettes?
YES.............1
NO..............2
46

45

PART M: ALCOHOLIC BEVERAGES

Now I would like to talk with you about drinking alcoholic beverages. Alcoholic beverages include liquor, such as whiskey, rum, gin or vodka, and beer and wine.

Begin M0

M-1. Have you had at least 12 drinks of any kind of alcoholic beverage in any one year?
YES.................. 1 (Q.M-3)
NO................... 2
11

M-2. What is your main reason for not drinking?
NO NEED/NOT NECESSARY........... 1 (PART N)
DON'T CARE TO/DISLIKE IT.......... 2 (PART N)
MEDICAL/HEALTH REASONS........... 3 (PART N)
RELIGIOUS/MORAL REASONS........... 4 (PART N)
BROUGHT UP NOT TO DRINK........... 5 (PART N)
OTHER (SPECIFY)....... 6 (PART N)
DK................... 8 (PART N)
12

M-3. Have you had at least one drink of beer, wine or liquor during the past year?
YES.................. 1 (Q.M-6)
NO................... 2
13

M-4. What is your main reason for not drinking during the past year?
NO NEED/NOT NECESSARY........... 1
DON'T CARE TO/ DISLIKE IT......... 2
MEDICAL/HEALTH REASONS........... 3
RELIGIOUS/MORAL REASONS........... 4
BROUGHT UP NOT TO DRINK........... 5
OTHER (SPECIFY)....... 6
DK................... 8
14

M-5. About how old were you when you quit drinking?
AGE: |_|_| 15-16
OR
DIDN'T QUIT......... 00 (Q.M-13)
DK................. 98 (Q.M-13)

M-6. On the average, how often do you drink alcoholic beverages, that is beer, wine or liquor?
DAYS A WEEK |_|_| 17-18
OR
DAYS A MONTH |_|_| 19
MORE THAN 3 BUT LESS THAN 12 TIMES A YEAR...... 95
NO MORE THAN 3 TIMES A YEAR...... 96

47

M-7. On the days that you have a drink, about how many drinks do you usually have?
OF DRINKS: |_|_| 20-21

M-8. In how many of the past 12 months did you have at least one drink of any alcoholic beverage, that is, beer, wine, or liquor?
MONTHS: |_|_| 22-23

M-9. During the past 12 months, on about how many days did you have 9 or more drinks of any alcoholic beverage, that is, beer, wine or liquor?
NONE.......... 000
DAYS: |_|_|_| 24-26
DK............ 998

M-10. During the past 12 months, on about how many days did you have at least 5 drinks of any alcoholic beverage. (Include those days already mentioned.)
NONE.......... 000
DAYS: |_|_|_| 27-29
DK............ 998

M-11. Do you now drink more, less or about the same as you did a year ago?
MORE........... 1
LESS........... 2
SAME........... 3
30

M-12. Do you now consider yourself a light, moderate or heavy drinker?
ABSTAINER........... 1
LIGHT............... 2
MODERATE............ 3
HEAVY............... 4
31

(GO TO SELF-ADMINISTRATION BOOKLET, PAGE 7; RECORD RESPONSES ON CHART.)

M-13. Now I would like you to think about your drinking at several different periods in your life. I am interested in your drinking patterns at these periods. Look at this card. Tell me the letter of the category which best describes your usual drinking pattern when you were about 25 years old.

HAND CARD 5 B

A.......... 01
B.......... 02
C.......... 03
D.......... 04
E.......... 05
F.......... 06
G.......... 07
DK......... 98
32-33

M-14. (IF S IS 36 OR OLDER, ASK:)
How about when you were 35?
A.......... 01
B.......... 02
C.......... 03
D.......... 04
E.......... 05
F.......... 06
G.......... 07
DK......... 98
34-35

M-15. (IF S 46 OR OLDER, ASK:) And when you were 45?
A.......... 01
B.......... 02
C.......... 03
D.......... 04
E.......... 05
F.......... 06
G.......... 07
DK......... 98
36-37

48

TIME BEGAN: _____ AM
PM

PART N: NUTRITION

In this part of the interview I'm going to ask you some questions about how often you eat certain foods and how your food is usually prepared. In answering these questions, think about your eating pattern over the past year.

You can answer by telling me the number of times per day, per week, per month or per year that you eat each food. If you haven't eaten that food in the past year the answer would be "never."

```
+-----------------------------------------------------------+
| NURSING HOME INSTRUCTIONS: CIRCLE ONE:                    |
| RESPONDENT CAN ANSWER THIS SECTION. . . . . . 1           |
| RESPONDENT CANNOT ANSWER THIS SECTION                     |
| ASK OF NURSING HOME STAFF . . . . . . 2 (PART O)          |
+-----------------------------------------------------------+
```

```
+-----------------------------------------------------------+
|                  CODING GUIDE                             |
| THESE SYMBOLS ARE USED IN THIS SECTION                    |
|   D = A DAY          Y = A YEAR                           |
|   W = A WEEK         N = NEVER                            |
|   M = A MONTH        DK = DON'T KNOW FREQUENCY            |
+-----------------------------------------------------------+
```

Begin N1

N-1. How often do you have the following dairy products? Include use as a beverage or on cereal but not in coffee or tea.

	# OF TIMES	D	W	M	Y	N	DK
a. lowfat milk, skim milk, buttermilk or dry milk?	a. |__|	1	2	3	4	5	8	11-13
b. whole milk or evaporated milk?	b. |__|	1	2	3	4	5	8	14-16
c. any kind of yogurt?	c. |__|	1	2	3	4	5	8	17-19
d. cottage cheese?	d. |__|	1	2	3	4	5	8	20-22
e. hard or soft cheese including cheese dishes such as macaroni and cheese?	e. |__|	1	2	3	4	5	8	23-25
f. ice cream?	f. |__|	1	2	3	4	5	8	26-28
g. cream, half and half, or sour cream?	g. |__|	1	2	3	4	5	8	29-31

N-2. About how many servings per week do you have of meat, fish or poultry? Include all meals and snacks.

N-2 # PER WEEK: \|__\| 32-33
DOESN'T EAT MEAT, FISH OR POULTRY...96 (Q.N-11)
DK......................98

N-3. How often do you eat poultry including chicken, turkey, duck, and game birds, either plain or in salads, casseroles, or stews?

N-3 # OF TIMES: \|__\| 34-35
A DAY....................1
A WEEK...................2
A MONTH..................3
A YEAR...................4
NEVER....................5 (Q.N-5)
DK.......................8

N-4. Do you usually eat poultry with or without the skin?

N-4 WITH SKIN............1 36
WITHOUT SKIN.........2
DK..................8 37

50

M-16. (IF S 56 OR OLDER, ASK:) And when you were 55?

M-16 A................01
B................02
C................03
D................04
E................05
F................06
G................07
DK..............98 38-39

M-17. (IF S 66 OR OLDER, ASK:) And when you were 65?

M-17 A................01
B................02
C................03
D................04
E................05
F................06
G................07
DK..............98 40-41

M-18. (IF S 76 OR OLDER, ASK:) And when you were 75?

M-18 A................01
B................02
C................03
D................04
E................05
F................06
G................07
DK..............98 42-43

(SHOW S THE HIGHEST POINT ON THE CHART AND ASK QUESTION M-19)

M-19. Did you ever drink more than the amount you drank when you were ___(AGE)___ for 3 months or longer?

M-19 YES....................1
NO....................2 (PART N)
DK..................8 (PART N) 44

(IF HIGHEST POINT IS A, CIRCLE 97)

M-20. Which of the categories on the chart best describes your drinking during that period?

M-20 A................01
B................02
C................03
D................04
E................05
F................06
G................07
DK..............98 45-46
HIGHEST PT. IS A. 97

M-21. About how old were you when you started drinking that amount?

M-21 AGE: \|__\|
DK..............98 47-48

M-22. For about how long was this typical of your drinking?

M-22 # YEARS: \|__\|
OR
MONTHS: \|__\|
DK..............98 49-50

TIME ENDED: _____ AM
PM 51

49

N-5. How often do you eat beef of all kinds including hamburger, steak, roast beef or beef stew?

N-5   # OF TIMES: |_|_|
A DAY............1
A WEEK...........2
A MONTH..........3
A YEAR...........4
NEVER............5 (Q.N-7)
DK...............8

38-39
40

N-6. When you eat ground beef do you usually buy regular, lean or extra lean?

N-6
REGULAR..........1
LEAN.............2
EXTRA LEAN.......3
DOESN'T EAT......4
DK...............8

41

N-7. How often do you eat......

# OF TIMES	D	W	M	Y	N	DK	
	1	2	3	4	5	8	
a. beef or chicken liver? |_|_|							*42-44*
b. liverwurst or liver sausage? |_|_|	1	2	3	4	5	8	*45-47*
c. sandwich or packaged luncheon meats, hot dogs and meat spreads? |_|_|							*48-50*
d. roast pork, pork chops, fresh ham or spare ribs? |_|_|	1	2	3	4	5	8	*51-53*
e. bacon or pork sausage? |_|_|	1	2	3	4	5	8	*54-56*

BOX L

INTERVIEWER: CHECK N-5 AND N-7d AND CIRCLE ONE:

S NEVER EATS BEEF AND PORK (N-5 and N-7d = 5) . . 1(Q.N-9)

OTHERWISE . . . . 2(Q.N-8)

N-8. Do you usually eat the fat on beef or pork?

N-8
YES..............1
NO...............2
DK...............8

57

N-9. How often do you eat......

# OF TIMES	D	W	M	Y	N	DK	
	1	2	3	4	5	8	
a. shellfish, including shrimp, clams, oysters, crab or lobster? |_|_|	1	2	3	4	5	8	*58-60*
b. fresh or frozen fish, including fish sticks? |_|_|	1	2	3	4	5	8	*61-63*
c. canned fish such as tuna fish, sardines and herring? |_|_|	1	2	3	4	5	8	*64-66*

51

N-10. How often do you eat......

# OF TIMES	D	W	M	Y	N	DK	IF ONLY CERTAIN TIMES (✓)	
	1	2	3	4	5	8		
a. chicken, fish or meat that has been fried or deep fat fried? |_|_|	1	2	3	4	5	8	( )	*67-70*
b. chicken, fish or meat that has been charcoal grilled? |_|_|	1	2	3	4	5	8	( )	*71-74*
c. chicken, fish or meat that has been broiled? |_|_|	1	2	3	4	5	8	( )	*75-78*

N-11. How often do you eat peanuts or peanut butter?

# OF TIMES	D	W	M	Y	N	DK
|_|_|	1	2	3	4	5	8

79-81

N-12. How often do you eat other nuts of all types?

# OF TIMES	D	W	M	Y	N	DK
|_|_|	1	2	3	4	5	8

82-84

N-13. Do you eat cold cereal all year round, mainly in certain seasons, or not at all?

ALL YEAR ROUND.....1
MAINLY IN CERTAIN SEASONS.........2
NOT AT ALL..........3 (Q.N-16)

85

N-14. (In those seasons) How often do you eat cold cereal?

# OF TIMES	D	W	M	Y	N	DK
|_|_|	1	2	3	4	5	8

86-88

N-15. What is the name of cold cereal that you eat most often? Looking at this card may help you. Please just tell me the number.

HAND CARD C

CODE #:|_|_|

OTHER (SPECIFY)

89-90

N-16. Do you eat hot cereal or grits all year round, mainly in certain seasons, or not at all?

ALL YEAR ROUND.....1
MAINLY IN CERTAIN SEASONS.........2
NOT AT ALL..........3 (Q.N-19)

91

N-17. (In those seasons) How often do you eat hot cereal?

# OF TIMES	D	W	M	Y	N	DK
|_|_|	1	2	3	4	5	8

92-94

52

N-18. What kind of hot cereal do you usually eat? This list may make it easier to remember.

HAND CARD D

N-18	
CREAM OF WHEAT/FARINA	01
OATMEAL	02
DARK FARINA/RALSTON	03
GRITS	04
OTHER (SPECIFY)	05
DK	98

91–96

N-19. How often do you eat.....

OF TIMES

		D	W	M	Y	N	DK
a.	any kind of rice?	1	2	3	4	5	8
b.	pasta such as spaghetti, noodles, macaroni?	1	2	3	4	5	8

97–99
100–102

N-20. How often do you eat.....

OF TIMES

		D	W	M	Y	N	DK
a.	whole grain bread or rolls such as whole wheat, bran, rye, or pumpernickel?	1	2	3	4	5	8
b.	white bread, rolls, or other yeast breads including bagels and English muffins?	1	2	3	4	5	8
c.	quick breads such as muffins, or biscuits, or flour tortillas?	1	2	3	4	5	8
d.	corn bread or hush puppies?	1	2	3	4	5	8
e.	corn tortillas?	1	2	3	4	5	8
f.	toaster tarts, breakfast bars or instant breakfast?	1	2	3	4	5	8

103–105
106–108
109–111
112–114
115–117
118–120

N-21. Now I'd like to ask you about fruits and vegetables of all kinds. This includes fresh, canned, dried, frozen, cooked, raw or juices. About how many servings of fruits and vegetables do you have per day or per week?

N-21	
# PER DAY: |_|_|	
OR	
# PER WEEK: |_|_|	
DOESN'T EAT FRUIT OR VEGETABLES	96 (Q.N-27)
DK	98

121–122
123

53

N-22. Now I'm going to ask you how often you eat the following fruits. First, tell me if you eat each fruit primarily during certain parts of the year. Second, tell me how often you eat that fruit when you eat it. It may be easier if you follow along on this card.

HANDS CARD E

Begin N2

		IF ONLY CERTAIN TIMES (✓)	# OF TIMES	D	W	M	Y	N	DK	
a.	fresh apples?	( )	|_|_|	1	2	3	4	5	8	( ) 11–14
b.	fresh pears?	( )	|_|_|	1	2	3	4	5	8	( )
c.	bananas?	( )	|_|_|	1	2	3	4	5	8	( )
d.	fresh oranges or tangerines?	( )	|_|_|	1	2	3	4	5	8	( )
e.	orange juice?	( )	|_|_|	1	2	3	4	5	8	( )
f.	powdered orange juice substitutes such as Tang?	( )	|_|_|	1	2	3	4	5	8	( )
g.	fresh grapefruit?	( )	|_|_|	1	2	3	4	5	8	( )
h.	grapefruit juice?	( )	|_|_|	1	2	3	4	5	8	( )
i.	Vitamin C enriched fruit drinks?	( )	|_|_|	1	2	3	4	5	8	( ) 43–46
j.	fresh or canned peaches or nectarines?	( )	|_|_|	1	2	3	4	5	8	( )
k.	cantaloupe?	( )	|_|_|	1	2	3	4	5	8	( )
l.	watermelon?	( )	|_|_|	1	2	3	4	5	8	( )
m.	fresh plums?	( )	|_|_|	1	2	3	4	5	8	( )
n.	fresh or frozen strawberries?	( )	|_|_|	1	2	3	4	5	8	( )
o.	fresh, canned or dried apricots including nectar?	( )	|_|_|	1	2	3	4	5	8	( )
p.	cooked or dried prunes including prune juice?	( )	|_|_|	1	2	3	4	5	8	( ) 71–74
q.	all canned fruit such as canned pears, pineapple, fruit cocktail or apple sauce?	( )	|_|_|	1	2	3	4	5	8	( ) 75–78

79–80

N-23. How often do you eat raw vegetables, green or mixed salads or cole slaw?

N-23	# OF TIMES: |_|_|	
	A DAY	1
	A WEEK	2
	A MONTH	3
	A YEAR	4
	NEVER	5 (Q.N-26)
	DK	8

81

N-24. How often do you use salad dressing of any kind?

N-24	# OF TIMES: |_|_|	
	A DAY	1
	A WEEK	2
	A MONTH	3
	A YEAR	4
	NEVER	5 (Q.N-26)
	DK	8

82–83
84

N-25. Do you usually use oil and vinegar alone as a dressing, low calorie dressing, or some other dressing?

N-25	OIL AND VINEGAR	1
	LOW CALORIE	2
	SOME OTHER KIND	3

85

54

N-26. Now I'm going to ask you how often you eat the following vegetables. First, tell me if you eat each vegetable primarily during certain parts of the year. Second, tell me how often you eat that vegetable when you eat it. It may be easier if you follow along on this card.

HANDS CARD F

Column headers: # OF TIMES | D(1) W(2) M(3) Y(4) N(5) DK(8) | IF ONLY CERTAIN TIMES (✓)

a. green peas?
b. green beans, green lima beans or string beans?
c. other beans or peas such as kidney or pinto beans, and blackeyed or chick peas?
d. okra?
e. broccoli?
f. cauliflower?
g. brussel sprouts?
h. corn?
i. summer squash such as zucchini, or yellow crook-neck?
j. winter squash such as acorn, butternut, hubbard or pumpkin?
k. raw or cooked carrots?
l. cucumber?
m. sweet red peppers?
n. sweet green peppers?
o. iceberg or head lettuce in a salad?
p. leaf lettuce in a salad?
q. cabbage including cole slaw?
r. raw or cooked greens, for example spinach, collards or turnip greens?
s. sweet potatoes or yellow yams?
t. instant or dehydrated potatoes?
u. baked, boiled or mashed white potatoes?
v. fried or hash brown potatoes?
w. fresh tomatoes?
x. cooked tomatoes, tomato soup, juice, sauce, or canned tomatoes?
y. vegetable soup?

Begin N3

N-27. How often do you eat all kinds of sweets and desserts such as cakes, donuts, cookies, pies, and candy?
OF TIMES | D(1) W(2) M(3) Y(4) N(5) DK(8)

55

N-28. How often do you eat chocolate in the form of candy, cakes, ice cream, cookies or fudge?
OF TIMES | D W M Y N DK (1 2 3 4 5 8)

N-29. How often do you eat salty snacks such as potato chips, pretzels, crackers, salted nuts, etc.?
OF TIMES | D W M Y N DK (1 2 3 4 5 8)

N-30. On the average, how many eggs do you usually eat per week including dishes such as omelettes and egg salad?
LESS THAN ONE A WEEK...00
OF EGGS PER WEEK:|__|
DOESN'T USE.........96

N-31. How often do you eat TV type dinners or other commercially prepared frozen dinners?
OF TIMES | D W M Y N DK (1 2 3 4 5 8)

N-32. On the average, about how often do you eat commercial fast food; for example, hamburgers, fried chicken, or pizza?
OF TIMES | D W M Y N DK (1 2 3 4 5 8)

N-33. How often do you eat any combination dishes with meat or cheese such as spaghetti and meat balls, macaroni and cheese, pizza, pork and beans, and enchiladas?
OF TIMES | D W M Y N DK (1 2 3 4 5 8)

N-34. How often do you use...
OF TIMES | D W M Y N DK (1 2 3 4 5 8)
a. ketchup or tomato chili sauce?
b. chili powder or hot red chili peppers?
c. soy sauce?
d. pickles or olives?

N-35. How often do you use cheese sauce, white sauce or other thick gravies?
OF TIMES | D W M Y N DK (1 2 3 4 5 8)

N-36. At how many meals per day or per week do you add butter or margarine to foods?
OF MEALS
PER DAY: |__|
OR
PER WEEK: |__|
DOESN'T USE.........96 (Q.N-38)

N-37. When you use it, do you usually use butter, margarine in a stick, margarine in a tub, or something else?
BUTTER............1
MARGARINE IN A STICK............2
MARGARINE IN A TUB.3
OTHER (SPECIFY)....4
DK................8

56

N-38. Not including potatoes, how often do you eat vegetables.....

		# OF TIMES	D	W	M	Y	N	DK	
a.	that are cooked or boiled in a little water?	|_|_|	1	2	3	4	5	8	111-116
b.	steamed or blanched?	|_|_|	1	2	3	4	5	8	117-119
c.	cooked or boiled in a lot of water?	|_|_|	1	2	3	4	5	6	120-122
d.	stir-fried or sauteed in butter or oil?	|_|_|	1	2	3	4	5	8	123-125
e.	baked in a stew, casserole, or in a soup?	|_|_|	1	2	3	4	5	8	126-128
f.	fried?	|_|_|	1	2	3	4	5	8	129-131

Begin N4

N-39. How often do you eat.....

		# OF TIMES	D	W	M	Y	N	DK	
a.	canned vegetables?	|_|_|	1	2	3	4	5	8	11-13
b.	fresh or frozen vegetables?	|_|_|	1	2	3	4	5	8	14-16

N-40. Look at the following list of fats and oils. What type of oil or fat do you usually use when frying foods at home?

HANDS CARD G

N-40 | OLIVE OIL.............................01
| LIQUID OIL OTHER THAN OLIVE OIL......02
| SOLID SHORTENING.....................03
| MARGARINE IN A STICK.................04
| MARGARINE IN A TUB...................05
| BUTTER...............................06
| LARD.................................07
| BACON GREASE OR PORK FAT.............08
| OTHER (SPECIFY)......................09
| DON'T KNOW...........................98
| NEVER FRY FOOD AT HOME...............96   17-18

N-41. On the average, how many (a - e) do you drink per day, week, month or year?

		# OF DRINKS	D	W	M	Y	N	DK	IF ONLY CERTAIN TIMES (✓)	
a.	glasses or cans of cola type soda, regular or diet	|_|_|	1	2	3	4	5	8	( )	19-22
b.	cans or bottles of beer	|_|_|	1	2	3	4	5	8	( )	23-26
c.	glasses of wine	|_|_|	1	2	3	4	5	8	( )	27-30
d.	shots or drinks of hard liquor, either straight or in a mixed drink	|_|_|	1	2	3	4	5	8	( )	31-34
e.	glasses or cans of diet soda, including cola, or any other artificially sweetened drink	|_|_|	1	2	3	4	5	8	( )	35-38

57

N-42. How often do you eat artificially sweetened foods or candies or add artificial sweeteners to beverages or foods?

# OF TIMES	D	W	M	Y	N	DK	
|_|_|	1	2	3	4	5	8	39-41

N-43. Do you drink coffee?

N-43 | YES.................1 | 42
| NO..................2 (Q.N-44e)

N-44. On the average how many (a - f) do you drink per day, week, month or year?

		# OF CUPS	D	W	M	Y	N	DK	
a.	cups of instant decaffeinated coffee	|_|_|	1	2	3	4	5	8	43-45
b.	cups of other instant coffee	|_|_|	1	2	3	4	5	8	46-48
c.	cups of ground decaffeinated coffee	|_|_|	1	2	3	4	5	8	49-51
d.	cups of other ground coffee	|_|_|	1	2	3	4	5	8	52-54
e.	cups of herb tea	|_|_|	1	2	3	4	5	8	55-57
f.	cups of regular tea, including iced tea	|_|_|	1	2	3	4	5	8	58-60

BOX H

INTERVIEWER: REVIEW N-43, N-44e, AND N-44f AND CIRCLE ONE:

SUBJECT DOES NOT DRINK COFFEE OR TEA [N-43 = NO (2) AND N-44e AND N-44f = NEVER (5)]...............1 (Q.N-46)
OTHERWISE.......................................2 (Q.N-45)

N-45. Which of these milk products do you usually put in your coffee or tea -- whole milk, skim milk, low fat milk, half and half, cream or non dairy creamer?

HANDS CARD H

N-45 | WHOLE MILK.........01
| SKIM MILK..........02
| LOW FAT MILK.......03
| HALF AND HALF......04
| CREAM..............05
| NONDAIRY CREAMER...06
| OTHER (SPECIFY)....07
| DOESN'T ADD MILK PRODUCT.........96
| DK.................98   61-62

N-46. Are you on any type of a special diet?

N-46 | YES.................1
| NO..................2 (Q.N-50)   63

N-47. Was this diet prescribed for you by a doctor, nurse or dietician?

N-47 | YES.................1
| NO..................2   64

58

N-48. Are you on this diet because of...

	Y	N	DK	
a. high blood pressure?	1	2	8	65
b. diabetes?	1	2	8	66
c. to lose weight?	1	2	8	67
d. food allergies?	1	2	8	68
e. heart disease?	1	2	8	69
f. something else?	1	2	8	70

(SPECIFY) |__|__| 71-72

N-49. What kind of diet is it...

	Y	N	DK	
a. low or no salt?	1	2	8	73
b. low sugar?	1	2	8	74
c. low calorie?	1	2	8	75
d. low fat?	1	2	8	76
e. something else?	1	2	8	77

(SPECIFY) |__|__| 78-79

N-50. Are there some foods that you are unable to eat because you have trouble chewing or biting?

YES................1
NO.................2
80

N-51. Do any of the following problems prevent you from eating the food that you need...

	Y	N	DK	
a. problems getting to the store?	1	2	8	81
b. problems purchasing groceries?	1	2	8	82
c. problems storing food?	1	2	8	83

N-52. Do you usually eat your main meal alone or with other people?

ALONE..............1
OTHER PEOPLE.......2
84

N-53. How often do you eat breakfast — almost everyday, sometimes, rarely or never?

ALMOST EVERYDAY....1
SOMETIMES.........2
RARELY OR NEVER....3
85

N-54. Including evening snacks, how many between meal snacks do you have per day?

OF SNACKS: |__|__| 86-87

N-55. How many meals do you usually eat a day?

OF MEALS: |__|__| 88-89

N-56. Do you use salt at the table or in cooking?

N-56 YES................1
NO.................2 (PART D)
90

N-57. Is it iodized?

N-57 YES................1
NO.................2
DK.................8
91

N-58. How frequently do you use salt at the table?

OF TIMES
|__|__|

D	W	M	Y	N	DK
1	2	3	4	5	8

92-94

TIME ENDED: _____ AM
PM

PART O: SLEEP

_____ PM

Now I'd like some information about how you sleep.

Begin OO

O-1. Please look at Column I on this card.

How often do you have trouble falling asleep? Would you say it is never, rarely, sometimes, often, or almost always?

HAND 5 CARD I

O-1
NEVER............ 1
RARELY........... 2
SOMETIMES........ 3
OFTEN............ 4
ALMOST ALWAYS.... 5
DK............... 8

11

O-2. How often do you have trouble with waking up during the night? (Would you say it was never, rarely, sometimes, often, or almost always?)

O-2
NEVER............ 1
RARELY........... 2
SOMETIMES........ 3
OFTEN............ 4
ALMOST ALWAYS.... 5
DK............... 8

12

O-3. How often do you have trouble with waking up too early and not being able to fall asleep again? (Would you say it is never, rarely, sometimes, often, or almost always?)

O-3
NEVER............ 1
RARELY........... 2
SOMETIMES........ 3
OFTEN............ 4
ALMOST ALWAYS.... 5
DK............... 8

13

O-4. How often do you get so sleepy during the day or evening that you have to take a nap? (Is it never, rarely, sometimes, often, or almost always?)

O-4
NEVER............ 1
RARELY........... 2
SOMETIMES........ 3
OFTEN............ 4
ALMOST ALWAYS.... 5
DK............... 8

14

Now look at Column II.

O-5. Compared to one year ago, do you have sleep problems much more now, somewhat more now, somewhat less now, much less now or is your sleeping pattern about the same?

O-5
MUCH MORE NOW...... 1
SOMEWHAT MORE NOW.. 2
SOMEWHAT LESS NOW.. 3
MUCH LESS NOW...... 4
ABOUT THE SAME..... 5
DK................. 8

15

O-6. How often do you usually take a sedative or sleeping pill that has been prescribed by a doctor to help you sleep?

O-6
NEVER............ 00 |__|__|
TIMES:
(CIRCLE ONE)
WEEKLY........... 1
MONTHLY.......... 2
YEARLY........... 3
DK............... 8

16-17

O-7. How many hours of sleep do you usually get a night (or when you usually sleep)?

O-7
HOURS: |__|__|

18

19-20

61

Begin PO

P-1. Sometimes people have things they want to do but they just feel too weak, too tired or they don't have enough energy to do them. How often do you feel this way -- a lot of the time, some of the time, once in awhile, or do you never feel this way?

P-1
A LOT OF THE TIME. 1
SOME OF THE TIME.. 2
ONCE IN AWHILE.... 3
NEVER............ 4

11

Now I'm going to read you some traits some people have. Using the categories on this card, please tell me how well these traits describe you. The first trait is.....

HAND 5 CARD J

	VERY WELL	FAIRLY WELL	SOME-WHAT	NOT AT ALL	DK
P-2. Having a strong need to excel or be best in most things.	1	2	3	4	8
P-3. Usually feeling pressed for time.	1	2	3	4	8
P-4. Being hard driving and competitive.	1	2	3	4	8
P-5. Eating too quickly.	1	2	3	4	8
P-6. Getting upset when you have to wait in line?	1	2	3	4	8

12
13
14
15
16

Now I'm going to read some statements. Don't worry about the exact meaning of these statements, just give me your first impressions. Using the categories on this card, I'd like you to tell me if you strongly disagree, disagree, feel neutral, agree, or strongly agree with each statement.

P-7. I like to have a lot of people around me.

HAND 5 CARD K

P-7
STRONGLY DISAGREE. 1
DISAGREE......... 2
FEEL NEUTRAL..... 3
AGREE............ 4
STRONGLY AGREE... 5

17

62

P-8. I am a cheerful, high-spirited person.

P-8 STRONGLY DISAGREE. 1
DISAGREE............ 2
FEEL NEUTRAL....... 3
AGREE.............. 4
STRONGLY AGREE.... 5

18

P-9. I don't get much pleasure from chatting with people.

P-9 STRONGLY DISAGREE. 1
DISAGREE............ 2
FEEL NEUTRAL....... 3
AGREE.............. 4
STRONGLY AGREE.... 5

19

P-10. I am a very active person.

P-10 STRONGLY DISAGREE. 1
DISAGREE............ 2
FEEL NEUTRAL....... 3
AGREE.............. 4
STRONGLY AGREE.... 5

20

P-11. I prefer jobs that let me work without being bothered by other people.

P-11 STRONGLY DISAGREE. 1
DISAGREE............ 2
FEEL NEUTRAL....... 3
AGREE.............. 4
STRONGLY AGREE.... 5

21

P-12. I have strong emotional attachments to my friends.

P-12 STRONGLY DISAGREE. 1
DISAGREE............ 2
FEEL NEUTRAL....... 3
AGREE.............. 4
STRONGLY AGREE.... 5

22

P-13. I am dominant, forceful, and assertive.

P-13 STRONGLY DISAGREE. 1
DISAGREE............ 2
FEEL NEUTRAL....... 3
AGREE.............. 4
STRONGLY AGREE.... 5

23

P-14. I have sometimes done things just for "kicks" or "thrills."

P-14 STRONGLY DISAGREE. 1
DISAGREE............ 2
FEEL NEUTRAL....... 3
AGREE.............. 4
STRONGLY AGREE.... 5

24

P-15. I don't like to waste my time day-dreaming.

P-15 STRONGLY DISAGREE. 1
DISAGREE............ 2
FEEL NEUTRAL....... 3
AGREE.............. 4
STRONGLY AGREE.... 5

25

P-16. Poetry has little or no affect on me.

P-16 STRONGLY DISAGREE..1
DISAGREE............2
FEEL NEUTRAL.......3
AGREE..............4
STRONGLY AGREE.....5

26

P-17. I often try new and foreign foods.

P-17 STRONGLY DISAGREE..1
DISAGREE............2
FEEL NEUTRAL.......3
AGREE..............4
STRONGLY AGREE.....5

27

P-18. I'm pretty set in my ways.

P-18 STRONGLY DISAGREE..1
DISAGREE............2
FEEL NEUTRAL.......3
AGREE..............4
STRONGLY AGREE.....5

28

P-19. I enjoy solving problems or puzzles.

P-19 STRONGLY DISAGREE..1
DISAGREE............2
FEEL NEUTRAL.......3
AGREE..............4
STRONGLY AGREE.....5

29

P-20. I have a very active imagination.

P-20 STRONGLY DISAGREE..1
DISAGREE............2
FEEL NEUTRAL.......3
AGREE..............4
STRONGLY AGREE.....5

30

PHYSICAL MEASUREMENT INTRODUCTION

I mentioned earlier that I would be measuring your pulse, blood pressure, and weight as a part of the interview. I would like to start the procedure now. As part of this procedure, you need to remain relaxed and seated for about fifteen (15) minutes. During this time, we will finish the questionnaire. If there are things you need to do before we start, such as going to the bathroom, I would like you to do that now. I would also suggest that should the phone or doorbell ring that I answer it for you. Would that be all right? [IF NECESSARY, ASK S TO MOVE TO A SUITABLE LOCATION TO TAKE THE BLOOD PRESSURE READING.]

Various factors such as smoking, drinking alcohol and drinking coffee can affect your pulse and blood pressure. Therefore, I would like to request that you do not smoke or drink coffee (or alcohol) during this time. Also, have you had any alcoholic beverages within the last 24 hours? [RECORD ON PMR.]

Now, I would like to explain what I am going to do. First, I will find the pulse in your right arm. Next, I will wrap the blood pressure cuff around your arm. At this point, we will finish the questionnaire. At the end of the interview, I will take your pulse and then inflate the cuff. You will feel a sensation of pressure on the arm when the cuff is inflated, and I will be inflating the cuff a maximum of five times. While I am measuring your blood pressure, I would like to avoid any conversation. I will be happy to answer your questions before or after measurements are taken.

Is there any medical reason you know of why this procedure should not be done?

[IF YES, RECORD ON PMR AND DISCONTINUE PROCEDURE AND CONTINUE WITH THE QUESTIONNAIRE.

OTHERWISE, ASK S TO REMOVE ANY OUTER CLOTHING/JEWELRY AND TO ROLL UP SLEEVE. OBSERVE SUBJECT'S ARM FOR CONDITIONS PREVENTING MEASUREMENT. IF CONDITIONS ARE PRESENT, RECORD ON PMR AND DISCONTINUE PROCEDURE.]

Have you had any needles or tubes in any veins in your arms in the last week? [IF YES, RECORD ON PMR AND DISCONTINUE IF BOTH ARMS ARE AFFECTED.]

Then I will go ahead and locate your pulse and place the cuff now.

[PLACE CUFF.]

Begin QQ

INTERVIEWER: BOX N

IF S IS UNABLE TO WALK CHECK THIS BOX ☐ AND GO TO PART R; OTHERWISE CONTINUE. 11

These next few questions concern physical activity.

Q-1. In things you do for recreation, for example, sports, hiking, dancing, etc., do you get much exercise, moderate exercise, little or no exercise?

MUCH EXERCISE............1
MODERATE EXERCISE........2
LITTLE OR NO EXERCISE....3   12

Q-2. In your usual day, aside from recreation, are you physically very active, moderately active, or quite inactive?

VERY ACTIVE..............1
MODERATELY ACTIVE........2
QUITE INACTIVE...........3   13

Q-3. Do you follow a regular program of physical exercise?

YES..................1
NO...............2 (PART R)   14

Q-4. Do you regularly jog as part of this program?

YES..................1
NO...............2 (PART R)   15

Q-5. On the average, how many miles per week do you jog?

MILES/WK: |__|__|__|
DK..............998   16-18

PART R: TEETH

These next questions are about your teeth.

Begin R0

R-1. Have you lost all your teeth from your upper jaw?
YES............... 1
NO............... 2 (Q.R-4)   11

R-2. Do you have a plate or false teeth for your upper jaw?
YES............... 1 (Q.R-4)
NO............... 2   12

R-3. How long has it been since you have had any teeth to chew with, natural or false, in your upper jaw? (READ CATEGORIES IF NECESSARY.)
LESS THAN A YEAR........ 0
1 BUT LESS THAN 5 YEARS.. 1
5 BUT LESS THAN 10 YEARS............ 2
10 BUT LESS THAN 20 YEARS............ 3
20 OR MORE............ 4
DK............ 8   13

R-4. Have you lost all your teeth from your lower jaw?
YES............... 1
NO............... 2 (BOX O)   14

R-5. Do you have a plate or false teeth for your lower jaw?
YES............... 1 (BOX O)
NO............... 2   15

R-6. How long has it been since you have had any teeth to chew with, natural or false, in your lower jaw? (READ CATEGORIES IF NECESSARY.)
LESS THAN A YEAR........ 1
1 BUT LESS THAN 5 YEARS.. 2
5 BUT LESS THAN 10 YEARS............ 3
10 BUT LESS THAN 20 YEARS............ 4
20 OR MORE............ 5
DK............ 8   16

BOX O

INTERVIEWER: CHECK Q.R-2 AND R-5 TO SEE IF S HAS DENTAL PLATES AND CIRCLE ONE:
R-2 OR R-5 = YES (1) 1 (Q.R-7)
OTHERWISE. 2 (Q.R-8)

R-7. Do you think that you need (a) new dental plate(s) or that the one(s) you have need(s) refitting?
YES, NEED NEW PLATE.. 1 (PART S)
YES, NEED REFITTING.. 2 (PART S)
NO................ 3 (PART S)
DK................ 8 (PART S)   17

R-8. Do you use fluoridated toothpaste?
YES............... 1
NO............... 2   18

PART S: HEARING

Now I'm going to ask you some questions about your hearing.

Begin S0

S-1. At any time over the past few years, have you ever noticed a ringing in your ears?
YES............... 1
NO............... 2 (Q.S-4)   11

S-2. Do you notice this ringing all the time, every few days or less often?
ALL THE TIME...... 1
EVERY FEW DAYS.... 2
LESS OFTEN........ 3   12

S-3. When it does occur, does it bother you quite a bit, just a little or not at all?
QUITE A BIT....... 1
JUST A LITTLE..... 2
NOT AT ALL........ 3   13

S-4. Have you ever used a hearing aid?
YES............... 1
NO............... 2 (Q.S-8)   14

S-5. Have you ever used a hearing aid for your left ear, right ear or both ears?
LEFT EAR.......... 1
RIGHT EAR......... 2
BOTH.............. 3   15

S-6. Do you use a hearing aid now?
YES............... 1
NO............... 2   16

S-7. (Does/Did) it improve your hearing not very much, somewhat or very much?
NOT VERY MUCH..... 1
SOMEWHAT.......... 2
VERY MUCH......... 3   17

S-8. In a normal conversation with several persons, are you able to hear well enough to understand what is said, without difficulty, with some difficulty, with much difficulty, or are you unable to understand at all (even using your hearing aid)?
WITH NO DIFFICULTY... 1
WITH SOME DIFFICULTY. 2
WITH MUCH DIFFICULTY. 3
UNABLE.............. 4   18

S-9. (Without a hearing aid), can you usually hear and understand what a person says without seeing his or, her face?

	YES	NO	DK
a. If that person whispers to you from across a quiet room?	1 (PART T)	2	8	19
b. If that person talks in a normal voice to you from across a quiet room?	1 (PART T)	2	8	20
c. If that person shouts to you from across a quiet room?	1 (PART T)	2	8	21
d. If that person speaks loudly into your better ear?	1 (PART T)	2	8	22

S-10. (Without a hearing aid), can you usually...

		YES	NO	DK	
a.	Tell the sound of speech from other sounds or noises?	a	1 (PART T)	2	8	23
b.	Tell one kind of noise from another?	b	1 (PART T)	2	8	24
c.	Hear loud noises?	c	1	2	8	25

Now, I am going to ask you questions concerning your vision.

Begin T0

T-1	Are you totally blind in either eye?	YES.............1 NO..............2 (Q.T-3) DK..............8 (Q.T-3)	11
T-2	Which one?	RIGHT...........1 LEFT............2 BOTH............3 (PART U)	12
T-3	Do you wear eyeglasses or contact lenses?	YES.............1 NO..............2 (Q.T-5)	13
T-4	How old were you when you first started wearing glasses or contact lenses?	AGE: |__|__| DK............98	14-15
T-5	Do you use a magnifying glass for reading?	YES.............1 NO..............2 (Q.T-7)	16
T-6	Do you use a magnifying glass for reading all the time, most of the time, some of the time or hardly ever?	ALL THE TIME.......1 MOST OF THE TIME...2 SOME OF THE TIME...3 HARDLY EVER........4	17

T-7. (When wearing eyeglasses/contact lenses) can you see well enough to recognize a friend...

T-7		YES	NO	DK	
	a. across the street?	a	1 (Q.T-8)	2	8	18
	b. across the room?	b	1	2	8	19
	c. at arms length?	c	1	2	8	20

T-8. (When wearing eyeglasses/contact lenses) can you see well enough...

T-8		YES	NO	DK	
	a. to recognize the letters in ordinary newspaper print?	a	1 (PART U)	2	8	21
	b. to recognize the letters in a headline?	b	1 (PART U)	2	8	22
	c. to tell if a light is on or off in a room?	c	1	2	8	23

PART U: BACKGROUND INFORMATION

In this section I'm going to ask you some questions about your background.

Begin t0

U-1. Most people in the United States have ancestors who came from other parts of the world. Here is a card listing some ethnic backgrounds. Which of these groups best describe your ethnic background? (RECORD ALL THAT APPLY.)

HAND S CARD L

01 02 03 04 05 06 07	
08 09 10 11 12 13 14	
15 16 17 18 19 20 21	
22 23 24 25 26 27	
OTHER (SPEC:FY).. 28	|_|_|11-12
	|_|_|13-14
	|_|_|15-16
DK............... 98	|_|_|17-18

U-2. Look at this card. Which of these categories best describes you?

HAND S CARD M

ALEUT, ESKIMO or AMERICAN INDIAN............. 1
ASIAN/PACIFIC ISLANDER.. 2
BLACK................ 3
WHITE................ 4
OTHER (SPECIFY)...... 5

19

U-3. Are you now married, widowed, divorced, separated or have you never been married?

MARRIED.......... 1
WIDOWED.......... 2
DIVORCED......... 3
SEPARATED........ 4
NEVER MARRIED.... 5

20

U-4. Would you say that you have lived most of your life in a rural area, in the city or in the city suburbs?

RURAL.............. 1
CITY.............. 2 (Q.U-6)
CITY SUBURBS...... 3 (Q.U-6)

21

U-5. When you lived in a rural area did you live on a farm?

YES.............. 1
NO............... 2

22

U-6. In the area where you lived most of your life, what was your primary source of drinking water: a community supply, a private well, a spring or some other source?

COMMUNITY......... 1
PRIVATE WELL...... 2
SPRING............ 3
OTHER (SPECIFY)... 4

23

U-7. In what state were you born?

STATE: _____

U-8. Have you ever worked at a job or a business full time or part time for a total of more than a year?

YES.............. 1
NO............... 2 (Q.U-21)

24

U-9. What kind of work have you done for the longest period of time? What was your occupation or complete job title? For example, carpenter, secretary, electrical engineer.

OCCUPATION/JOB TITLE: _____

\|_\|_\|25-27

U-10. What were your most important activities or duties as a(n) (OCCUPATION): for example, sell cars, keep account books, sweep floors?

DUTIES: _____

28-29

U-11. For how many years have you worked as a(n) (OCCUPATION)?

YRS: \|_\|_\|

30-32

U-12. While employed as a(n) (OCCUPATION), what was the name of the employer for whom you worked the longest?

EMPLOYER: _____

SELF EMPLOYED.......... \|_\|

33

U-13. What kind of business or industry was that employer in, that is, what does the company or your part of the company do or make? For example, automobile manufacturing, state labor dept., dairy farming, retail shoe sales?

BUSINESS/INDUSTRY: _____

34

U-14. Do you still work for (EMPLOYER) as a(n) (OCCUPATION)?

YES.............. 1 (Q.U-27)
NO............... 2

35-38

U-15. Have you stopped working at or retired from your usual job or occupation?

YES.............. 1
NO............... 2 (Q.U-21)

U-16. In what year was that?

YR: \|1\|9\|_\|_\|

39

U-17. Did you stop working because of reasons related to your health?

YES.............. 1
NO............... 2 (Q.U-20)

40

U-18. Did you receive disability benefits from Social Security at that time?

YES.............. 1
NO............... 2 (Q.U-20)

41

U-19. Are you still getting them?

YES.............. 1
NO............... 2

42

U-20. Did you stop work at your usual occupation voluntarily?

YES.............. 1
NO............... 2

U-21. These next questions are about your current status. During the last three months what have you been doing most: working, retired, keeping house, going to school or looking for work?

WORKING............. 1 (Q.U-23)
RETIRED............. 2
KEEPING HOUSE....... 3
STUDENT............. 4
LOOKING FOR WORK.... 5
OTHER (SPECIFY)..... 6

43

U-22. During the last three months, have you worked at all at a job or business?

YES...............1
NO................2 (BOX P)

44

U-23. What kind of work are you doing? What is your occupation or complete job title? For example, carpenter, secretary, electrical engineer.

OCCUPATION/JOB TITLE:

45-47

U-24. What are your most important activities or duties? For example, sell cars, keep account books, sweep floors.

DUTIES:

U-25. What is the name of your employer?

EMPLOYER:

SELF EMPLOYED.........

48-50

U-26. What kind of business or industry is that employer in, that is, what does the company or your part of the company, do or make? For example, automobile manufacturing, state labor dept., dairy farming, retail shoe sales.

BUSINESS/INDUSTRY:

51-52

U-27. On the average, how many hours a week do you work as a(n) (OCCUPATION)?

HR/WK:

BOX P

INTERVIEWER: CHECK Q.U-8 AND CIRCLE ONE:

Q.U-8 = YES (1)..........1 (Q.U-28)

Q.U-8 = NO (2)..........2 (Q.U-29)

U-28. Have you ever worked at an occupation in which you were heavily exposed to dusts, fumes, or vapors?

YES...............1
NO................2
DK................8

53

U-29. Have you ever had a hobby in which you were heavily exposed to dusts, fumes, or vapors?

YES...............1
NO................2
DK................8

54

73

U-30. Please look at this card. Which of these income groups represents your total combined family income for the past 12 months? Include income from all sources such as wages, salaries, social security or retirement benefits, help from relatives, rent from property and so forth.

HAND S CARD N

A...01
B...02
C...03
D...04
E...05
F...06
G...07
H...08
I...09
J...10
K...11
L...12
M...13
N...14
DK..98

55-56

U-31. Please look at this card again. Which of these income groups represents your personal income for the past 12 months? Again include income from all sources such as wages, salaries, social security or retirement benefits, help from relatives, rent from property and so forth.

A...01
B...02
C...03
D...04
E...05
F...06
G...07
H...08
I...09
J...10
K...11
L...12
M...13
N...14
DK..98

57-58

U-32. During the past 12 months, did you receive personal income from the following sources?

		YES	NO	DK	
a. Wages or salary?	a	1	2	8	59
b. Social security or railroad retirement?	b	1	2	8	60
c. Welfare payments or other public assistance such as aid to families with dependent children, old age assistance or aid to the blind or totally disabled?	c	1	2	8	61
d. Unemployment compensation or workmen's compensation?	d	1	2	8	62
e. Government employee pensions or private pensions?	e	1	2	8	63
f. Net income from a farm?	f	1	2	8	64
g. Veterans' payments?	g	1	2	8	65
h. Alimony or child support?	h	1	2	8	66
i. Other money contributed from persons not living in the household?	i	1	2	8	67
j. Investments?	j	1	2	8	68
k. Anything else?	k	1	2	8	69

(SPECIFY)

70

U-33. (IF S IS FEMALE, ASK:) Please tell me your father's last name? NAME:

71-85

74

OBSERVATION SHEET

INTERVIEWER: COMPLETE AT CONCLUSION OF INTERVIEW

OS-1. Do you feel that the information provided by the Subject or Proxy was satisfactory?

YES. 1 (Q.0S-3)
NO 2   105

OS-2. If not, why not?

OS-3. Please circle the number that best describes the subject's awareness level during the interview.

1   2   3   4   5
Very   Very
Alert   Confused

OR

SUBJECT NOT OBSERVED BY INTERVIEWER 0   106

COMMENTS:

OS-4. In regard to the questionnaire do you feel the questionnaire:

	YES	NO
a. held the respondent's attention throughout the interview?.	1	2
b. was upsetting or depressing to the respondent?.	1	2
c. was boring or uninteresting to the respondent?.	1	2

(IF YES TO b OR c):

OS-5. Was there a section that seemed to be particularly upsetting or problematic for the respondent? If so, note below.

OS-6. Record any relevant observations, comments or impressions you may have had about this interview.

76

U-34. My supervisor, as part of a validation procedure, may be contacting you in the near future to make sure that I conducted this interview. I'd like to (confirm/have) your telephone number, starting with the area code. (IF NO PHONE, RECORD AREA CODE.)

U-34 |_|_|_|_|_|_|_|_|_|_| 81-90

REFUSE: 9999999996

BOX Q

INTERVIEWER: CHECK PRIMARY RESPONDENT AND IF P OR S WITH ASSISTANCE, RECORD NAME, RELATIONSHIP AND TELEPHONE NUMBER AND WHY PROXY/ASSISTANCE WAS USED.

NAME	RELATION-SHIP TO S	TELEPHONE	PRIMARY (✓)
S		( )	( )
P #1		( )	( )
P #2		( )	( )
S WITH ASSISTANCE #1		( )	( )
S WITH ASSISTANCE #2		( )	( )

IF PROXY OR ASSISTANCE: STATE REASON WHY PROXY/ASSISTANCE WAS NEEDED:

TIME ENDED _____ AM PM   96-100

AUTHORIZATION FORM STATEMENT

"Thank you very much for taking the time to participate in this interview. In connection with the medical history that you have given us, as part of this survey, it may be necessary to obtain additional or more technical information from staff or records in hospitals or other in-patient facilities. This form authorizes the U.S. Public Health Service to obtain this information. As with all of the information you have given us, this information will be kept confidential and used only for statistical purposes." (HAVE S SIGN FORM)

[TAKE PHYSICAL MEASUREMENT READINGS]

OFFICE USE ONLY:

PR: |_|_| 101
REL: |_|_|_| 102-103
|_| 104

CHECK LIST FOR PHYSICAL MEASUREMENTS

Pulse & Blood Pressure Preparation

1. Read the Physical Measurements Introduction. Ask subject if has any problems that would inhibit the reading.

2. Position the subject.

3. Locate radial and brachial pulse.

4. Select and place the cuff.

5. Continue interview for fifteen minutes.

Pulse & Blood Pressure Measurement

6. Obtain resting pulse and record.

7. Obtain MIL, deflate rapidly, disconnect the manometer tubing and record.

8. Wait thirty seconds.

9. Place stethoscope in ears, ear pieces turned forward, and diaphragm over brachial pulse point.

10. Inflate rapidly to MIL.

11. Deflate 2mm Hg per second, eyes level with midpoint of the manometer column. Read the point on the manometer when the first sound is heard (systolic) and sound disappears (diastolic).

12. Continue deflation to 10mm Hg below last sound.

13. Deflate rapidly to zero.

14. Remove stethoscope from ears.

15. Disconnect manometer tubing.

16. Record readings on PMR.

17. Wait thirty seconds.

18. Repeat steps 9-17 for two more readings.

Weight

1. Place scale on hard surfaced floor and adjust to zero if necessary.

2. Stand to one side of scale looking directly down onto face of scale.

3. Record weight on PMR.

Reporting to Subject

1. Record readings and identifying information on the Report of Physical Measurement Finding and, using the Blood Pressure Value box, determine which statement to read to the subject.

2. Ask subject to sign form and give the top copy to the subject to keep.

BLOOD PRESSURE VALUE BOX

Elevated systolic blood pressure of 230 by palpation of radial pulse only. 4

Systolic		Diastolic			
	Under 90	90 - 94	95 - 114	115 - 129	130 or More
Under 150	1	2	3	4	5
150-159	2	2	3	4	5
160-239	3	3	3	4	5
240 or more	5	5	5	5	5

PART C

INTERVIEWER: READ INSTRUCTIONS TO RESPONDENT.

These next questions are about your pregnancy and menstrual history. I can read these questions to you or you can fill them out yourself. Which would you prefer? (IF SELF ADMINISTERED): Please circle one number next to the answer that you choose or write in the correct response. A "GO TO" statement will tell you which question to go to next. If there is no "GO TO" statement just go to the next question. If you need any help ask me for assistance.

C-1. Have you ever been pregnant? Include live births, stillbirths, miscarriages and abortions.
1 Yes (GO TO C-2)
2 No (GO TO C-8)

C-2. Are you pregnant now?
1 Yes
2 No

C-3. How old were you when your first child was born? This means the first child born alive or stillborn.
Age: _____ (GO TO C-4)
OR
0 I had no births (GO TO C-6)

C-4. How old were you when your last child was born? Include stillbirths.
Age: _____

C-5. How many live births have you had?
Number of Live Births: _____
OR
0 I had no live births

C-6. Have you ever had a miscarriage?
1 Yes (GO TO C-7)
2 No (GO TO C-8)

C-7. How many miscarriages have you had?
Number of Miscarriages: _____

C-8. Are you still having periods?
1 Yes (GO TO C-9)
2 I am pregnant now (GO TO C-9)
3 No (GO TO C-11)

C-9. Are your periods regular or irregular? By regular we mean your periods come about once a month. You can usually predict when they will come and they usually last about the same number of days.
1 My periods are regular (GO TO C-21)
2 My periods are irregular (GO TO C-10)

C-10. Are they irregular because you are going through the change of life or for some other reason?
1 My periods are irregular because of the change of life (GO TO C-15)
2 My periods are irregular for some other reason (GO TO C-21)

C-11. At what age did you have your last period?
Age: _____

[GO TO NEXT PAGE]

OMB No. 0925-0161
Approval Expires 12-31-83

ID NUMBER

U.S. DEPARTMENT OF HEALTH AND HUMAN SERVICES
PUBLIC HEALTH SERVICE
NATIONAL CENTER FOR HEALTH STATISTICS
NATIONAL INSTITUTE ON AGING
NATIONAL INSTITUTES OF HEALTH

NHANES I EPIDEMIOLOGIC FOLLOWUP SURVEY

SUBJECT QUESTIONNAIRE

ASSURANCE OF CONFIDENTIALITY

PHS-T-574
(7-82)

C-12. Did your periods stop naturally, because you had surgery or for some other reason?

1 My periods stopped naturally (GO TO C-14)

2 My periods stopped because of surgery (GO TO C-14)

3 My periods stopped for some other reason (GO TO C-13)

C-13. What was the reason?

REASON: _____

C-14. Do you still have your womb or uterus?

1 Yes

2 No

C-15. Do you still have <u>both</u> your ovaries?

1 Yes (GO TO C-17)

2 No (GO TO C-16)

C-16. Do you still have <u>one</u> ovary?

1 Yes

2 No

C-17. Did you ever take female hormone pills for reasons related to menopause, including hot flashes or mood changes around the time you were beginning the change of life? This would include hormone pills taken for natural change of life or because your periods stopped due to an operation.

1 Yes (GO TO C-18)

2 No (GO TO C-23)

C-18. How old were you when you <u>first</u> took hormone pills?

Age: _____

C-19. How old were you when you <u>last</u> took hormone pills?

Age: _____

OR

1 I am taking hormone pills now

C-20. Altogether for about how many years have you taken hormone pills?

Years: _____ (GO TO C-23)

OR

Months: _____ (GO TO C-23)

[GO TO NEXT PAGE]

4

C-21. Do you still have <u>both</u> your ovaries?

1 Yes (GO TO C-23)

2 No (GO TO C-22)

C-22. Do you still have <u>one</u> ovary?

1 Yes

2 No

C-23. Have you ever taken birth control pills for any reason?

1 Yes (GO TO C-24)

2 No (STOP. RETURN BOOKLET TO INTERVIEWER.)

C-24. How old were you when you <u>first</u> took birth control pills?

Age: _____

C-25. How old were you when you <u>last</u> took birth control pills?

Age: _____

OR

1 I am taking birth control pills now

C-26. Altogether for about how many years have you taken birth control pills?

I took birth control pills for:

Years: _____

OR

Months: _____

C-27. Which of these answers best describes the reason or reasons that you took birth control pills: for birth control; irregular periods; change of life or for some other reason?

1 For birth control

2 Irregular periods

3 Change of life

4 Some other reason (What?)

_____

_____

[STOP. RETURN BOOKLET TO INTERVIEWER]

5

ALCOHOL CHART
(SUBJECT)
LIFETIME DRINKING PATTERN
RESPONSES TO QUESTIONS M-13 THROUGH M-18

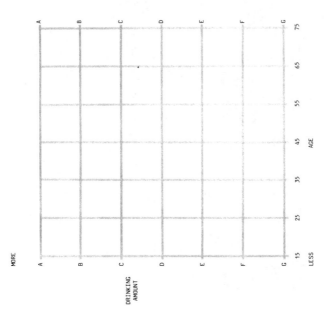

RESPONSE TO QUESTION D-17

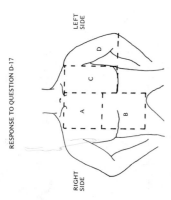

RESPONSE TO QUESTION E-100

INSTRUCTIONS: Place "x" on the line to indicate the severity of pain. On the scale, the left side is no pain and the right side is very severe pain.

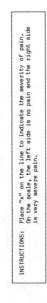

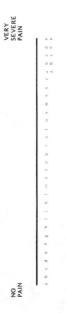

INSTRUCTIONS: Please circle one number for each question I-21 through I-39 which best answers or describes your feelings -- DURING THE PAST MONTH.

I-21. How have you been feeling in general, during the past month?
1 In excellent spirits
2 In very good spirits
3 In good spirits mostly
4 I have been up and down in spirits a lot
5 In low spirits mostly
6 In very low spirits

I-22. Have you been under or felt you were under any strain, stress, or pressure, during the past month?
1 Yes -- almost more than I could bear or stand
2 Yes -- quite a bit of pressure
3 Yes -- some -- more than usual
4 Yes -- some -- but about usual
5 Yes -- a little
6 Not at all

I-23. How happy, satisfied, or pleased have you been with your personal life, during the past month?
1 Extremely happy -- could not have been more satisfied or pleased
2 Very happy
3 Fairly happy
4 Satisfied -- pleased
5 Somewhat dissatisfied
6 Very dissatisfied

I-24. Have you been anxious, worried or upset, during the past month?
1 Extremely so -- to the point of being sick or almost sick
2 Very much so
3 Quite a bit
4 Some -- enough to bother me
5 A little bit
6 Not at all

I-25. Have you been bothered by any illness, bodily disorder, pains, or fears about your health, during the past month?
1 All the time
2 Most of the time
3 A good bit of the time
4 Some of the time
5 A little of the time
6 None of the time

I-26. Have you been feeling emotionally stable and sure of yourself, during the past month?
1 All the time
2 Most of the time
3 A good bit of the time
4 Some of the time
5 A little of the time
6 None of the time

9

INSTRUCTIONS: Please circle one number for each statement (Questions I-1 through I-20) which best describes how often you felt or behaved this way -- DURING THE PAST WEEK.

DURING THE PAST WEEK:

	Rarely or none of the time (less than 1 day)	Some or a little of the time (1-2 days)	Occasionally or a moderate amount of time (3-4 days)	Most or all of the time (5-7 days)
I-1. I was bothered by things that usually don't bother me.	0	1	2	3
I-2. I did not feel like eating; my appetite was poor.	0	1	2	3
I-3. I felt that I could not shake off the blues even with help from my family or friends.	0	1	2	3
I-4. I felt that I was just as good as other people.	0	1	2	3
I-5. I had trouble keeping my mind on what I was doing.	0	1	2	3
I-6. I felt depressed.	0	1	2	3
I-7. I felt that everything I did was an effort.	0	1	2	3
I-8. I felt hopeful about the future.	0	1	2	3
I-9. I thought my life had been a failure.	0	1	2	3
I-10. I felt fearful.	0	1	2	3
I-11. My sleep was restless.	0	1	2	3
I-12. I was happy.	0	1	2	3
I-13. I talked less than usual.	0	1	2	3
I-14. I felt lonely.	0	1	2	3
I-15. People were unfriendly.	0	1	2	3
I-16. I enjoyed life.	0	1	2	3
I-17. I had crying spells.	0	1	2	3
I-18. I felt sad.	0	1	2	3
I-19. I felt that people disliked me.	0	1	2	3
I-20. I could not get "going".	0	1	2	3

[GO TO NEXT PAGE]

PART J

INSTRUCTIONS: These next questions are about bowel and bladder habits. For each question, please circle the number next to the answer that best describes your situation.

J-1. Do you have trouble with your bowels which makes you con-stipated or gives you diarrhea?
1 I get constipated
2 I get diarrhea
3 I do not have trouble with my bowels

J-2. How often do you usually have a bowel movement?
1 Once a week or less often
2 Two or three times a week
3 Four to six times a week
4 Once a day
5 Two or three times a day
6 Four or more times a day

J-3. Which of the following best describes your usual bowel movement; is it normal, loose or watery, or hard or very firm?
1 Normal
2 Loose or watery
3 Hard or firm

J-4. During the past few months, how often have you lost control over your bowels or had an accident; often, occasionally, or never?
1 Often
2 Occasionally
3 Never

J-5. How often do you use a laxative or stool softener?
1 Every day
2 Every other day
3 Once or twice a week
4 Once or twice a month
5 Less than once a month
6 Never

J-6. During the past few months, how often have you lost control over your urine; often, occasionally, or never?
1 Often
2 Occasionally
3 Never

J-7. How often do you dribble, leak, or lose urine when you laugh, strain, or cough; often, occasionally or never?
1 Often
2 Occasionally
3 Never (STOP. RETURN BOOKLET TO INTERVIEWER.)

J-8. Do you dribble or leak urine only when you laugh, strain, or cough?
1 Yes
2 No, I dribble or leak urine at other times

OFFICE USE ONLY
FILLED OUT BY: SUBJECT. 1
SUBJECT WITH ASSISTANCE . 2
INTERVIEWER. 3
PROXY. 4

PART I (continued)

INSTRUCTIONS: For questions I-27 through I-30 please circle the number which best indicates your feelings -- DURING THE PAST MONTH.

I-27. How concerned or worried about your HEALTH have you been, during the past month?
0 1 2 3 4 5 6 7 8 9 10
Not concerned at all ... Very concerned

I-28. How RELAXED or TENSE have you been, during the past month?
0 1 2 3 4 5 6 7 8 9 10
Very relaxed ... Very tense

I-29. How much ENERGY, PEP, VITALITY have you felt, during the past month?
0 1 2 3 4 5 6 7 8 9 10
No energy at all, listless ... Very energetic dynamic

I-30. How DEPRESSED or CHEERFUL have you been, during the past month?
0 1 2 3 4 5 6 7 8 9 10
Very depressed ... Very cheerful

INSTRUCTIONS: Please circle the number that is next to the answer that best describes your situation.

I-31. In general, about how many relatives and friends do you have that you feel close to? These are people with whom you feel at ease, can talk to about private matters, and can call on for help.
0 None
1 One person
2 Two people
3 Three or four people
4 Five to nine people
5 Ten to nineteen people
6 Twenty or more people

HOSPITAL AND HEALTH CARE FACILITY CHART
(SUBJECT)

1. QUES #: _____ CONDITION: _____ YEAR: _____
   FACILITY NAME: _____ TYPE: _____ |__|__|__|
   ADDRESS: _____
            STREET   CITY   STATE |__|__|__|
   COMMENTS: _____

2. QUES #: _____ CONDITION: _____ YEAR: _____
   FACILITY NAME: _____ TYPE: _____ |__|__|__|
   ADDRESS: _____
            STREET   CITY   STATE |__|__|__|
   COMMENTS: _____

3. QUES #: _____ CONDITION: _____ YEAR: _____
   FACILITY NAME: _____ TYPE: _____ |__|__|__|
   ADDRESS: _____
            STREET   CITY   STATE |__|__|__|
   COMMENTS: _____

4. QUES #: _____ CONDITION: _____ YEAR: _____
   FACILITY NAME: _____ TYPE: _____ |__|__|__|
   ADDRESS: _____
            STREET   CITY   STATE |__|__|__|
   COMMENTS: _____

5. QUES #: _____ CONDITION: _____ YEAR: _____
   FACILITY NAME: _____ TYPE: _____ |__|__|__|
   ADDRESS: _____
            STREET   CITY   STATE |__|__|__|
   COMMENTS: _____

6. QUES #: _____ CONDITION: _____ YEAR: _____
   FACILITY NAME: _____ TYPE: _____ |__|__|__|
   ADDRESS: _____
            STREET   CITY   STATE |__|__|__|
   COMMENTS: _____

U.S. GOVERNMENT PRINTING OFFICE: 1982 O - 393-367

NHANES I FOLLOWUP
HAND CARDS

SUBJECT QUESTIONNAIRE

CARD A

NO DIFFICULTY

SOME DIFFICULTY

MUCH DIFFICULTY

UNABLE TO DO

CARD B (DRINKING PATTERNS)

A { 9 OR MORE DRINKS A DAY
      OR
      60 OR MORE DRINKS A WEEK

B { ABOUT 6 TO 8 DRINKS A DAY
      OR
      40 TO 59 DRINKS A WEEK

C { ABOUT 4 OR 5 DRINKS A DAY
      OR
      25 TO 39 DRINKS A WEEK

D { ABOUT 2 OR 3 DRINKS A DAY
      OR
      10 TO 24 DRINKS A WEEK

E   1 TO 9 DRINKS A WEEK

F   LESS THAN 1 DRINK A WEEK

G   DID NOT DRINK

CARD C

01 = ALL BRAN
02 = BRAN BUDS
03 = BRAN CHEX
04 = BRAN FLAKES
05 = BUC WHEATS
06 = CHEERIOS
07 = CORN BRAN
08 = CORN CHEX
09 = CORN FLAKES
10 = CRACKLIN BRAN
11 = CRISPY WHEATS
     AND RAISINS
12 = FRUIT AND FIBER
13 = GRANOLA
14 = GRAPE NUTS
15 = GRAPE NUTS FLAKES
16 = GOLDEN CHARMS
17 = HEARTLAND CEREAL
18 = LIFE
19 = MOST
20 = NUTRI-GRAIN
21 = PRODUCT 19
22 = PUFFED RICE
23 = PUFFED WHEAT
24 = QUAKER 100%
     NATURAL CEREAL
25 = RAISIN BRAN
26 = RAISIN, RICE
     AND RYE
27 = RICE CHEX
28 = RICE KRISPIES
29 = SHREDDED WHEAT
30 = SPECIAL K
31 = TEAM
32 = TOTAL
33 = WHEAT CHEX
34 = WHEATIES

CARD D

01 = CREAM OF WHEAT/FARINA

02 = OATMEAL

03 = DARK FARINA/RALSTON

04 = GRITS

05 = OTHER (SPECIFY)

CARD E

A. FRESH APPLES
B. FRESH PEARS
C. BANANAS
D. FRESH ORANGES OR TANGERINES
E. ORANGE JUICE
F. POWDERED ORANGE JUICE SUBSTITUTES SUCH AS TANG
G. FRESH GRAPEFRUIT
H. GRAPEFRUIT JUICE
I. VITAMIN C ENRICHED FRUIT DRINKS
J. FRESH OR CANNED PEACHES OR NECTARINES
K. CANTALOUPE
L. WATERMELON
M. FRESH PLUMS
N. FRESH OR FROZEN STRAWBERRIES
O. FRESH, CANNED OR DRIED APRICOTS
P. COOKED OR DRIED PRUNES INCLUDING PRUNE JUICE
Q. ALL CANNED FRUIT SUCH AS CANNED PEARS, PINEAPPLE, FRUIT COCKTAIL OR APPLE SAUCE

CARD F

A. GREEN PEAS
B. GREEN BEANS, GREEN LIMA BEANS OR STRING BEANS
C. OTHER BEANS OR PEAS, I.E., KIDNEY OR PINTO BEANS, AND BLACKEYED OR CHICK PEAS
D. OKRA
E. BROCCOLI
F. CAULIFLOWER
G. BRUSSEL SPROUTS
H. CORN
I. SUMMER SQUASH SUCH AS ZUCCHINI, YELLOW, OR CROOKNECK
J. WINTER SQUASH SUCH AS ACORN, BUTTERNUT, HUBBARD OR PUMPKIN
K. RAW OR COOKED CARROTS
L. CUCUMBER
M. SWEET RED PEPPERS
N. SWEET GREEN PEPPERS
O. ICEBERG OR HEAD LETTUCE IN A SALAD
P. LEAF LETTUCE IN A SALAD
Q. CABBAGE INCLUDING COLE SLAW
R. RAW OR COOKED GREENS, E.G., SPINACH, COLLARDS OR TURNIP GREENS
S. SWEET POTATOES OR YELLOW YAMS
T. INSTANT OR DEHYDRATED POTATOES
U. BAKED, BOILED OR MASHED WHITE POTATOES
V. FRIED OR HASH BROWN POTATOES
W. FRESH TOMATOES
X. COOKED TOMATOES, TOMATO SOUP, JUICE, SAUCE OR CANNED TOMATOES
Y. VEGETABLE SOUP

CARD G

01 = OLIVE OIL

02 = LIQUID OIL OTHER THAN OLIVE OIL

03 = SOLID SHORTENING

04 = MARGARINE IN A STICK

05 = MARGARINE IN A TUB

06 = BUTTER

07 = LARD

08 = BACON GREASE OR PORK FAT

09 = OTHER (SPECIFY)

CARD I

COLUMN I	COLUMN II
NEVER	MUCH MORE NOW
RARELY	SOMEWHAT MORE NOW
SOMETIMES	SOMEWHAT LESS NOW
OFTEN	MUCH LESS NOW
ALMOST ALWAYS	ABOUT THE SAME

CARD J

DESCRIBES ME VERY WELL

DESCRIBES ME FAIRLY WELL

DESCRIBES ME SOMEWHAT

DESCRIBES ME NOT AT ALL

COFFEE CARD

CUPS OF;

A. INSTANT DECAFFEINATED COFFEE

B. OTHER INSTANT COFFEE

C. GROUND DECAFFEINATED COFFEE

D. OTHER GROUND COFFEE

E. HERB TEA

F. REGULAR TEA, INCLUDING ICED TEA

CARD H

1 = WHOLE MILK

2 = SKIM MILK

3 = LOW FAT MILK

4 = HALF AND HALF

5 = CREAM

6 = NONDAIRY CREAMER

CARD K

STRONGLY DISAGREE

DISAGREE

FEEL NEUTRAL

AGREE

STRONGLY AGREE

CARD L

01 = English, Welsh	15 = African
02 = Irish	16 = Middle Eastern
03 = Scottish	17 = Indian, Pakistani
04 = Canadian	18 = Chinese
05 = German	19 = Japanese
06 = French	20 = Pacific Islands, Polynesian
07 = Italian	21 = Aleut, Eskimo or American Indian
08 = Dutch	22 = Mexican
09 = Greek	23 = Puerto Rican
10 = Portuguese	24 = Cuban
11 = Russian	25 = Spain
12 = Czechoslovakian	26 = All other Spanish (Central or
13 = Other Eastern European	South American)
(Polish, Hungarian)	27 = Black
14 = Scandinavian (Norwegian,	28 = Other
Swedish, Finnish, Danish)	

CARD M

01 = ALEUT, ESKIMO OR AMERICAN INDIAN

02 = ASIAN/PACIFIC ISLANDER

03 = BLACK

04 = WHITE

CARD N
INCOME

Under $3,000.	. . . . .	.	A
$3,000 -	$3,999	. . . .	B
$4,000 -	$4,999	. . . .	C
$5,000 -	$5,999	. . . .	D
$6,000 -	$6,999	. . . .	E
$7,000 -	$9,999	. . . .	F
$10,000 -	$14,999	. . . .	G
$15,000 -	$19,999	. . . .	H
$20,000 -	$24,999	. . . .	I
$25,000 -	$34,999	. . . .	J
$35,000 -	$49,999	. . . .	K
$50,000 -	$74,999	. . . .	L
$75,000 -	$100,000	. . . .	M
Over $100,000.	. . . . .	.	N

APPENDIX B

Hospital Record Form

OMB No.: 0925-0161
Expiration Date: 12/31/83

NOTICE — Information contained on this form which would permit identification of an individual or establishment has been collected with a guarantee that it will be held in strict confidence, will be used only for purposes stated for this study, and will not be disclosed or released to others without the consent of the individual or the establishment in accordance with Section 308(d) of the Public Health Service Act (42 USC 242m).

ID#: _____

PATIENT NAME: _____

☐ INFORMATION SHOWN ON LABEL
☐ AGREES WITH HOSPITAL RECORDS
☐ OTHER (SPECIFY) _____

U.S. Department of Health and Human Services
National Center for Health Statistics
National Institute on Aging
NHANES I Epidemiologic Followup Survey

HOSPITAL RECORD FORM
TO BE FILLED OUT BY MEDICAL RECORDS DEPARTMENT

1. PATIENT MEDICAL RECORD NUMBER _____

2. DATE OF ADMISSION ___/___/___ DATE OF DISCHARGE ___/___/___
   MONTH / DAY / YEAR   MONTH / DAY / YEAR

3. WAS THE PATIENT IN: CARDIAC INTENSIVE CARE UNIT
   ☐ Yes, _____ Days
        NUMBER
   ☐ No

   OTHER INTENSIVE CARE UNIT
   ☐ Yes, _____ Days
        NUMBER
   ☐ No

4. DISPOSITION OF PATIENT (Check One):
   ☐ Routine discharge/discharged home
   ☐ Left against medical advice
   ☐ Discharged/transferred to another facility or organization
   ☐ Discharged/referred to organized home care service
   ☐ Died
   ☐ Not stated

5. ANY OTHER HOSPITALS LISTED IN ADMISSION NOTES OR DISCHARGE SUMMARY
   Name: _____ City/State: _____ Year: _____
   Name: _____ City/State: _____ Year: _____
   Name: _____ City/State: _____ Year: _____

(PLEASE TURN THE PAGE)

6. WHAT WERE THE DIAGNOSES ESTABLISHED AT TIME OF DISCHARGE? (Principal diagnosis is the condition after study chiefly responsible for the hospital stay.) (If more space is needed for additional diagnoses, write the diagnoses and the Westat ID number on a separate sheet of paper and attach to this form.)

Principal Diagnosis:

1.) _____

Other Diagnoses:

2.) _____

3.) _____

4.) _____

5.) _____

6.) _____

OFFICE USE ONLY

7. WHAT WERE THE SURGICAL PROCEDURES PERFORMED DURING THIS ADMISSION? (Include all biopsy and surgical procedures discussed or listed in the discharge summary.)

SURGICAL PROCEDURES: Check (✓) if none ☐

1. _____
2. _____
3. _____
4. _____

OFFICE USE ONLY

8. PLEASE ATTACH A PHOTOCOPY OF THE FACE SHEET AND THE DISCHARGE SUMMARY FOR THIS INPATIENT STAY.
   PLEASE ATTACH A PHOTOCOPY OF THE THIRD DAY EKG IF MYOCARDIAL INFARCTION DIAGNOSED DURING THIS STAY.
   PLEASE ATTACH A PHOTOCOPY OF THE PATHOLOGY REPORT CONFIRMING THE DIAGNOSIS OF CANCER MADE DURING THIS STAY. (Write the Westat I.D. number on each photocopied page. If you do not have photo-copying capabilities, please transcribe the information from the face sheet, the discharge summary, EKG report, and pathology report onto a separate sheet, record the Westat ID Number on that sheet, and staple it to this form.)

	Yes	No	
a. Face Sheet	☐	☐	(Why not? _____)
b. Discharge Summary	☐	☐	(Why not? _____)
c. Pathology Report	☐	☐	(Why not? _____)
d. Third Day EKG	☐	☐	(Why not? _____)

COMPLETED BY _____ DATE _____

137

APPENDIX C

Nursing Home/Personal Care Home Record Form

MFI ID#: _____ WESTAT ID#: _____

OMB No.: 0925-0161
Expiration Date: 12/31/83

NURSING HOME NAME: _____

Please complete one form for each
inpatient care episode that terminated since January 1, ____
for:

NOTICE - Information contained on this form
which will permit identification of any individual or establishment has been collected with
a guarantee that it will be held in strict confidence, will be used only for purposes stated
for this study, and will not be disclosed or released to others without the consent of the
individual or establishment in accordance with
Section 308(d) of the Public Health Service Act
(42 USC 242m).

NAME: _____
BIRTHDATE: _____
SOCIAL SECURITY #: _____

☐ INFORMATION SHOWN ON LABEL
   AGREES WITH NURSING HOME RECORDS
☐ OTHER (SPECIFY) _____

U.S. Department of Health and Human Services
National Center for Health Statistics
National Institute on Aging
NHANES I Epidemiologic Followup Survey

NURSING HOME/PERSONAL CARE HOME RECORD FORM
TO BE FILLED OUT BY MEDICAL RECORDS DEPARTMENT

1. PATIENT MEDICAL RECORD # _____

2. DATE OF ADMISSION ___/___/___   DATE OF DISCHARGE ___/___/___
                     MONTH/DAY/YEAR   MONTH/DAY/YEAR

3. PATIENT ADMITTED FROM: (Check One)
   ☐ Private residence   ☐ Chronic disease hospital (SPECIFY BELOW)
   ☐ Acute care hospital (SPECIFY BELOW)   ☐ Other nursing home (SPECIFY BELOW)
   NAME OF FACILITY: _____   CITY/STATE: _____

4. OTHER HOSPITALS PROVIDING CARE DURING NURSING HOME/PERSONAL CARE HOME STAY
   Name: _____   City/State: _____   Year: _____
   Name: _____   City/State: _____   Year: _____
   Name: _____   City/State: _____   Year: _____

5. DISPOSITION OF PATIENT: (Check One)
   ☐ Not discharged/still inpatient   ☐ Died
   ☐ Discharged to private residence/   ☐ Discharged to private residence/
     referral to organized home care   no referral
     services

   Transferred to another health care facility (SPECIFY BELOW)
   ☐ Acute care hospital   ☐ Chronic disease hospital
   ☐ Other nursing home   ☐ Other (SPECIFY) _____
   NAME OF FACILITY: _____   CITY/STATE: _____

(PLEASE TURN PAGE)

6. WHAT WERE THE DIAGNOSES ESTABLISHED AT ADMISSION?

Principal Diagnosis at Admission:

1.) _____

Other Major Diseases or Conditions Present
at Time of Admission:

2.) _____

3.) _____

4.) _____

5.) _____

6.) _____

7. PLEASE ATTACH A PHOTOCOPY OF THE ADMISSION SHEET. (Write the Westat I.D. number on each photocopied
   page. If you do not have photocopying capabilities, please transcribe the information from the
   admission sheet onto a separate sheet, record the Westat ID Number on that sheet, and staple it
   to THIS form.)

                        Yes   No
   Admission Sheet   ☐   ☐   (Why not? _____)

COMPLETED BY _____   DATE _____

OFFICE USE ONLY

1. E
2. E
3.
4. E
5. E
6. E
   E

140

APPENDIX D

Scoring Keys for Psychological Scales

These keys employ the Question Numbers in the NHANES I Epidemiologic Follow-up Survey Questionnaire Coding Manual (September 1984).

GWB Scales: Valid responses for items I21 to I26 are 1 to 6; for items I27 to I30, 0 to 10. All other responses are treated as missing.

Neuroticism/Negative Affect = 21 (constant) − I22 − I24 + I26 + I28 − I30.

Positive Affect = 12 (constant) − I21 − I23 + I29.

Health Concern = 6 (constant) − I25 + I27.

Total GWB = 35 (constant) − I21 + I22 − I23 + I24 + I25 − I26 − I27 − I28 + I29 + I30. Or, Positive Affect − Neuroticism/Negative Affect − Health Concern + 50.

CES Depression: Valid responses for all items are 0 to 3. CES-D = 12 (constant) + I1 + I2 + I3 − I4 + I5 + I6 + I7 − I8 + I9 + I10 + I11 − I12 + I13 + I14 + I15 − I16 + I17 + I18 + I19 + I20.

Extraversion and Openness: Valid responses for all items are 1 to 5.
Extraversion = 4 (constant) + P7 + P8 − P9 + P10 − P11 + P12 + P13 + P14.
Openness to Experience = 12 (constant) − P15 − P16 + P17 − P18 + P19 + P20.

APPENDIX E

Modifications to the Scoring of the Walking Domain for Constructing the HAQ Disability Index

The Health Assessment Questionnaire (HAQ) instrument asked about the degree of difficulty in walking outdoors on flat ground, whereas the NHEFS instrument asked about the degree of difficulty in walking a quarter of a mile. If "much difficulty" or "unable to do" was reported in this question, then another question followed asking about the degree of difficulty in walking from one room to another on the same level. To project the degree of difficulty in walking outdoors on flat ground, "no difficulty" or "some difficulty" in walking a quarter of a mile substituted for "no difficulty" in walking outdoors; "much difficulty" or "unable" to walk a quarter mile but "no difficulty" in walking from room to room substituted for "some difficulty" in walking outdoors; "some difficulty" or "much difficulty" in walking from room to room substituted for "much difficulty" in walking outdoors; and "unable" to walk from room to room meant "unable" to walk outdoors. Table E–1 shows the percentage distributions for the degree of difficulty in the two NHEFS questions on walking and the projected levels for difficulty in walking outdoors; these data replace the NHEFS items included in the walking domain.

Table E–1 Degree of Difficulty in "Walking Outdoors on Flat Ground" Estimated According to Performance in Walking a 1/4 Mile and Walking from One Room to Another

	Walk room to room				
	No diff	Some	Much	Unable	Missing
Walk 1/4 mile: *n* (score)					
No difficulty	2325 (0)—skipped "walk room to room" question				
Some	474 (0)—skipped "walk room to room" question				
Much	116 (1)	45 (2)	9 (2)	—	11 (1)
Unable	161 (1)	85 (2)	62 (2)	84 (3)	12 (1)
Missing	55 (0)	8 (1)	1 (2)	—	20 (missing)

	Projected difficulty in walking outdoors			
Total*	No diff (0)	Some diff (1)	Much (2)	Unable (3)
n = 3448	2854	308	202	82
	82.8%	8.9%	5.9%	2.4%

*Does not include missing from both questions (*n* = 20) and those confined to bed (*n* = 49).

292

Index

Page numbers in *italics* indicate illustrations. Page numbers followed by *t* indicate tables.